Cyndi, 9-24-06

This looks like a great
resource book. I hope you
find some useful info.
     Love you—
          Chris

Breast Cancer

BEYOND CONVENTION

Breast Cancer

BEYOND CONVENTION

The World's Foremost Authorities
on Complementary and
Alternative Medicine Offer
Advice on Healing

Edited by Mary Tagliaferri, M.D., L.Ac.,
Isaac Cohen, O.M.D., L.Ac.,
and Debu Tripathy, M.D.

ATRIA BOOKS
New York London Toronto Sydney Singapore

The ideas, procedures, and suggestions in this book are not intended as a substitute for the medical advice of your trained health professional. All matters regarding your health require medical supervision. Consult your physician before adopting the suggestions in this book, as well as about any condition that may require diagnosis or medical attention. The author and publisher disclaim any liability arising directly or indirectly from the use of the book.

Library of Congress Cataloging-in-Publication Data

    Breast cancer : beyond convention : the world's foremost authorities on complementary and alternative medicine offer advice on healing / edited by Mary Tagliaferri, Isaac Cohen, and Debu Tripathy.
      p.   cm.
    Includes bibliographical references.
    ISBN 0-7434-1011-4 (alk. paper)
    1. Breast—Cancer—Alternative treatment. 2. Breast—Cancer—Popular works. I. Tagliaferri, Mary. II. Cohen, Isaac, O.M.D. III. Tripathy, Debu.

RC280.B8 B66566 2002
616.99'44906—dc21   2002016930

First Atria Books hardcover printing June 2002

10 9 8 7 6 5 4 3 2 1

ATRIA BOOKS is a trademark of Simon & Schuster, Inc.

For information regarding special discounts for bulk purchases please contact Simon & Schuster Special Sales at 1-800-456-6798 or business@simonandschuster.com

Printed in the U.S.A.

To my best friend, Lila Kahn, for helping me heal at home after surgery, and to one of my most cherished teachers, Lucero Dorado, for helping me learn home is where healing begins.

Mary Tagliaferri, M.D., L.Ac.

To all my patients, for without them I wouldn't have gained experience in medicine and humility about our limitations. In particular it was Gwen Gatewood whose ups and downs with breast cancer inspired me to research better options. I would also like to acknowledge three of my teachers: Wei Meifang, M.D., Alex Tiberi, L.Ac., and Master Chang Liengway, for without them I wouldn't know where to begin.

Isaac Cohen, O.M.D., L.Ac.

To Susan Claymon, who lived with metastatic breast cancer for eight years, and to Helene Smith, whose scientific credibility coupled with her boundless imagination spurred me to enter the field of alternative and complementary medicine research.

Debu Tripathy, M.D.

*A portion of the proceeds from the sale of this book
will be donated to the UCSF Carol Franc Buck Breast
Care Center Complementary and Alternative Medicine Program.*

Contents

Preface

In the summer of 1996, the three of us met at Dr. Debu Tripathy's office at the University of California, San Francisco, for the first time. Debu was already a seasoned breast oncologist, well known for his leading role in the clinical trials for Genentech's novel therapeutic agent, Herceptin, the first monoclonal antibody in the treatment of breast cancer. Isaac Cohen was a licensed acupuncturist and herbalist, who dedicated his practice to the treatment of breast cancer and was popular in the San Francisco Bay Area for integrating Western and Eastern medicine. I was a licensed acupuncturist and herbalist, who was diagnosed with breast cancer at age thirty. When I met with Debu and Isaac six years ago, I was recovering from six weeks of breast radiation and was relying on traditional Chinese medicine to abate the side effects of my Western medical treatments and to boost my immune system.

Coincidentally, at the same time, all three of us began to see the importance of generating scientific data regarding the use of herbal therapies for breast cancer. Through our own personal experiences, we became dedicated to this process. Isaac secured a seed grant from the

ARKAY Foundation in Carmel, California, to study the effects of traditional Chinese herbal medicine for the treatment of breast cancer. Debu was approached by Dr. Helene Smith, a close colleague diagnosed with breast cancer, to study Tibetan medicine. I challenged Dr. Laura Esserman, the director of the UCSF Breast Care Center, to begin a research program dedicated to studying the effects of traditional Chinese medicine as an anticancer therapy, to control the side effects of Western medical treatments, and to boost the immune system. All three of us had the same aims, but we were not quite sure where to begin. After several meetings that went late into the night, we agreed to study the clinical benefits of herbal therapies in clinical trials and to elucidate some of the biological mechanisms by which traditional Chinese herbs may affect cancer cells, the immune system, and hormonal regulation. In addition, Debu was very generous with his time, spending endless nights teaching Isaac and me how to design clinical trials using reliable outcome tools to appropriately answer our research questions. Our first task was to raise money for the new research program at the UCSF Breast Care Center. As the only full-time employee of the program, I began to write research grants to various government agencies. Isaac started an extensive literature search and developed meaningful research collaborations with Chinese authorities on cancer to find historical and modern justifications for our herbal medicine approaches.

Our program has grown to include breast surgeons, oncologists, gynecologists, immunologists, medical anthropologists, basic scientists, and licensed acupuncturists. We have completed one clinical trial that studied the effects of Tibetan medicine for metastatic breast cancer; it was featured on *Dateline* in January 2001. We have four other active clinical trials to evaluate the effects of traditional Chinese herbs on reducing the side effects from chemotherapy and on decreasing hot flashes and other unwanted symptoms of menopause, an anticancer study with one Chinese herb, and a trial comparing soy with tamoxifen for breast cancer prevention. In addition, we have several laboratory studies under way evaluating herbs as anticancer agents and as regulators of the hormonal system.

It has become clear to us through our research endeavors that there is no good resource or guidebook to help women make decisions about the use of alternative therapies for breast cancer. Moreover, most of the available literature justifies the use of complementary and alternative therapies based on the author's recommendations or experiences, not on scientific data. Our intention with this collaborative project is to provide women with the most up-to-date scientific findings that support the use of alternative therapies for breast cancer.

We believe that we have covered the most popular alternative therapies used by women with breast cancer, but we have certainly not covered them all. We are extremely proud of the team of experts who agreed to take time from their busy academic lives to write chapters that tackle the science with language that is easy to understand. We are grateful to the authors who provided insight into the deeper aspects of the healing journey that goes far beyond conventional care. This book would not have been completed without the outstanding editorial skills of Connie Hatch and Colleen Kapklein who made sure the chapters were easy to read and the science was clearly described in nonmedical jargon. We know we could never have found a better literary agent than Jandy Nelson at Manus and Associates, who understood the importance of this book and was willing to work tirelessly on making it happen. Emily Bestler, our editor at Pocket Books, was a phenomenal support, and the freedom she extended to us in putting together a collaborative project, with numerous expert voices, has been deeply appreciated.

Being diagnosed with breast cancer is overwhelming. Many people will make recommendations or suggestions for you to try various forms of alternative and complementary therapies. Now you have a guidebook at your side to help with this decision making process that extends beyond anecdotal evidence. We hope the chapters in our book will clarify many of the questions that may arise about the risks and benefits of treatments you encounter after being diagnosed with breast cancer. This is the book I dreamed of when I was diagnosed with breast cancer six years ago.

Mary Tagliaferri, M.D., L.Ac.

Foreword

I am delighted to write a foreword for this pioneering book on breast cancer. These wonderful essays span the entire range of options from conventional to alternative. Each author has made profound contributions to the medical community, and the expertise and experience they share in this book may help provide you with new hope and new choices.

They address not only the physical but also the psychological, emotional, and spiritual dimensions of curing and healing, suffering and transformation. Indeed, this book embodies an integrative approach that is both wise and far-reaching. Each contributor offers a different voice and point of view. Not all may be useful to you, and not all may ultimately be proved correct, but I hope you find them to be as interesting as I have.

Anyone who is faced with a life-threatening illness such as breast cancer has a natural tendency to want to get as much information and to do everything possible to get better. It is becoming increasingly apparent that while traditional Western, allopathic medicine (primarily chemotherapy, radiation, and surgery) offers much value and hope to people with breast cancer, many other options are also available. All systems of healing have limitations.

The problem is making sense of these myriad choices, which can feel especially overwhelming when a person is ill and in emotional and spiritual turmoil. Reading this book is like having a wise friend by your side.

I am a scientist as well as a clinician because I believe in the power of science to help sort out conflicting claims and to distinguish fact from fancy, what sounds plausible from what is real, what works and what doesn't, for whom, and under what circumstances.

Indeed, that is the whole point of science. As Tom Cruise playing Jerry Maguire might say if he were a scientist, "Show me the data!" The peer-reviewed scientific process is about people challenging each other to demonstrate scientific evidence, not just their opinions or beliefs, to support their positions. Dr. Denis Burkit once wrote, "Not everything that counts can be counted"—and not everything meaningful is measurable, but much is.

The question is not "Should Americans seek out alternative medicine practitioners?" because so many already are. Although there is relatively little hard scientific evidence proving the value of most alternative medicine approaches, several studies have revealed that as much money is spent out of pocket for complementary or alternative medicine as for traditional physicians' services. In most cases, these decisions are being made with inadequate scientific information to make informed and intelligent choices.

The editors of *The New England Journal of Medicine* stated, "There cannot be two kinds of medicine—conventional and alternative. There is only medicine that has been adequately tested and medicine that has not, medicine that works and medicine that may or may not work. Once a treatment has been tested rigorously, it no longer matters whether it was considered alternative at the outset. If it is found to be reasonably safe and effective, it will be accepted."[1]

But this presumes that funding is available to rigorously test complementary medicine. Also, conventional approaches such as drugs and surgery are not always held to the same scientific standards. Although research in alternative and mind-body medicine is important, it is often very difficult to obtain funding to do these studies. In my experience, it is often a catch-22: many funding agencies presume that these approaches have little value, so they are reluctant to fund studies to determine their effectiveness; yet, one cannot assess their effectiveness without funding to do the research. The National Center for Complementary and Alternative Medicine at the National Institutes of Health (NIH) is a good start, but it still provides only a fraction of the overall NIH budget.

Thus, just because data are not available does not mean an alternative treatment is ineffective, only that we don't yet know. The presumption that unstudied approaches have no value is itself unscientific until these approaches are scientifically studied and tested. At the same time, just because someone believes in the efficacy of their treatment doesn't mean it really works.

The medicine of the twenty-first century should integrate the best of traditional allopathic medicine and of complementary or alternative medicine. Our research has demonstrated that an integrated approach can be both medically effective and cost effective.

We tend to think of an advance in medicine as a new drug, a new surgical technique, a laser—something high-tech and expensive. We often have a hard time believing that the simple choices we make each day in our lives—for example, what we eat, how we respond to stress, whether or not we smoke, how much exercise we get, and the quality of our social and spiritual relationships—can make such a powerful difference in our health and well-being, even our survival. But they often do.

When we treat these underlying issues, we find that the body often has a remarkable capacity to begin healing itself—and much more quickly than had once been thought possible. But not always. On the other hand, if we just bypass the problem, literally with surgery or figuratively with drugs, without also addressing these underlying causes, then the same problem may recur or new problems may emerge. Often it can feel like mopping up the floor around an overflowing sink without also turning off the faucet.

For the past twenty-four years, my colleagues and I at the nonprofit Preventive Medicine Research Institute have conducted a series of scientific studies and randomized clinical trials demonstrating that the progression of even severe coronary heart disease can often be reversed by making comprehensive changes in diet and lifestyle, without coronary bypass surgery, angioplasty, or a lifetime of cholesterol-lowering drugs. These lifestyle changes include a very low-fat, plant-based, whole-foods diet; stress management techniques; moderate exercise; smoking cessation; and psychosocial support. We have published our findings in peer-reviewed medical and scientific journals.[2-8]

Our work is a model of a scientifically based approach that may be helpful to others in building bridges between the alternative and conventional medical communities. The idea that heart disease might be reversible was a radical concept when we began our first study; now, it has become mainstream and is generally accepted as true by most cardiologists and scientists. In our research, we use the latest high-tech, expensive, state-of-the-art medical techniques such as computer-analyzed quantitative coronary arteriography and cardiac position emission tomography to prove the power of ancient, low-tech, and inexpensive alternative and mind-body interventions.

I think we may be at a similar place with respect to the evidence linking diet and lifestyle with breast cancer, prostate cancer, and colon cancer to where we were in 1977 when we began studying coronary heart disease. There are data from animal studies, epidemiological surveys, and anecdotal case reports in humans suggesting that diet and lifestyle choices may play a role in the development of these illnesses. For example, the incidence of clinically significant prostate, breast, and colon cancers is much lower in parts of the world that eat a predominantly low-fat, whole-foods, plant-based diet. Subgroups of people in the United States who eat this diet also have much lower rates of these cancers than those who eat a typical American diet. However, randomized controlled trials have not yet been completed to see whether altering the diet may influence the progression of cancer. Many of these trials are currently under way.

Diet is only part of the story. For example, a randomized controlled trial of women with metastatic breast cancer has shown that women who received group support lived twice as long as those in the control group.[9] Other studies have shown that people who feel lonely, depressed, and isolated are many times more likely to get sick and die prematurely than those who have a strong sense of connection, community, and intimacy.[10]

In 1997, we began a randomized controlled trial in collaboration with Dr. Peter Carroll at the University of California, San Francisco, and

Dr. William Fair at Memorial Sloan-Kettering Cancer Center to determine whether prostate cancer can be affected by comprehensive changes in diet and lifestyle, without surgery, radiation, or drug (hormonal) treatments. Men with biopsy-proven prostate cancer who have elected not to be treated conventionally ("watchful waiting") were randomly assigned to an experimental group that was asked to make comprehensive lifestyle changes or to a control group that was not.

We have the opportunity to determine the effects of diet and comprehensive lifestyle changes on prostate cancer without confounding variables—a study that would not be ethically possible in breast cancer, colon cancer, or related illnesses. Whatever we show, the data may be of wide interest.

While it would be premature and unwise to draw any definitive conclusions from a study that is still in progress, our preliminary data are encouraging. An increasing number of scientists believe that what affects prostate cancer will likely affect breast cancer as well, so research in one area has direct implications for the other.

The authors of this book describe numerous innovative research strategies that will begin the process of illuminating the scientific and clinical basis of many alternative modalities that have been used for centuries or, in some cases, formulated more recently on the basis of theory and the observations of seasoned clinicians. It will require tenacity and imagination to adapt the investigative process to the individualized nature of alternative medicine while maintaining scientific validity.

Clearly, more good science is needed. What to do in the meantime?

In choosing any therapy, one considers what is called the risk/benefit ratio. In other words, if the risk is small and the potential benefit is great, then it is probably a choice worth making.

I suspect that the optimal treatment for breast cancer and prostate cancer will integrate the best of conventional and complementary therapies. For example, there is a significant risk of recurrence after the surgical removal of breast cancer or prostate cancer, even if it seems that the tumor was localized at the time of surgery, because of microscopic metastases. In this context, even though the data are not conclusive that changes in diet and lifestyle affect the progression of breast cancer or prostate cancer, there is enough evidence to suggest that they might.

Since the only side effects of eating a low-fat, whole-foods, plant-based diet (along with exercise, meditation, and support groups) are beneficial, one can make a persuasive case that it would be prudent to do all of these practices in addition to conventional treatments when these are chosen. Some alternative interventions do have risks, so one needs to exercise caution in these areas as well. Clearly, more scientific research is needed. This book can help you to find the right balance in making difficult choices.

Dean Ornish, M.D.
Founder and President, Preventive Medicine Research Institute
Clinical Professor of Medicine,
University of California, San Francisco

CHAPTER ONE

A Diagnosis of Breast Cancer: Taking Your First Steps

Susan Love, M.D., M.B.A.

SUSAN LOVE, M.D., M.B.A., is a researcher, author, activist, surgeon, and founder of LLuminari,^{SM} a multimedia women's-health content company, and www.SusanLoveMD.com. As author of *Dr. Susan Love's Breast Book* and *Dr. Susan Love's Hormone Book*, she has gained the trust of women worldwide. She is currently the medical director of the Susan Love, M.D., Breast Cancer Foundation, a nonprofit organization dedicated to the eradication of breast cancer, an adjunct professor of surgery at UCLA, a member of the National Cancer Advisory Board, and a director of the National Breast Cancer Coalition.

Hearing the words "you have breast cancer" is shocking. The shock can last for minutes to hours, and it is soon followed by questions: "How can this be?" "What does this mean?" "Am I going to die?" "What should I do?" Many people close at hand will try to answer your questions and direct you on a path of treatment. But over the years I have learned that treatment is not enough for most women. Most of us need to be healed as well. Treatment is pretty easy to get and pretty standardized, but to feel healed, you must put together a different plan that is unique to you. This often includes what some people term alternative and conventional therapies.

With a diagnosis of breast cancer you enter the world of the "sick." Your modesty goes first. Your dignity is also left at the exam room door as you walk around in a short hospital gown with your bare bottom exposed to the world. You reveal intimate details about your body to perfect strangers, over and over again—but they never once ask you questions about who you are as a person, who you love, and who loves you. You have ceased to be a unique contributing person in the world and have become a "case." The treatments of breast cancer, which I have called "slash, burn, and poison," are depersonalizing and cold: "one size fits all." They may well improve the statistics of survival, but they don't empower the woman who has to undergo them. In order to reclaim the process you have to take control of your treatment and control of how you are treated. You need to find ways that work for you to heal yourself as well as treat this disease. You need to find your own way through the maze of breast cancer, its practitioners, its standard therapies, and its complementary treatments and form your own unique path to healing.

All this takes time and energy, of course; neither is plentiful when you have just been diagnosed with breast cancer. That is okay. You don't have to do everything at once. Besides, a diagnosis of breast cancer is not an emergency. Most breast cancers have been present for eight to ten years by the time you can see them on a mammogram or feel them. They have either spread microscopically, or not spread, by the time of diagnosis. Although you shouldn't spend the next six months studying the problem, you do have time to catch your breath, get a second opinion, and search out the options.

It is important to start with an understanding of the current hypothesis of breast cancer. Most breast cancer starts in the lining of the milk ducts. The breast consists of approximately six to eight ductal systems. The ductal system consists of lobules that make the milk and ducts that are the pipelines, carrying milk to the nipple. We think that breast cancer is the result of a series of steps. First there are an increased number of cells in the lining of the milk ducts, almost like rust. This is called hyperplasia. The cells then become "funny looking" and are then called atypical hyperplasia. After a time the cells actually resemble breast cancer cells, but they are completely contained by the ducts. This is called ductal carcinoma in situ, or DCIS (a similar progression can be outlined in the lobules). Finally the cells invade outside of the ducts into the surrounding fat and become invasive ductal cancer.

This is what we commonly call breast cancer. Once breast cancer is invasive, it has the ability to cause new blood vessels to grow in order to feed the tumor. Soon after, cancer cells have the ability to invade the blood vessels and travel throughout the body. The cells find a comfortable environment in other organs and form new colonies of breast cancer cells. In fact, it is the breast cancer cells elsewhere in the body that

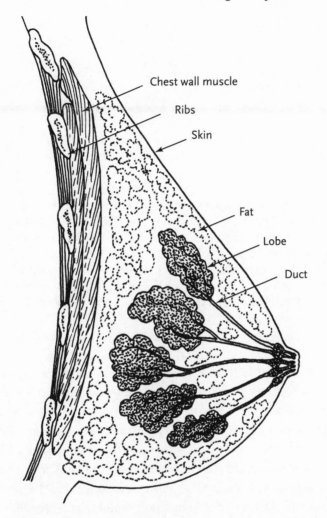

Chest wall muscle

Ribs

Skin

Fat

Lobe

Duct

FIGURE 1.1 Cross-section of the breast. Note that the breast consists of approximately 6–8 ducts that drain at the nipple. The ductal system consists of lobules that make the milk and then drain through the ducts.

are life threatening. If they start to grow they can interfere with vital functions in the liver, lungs, or brain and finally lead to death.

This whole process does not take place very rapidly. In fact, it is estimated that the average breast cancer has been present for eight to ten years by the time it can be felt as a lump or seen on a mammogram. It is also true that cancer cells and colonies of cancer do not grow continuously in the body; more likely they rest and grow over the years, depending in

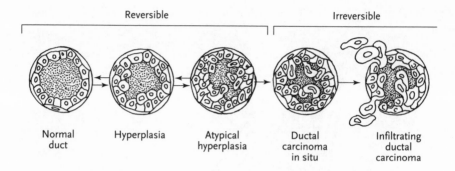

Reversible | Irreversible

| Normal duct | Hyperplasia | Atypical hyperplasia | Ductal carcinoma in situ | Infiltrating ductal carcinoma |

FIGURE 1.2 Steps in the process of breast cancer. First there is an increase in the number of epithelial cells lining the milk ducts called hyperplasia. As the epithelial cells continue to replicate and divide, they begin to look abnormal and are called atypical hyperplasia. When the cells actually resemble breast cancer cells but are contained within the ductal wall, it is called ductal carcinoma in situ. Once the cells break through the ductal wall to invade surrounding tissue, it is called infiltrating ductal carcinoma.

part on the environment in which they find themselves. What triggers cancer cells to grow and become detectable at one time rather than another? We really don't know, but we suspect that this is where such factors as stress and the immune system may act. Women often speak of getting cancer after a particularly stressful period of time, and wonder whether the stress caused the cancer. This is unlikely, as it takes a long time for the process to evolve. What is more likely is that the stress alters the hormonal balance of the body and possibly depresses the immune system. This imbalance may lead to stimulation of a quiescent colony of breast cancer cells, causing them to multiply, divide, and possibly spread to other parts of the body. This is what happens when a tumor re-emerges after a period of dormancy. What were those cells doing for ten years? They were asleep. What put them to sleep? What woke them up? It is highly likely that the general status of health and vitality in the person will have a major impact on the status of those cells.

Our belief that all cancer cells have to be killed may not be a good one after all. This notion of killing comes in part from thinking about breast cancer as a foreign invader that gets into the body and grows continuously until it takes over. In fact, breast cancer starts in your own cells, which develop mutations, allowing them to replicate without limit and invade outside their own territory. These cancer cells are not in isolation. The cells around them, and the general state of the body, influence their capacity to thrive. A criminal analogy might work here. Some criminals have severe character defects that cannot be changed, but many can be rehabilitated if they are put into another environment. Cancer cells may also be able to be rehabilitated, reversed, or controlled if the environment of cells, hormones, and the immune system around them is changed. This becomes important in our approach to treating breast cancer. When I first started in this field twenty-five years ago, we did not have chemotherapy. Instead, if a premenopausal woman was diagnosed with breast cancer, we would take out her ovaries. Interesting new studies have monitored these women, and it turns out that taking out a woman's ovaries is as effective as chemotherapy in premenopausal women with estrogen receptor–positive cancers. Why would putting a woman into menopause treat her breast cancer? It does not kill cells the way that chemotherapy does. What it does do is change the environment for the cells by changing the hormonal milieu. The cells are probably "put to sleep" and stay asleep unless something comes to wake them up.

All of this becomes important in the way we approach breast cancer therapy. Our current therapies of chemotherapy, surgery, and radiation therapy, albeit the best we have, are crude ways of dealing with the disease. They have been shown to make some difference in survival from breast cancer, but they are focused on killing cancer cells rather than changing their environment. Hormonal therapies, immune approaches, mind-body techniques, nutritional treatment, and other alternative treatments focus on strengthening the body and altering the immune system to make important changes in the internal environment.

With this understanding, it becomes obvious that we need to address newly diagnosed breast cancer on three different fronts. The first is to do something that will prevent breast cancer from recurring in the breast. This is called local therapy and usually involves surgery to remove the cancer, in combination with radiation therapy to clean up any microscopic cells that have been left behind. The surgery is usually a lumpectomy or wide excision around the original tumor, but it can be a mastectomy if the mass is so large that it cannot be removed any other way. It is very interesting that chemotherapy will not always take care of this bulk of cancer cells in the breast. It seems that systemic therapy, regardless of whether it is chemotherapy, hormone modulation, or alternative medicine, works better on microscopic cells than on chunks of cancer. In all of these situations, surgery still appears to be the best way to debulk, or remove, the chunks of cancer. Local therapy can be curative if—and it is a big if—the body has either taken care of all the cells that may have gotten out or reversed them.

The next phase is systemic therapy. We presume that cells from most cancers have escaped through the bloodstream and "gotten out." These cells will seed other organs, and they can grow and affect these distant organs later on. Systemic therapies are those which are given by mouth or vein, get into the bloodstream, and therefore have a chance of affecting these cells. The most common systemic therapy is chemotherapy, with drugs that interfere with cell division and, as such, poison cancer cells as well as some normal cells. Hormonal therapy with agents such as tamoxifen, by contrast, changes the environment of the cell and probably acts more to control or reverse cancers.

The third aspect of treatment is to strengthen the body and immune system so that they can better reverse or control the cancer cells. This is where nutrition, exercise, meditation, visualization, support groups, and other alternative techniques come in. They are as important as the drugs. We all know women who have small cancers, with good prognoses, who get all the standard traditional therapies, yet rapidly succumb to the disease. By contrast, some women whom we expect to do poorly live—to everyone's surprise. There is no question in my mind that these results are in part attributable to holistic approaches to disease. Data from new studies are showing that women who are overweight have a higher rate of recurrence than women who are not overweight. Exercise has been demonstrated to prevent breast cancer and may well help prevent recurrence. David Spiegel has demonstrated that women with metastatic disease who participated in support groups lived 18 months longer than women who did not.[1] Can alternative therapies cure cancer by themselves? I don't know, but I would not personally risk it. On the other hand, can standard therapies cure cancer by themselves? I don't know, but I certainly would not risk doing one without the other.

And what about metastatic disease? Metastasis occurs when the cancer has been treated and then returns in other organs of the body: lungs, liver, bones, or brain. Again, the standard therapies are limited. We try different hormonal and chemotherapy drugs as well as radiation in an attempt to get the cancer back into remission, but we are not generally able to cure breast cancer at this point. Can we control it? We certainly try—and again, it is here that complementary therapies are important. If we believe that a change in the environment of the body is what causes the cancer to wake up, then we certainly need a change in the environment of the body to put it back to sleep.

In addition to facing the shocking news of breast cancer and choosing specific treatment options, you still have to deal with the many debilitating side effects. In some ways, this is the most important time for women, since this is frequently when healing takes place. Tissues that have been damaged by chemotherapy, surgery, and radiation can be healed by nutrition and exercise. Acupuncture has been used successfully to treat postsurgical pain, chemotherapy-related nausea and vomiting, and the fatigue induced by radiation. Traditional Chinese medicine, herbs, and other therapies have been used to help women with breast cancer deal with the symptoms of premature menopause and the side effects of tamoxifen. The body clearly needs to be rebalanced after the assault from cancer therapy. Nutritional, physical, and spiritual rebalancing will make the difference.

How can a woman put together the best approach to treat her disease and heal herself? When she is newly diagnosed with breast cancer or discovers a recurrence, she needs to first put together a team of experts that includes a breast cancer specialist she can trust and work with, who will help guide her. This could be a surgeon, an oncologist, a radiation therapist, or even a primary care physician. It is important that each person feels comfortable with her care providers and acts as a partner in her team. This may mean shopping around.

Many medical doctors are scared of alternative therapies, probably because they don't know much about them. Many of their criticisms do not hold water when examined closely. Although they often cite an absence of scientific studies of alternative therapies, they will often suggest drugs that have yet to be proved effective by the "gold standard" of randomized controlled clinical trials. The recent experience when thirty thousand women underwent high-dose chemotherapy with stem cell rescue before studies demonstrated that it was not better than standard chemotherapy is a perfect example of how modern medicine is not always based on science. Some doctors complain that alternative therapy is not standardized; yet, these same physicians will argue that modern medicine cannot be dictated by insurance companies because it is not standardized. Finally, they suggest that alternative therapy is too personality driven, but at the same time, we often search for the "best" surgeon or oncologist with the understanding that the person delivering the care is as important as the care. In reality, these physicians are uncomfortable because they have not been trained in that tradition and do not feel knowledgeable about its use. By explaining to your physicians what you are doing, you can often educate them. Ask your alternative practitioners for information that you can share with your medical team. Your experience may well pave the way for the next woman with breast cancer who wants to explore a broader range of healing.

Not only is it important to find the right team of medical doctors, but you must find the right team of alternative practitioners as well. There is no advantage to walking into a health food store and picking herbs and supplements off the shelf and combining them willy-nilly. Different herbs have different effects and may or may not lend themselves to combinations. It is important that you see a trained herbalist, naturopath, or traditional Chinese medicine doctor who can guide you in this approach. Ask for their credentials and training; talk to people whom they have treated. Nutritionists and personal trainers will also be important in helping you revise your lifestyle in a more healthy manner. Look for a counselor experienced with breast cancer survivors and/or a support group to help your emotional healing. Find the best approach for your spiritual healing, whether in traditional religion, yoga, meditation, or your own personal journey. All of this is important. After a diagnosis of breast cancer, your life will never again be the same. But it can be better as you put together your approach to therapy and healing from this disease.

This is an individual journey—one that is unpredictable. We all desire magic: "If I just eat this, take this herb, and do this exercise, the cancer won't come back again." There is no magic. One of my patients had a very small tumor, with prognostic factors that were all good. She begged us to give her chemotherapy even though we had no statistical evidence that the medicine would benefit her. She just "felt" that she had a bad tumor and needed it. We finally gave in and treated her with our most aggressive regimen. She changed her life, but within two years she was dead of metastatic breast cancer. On the other hand, one of my very first patients was a young woman with a very aggressive type of breast cancer. Not only was the tumor large, but also she had twenty positive lymph nodes. She underwent standard chemotherapy and radiation before revamping her life. She left her husband, moved to Hawaii, and started a nutrition and spiritual program that completely changed her life. She is still alive and well twenty years later.

I tell these stories not because I think that we can control all cancers with alternative approaches, but rather because I think they demonstrate how little we understand about this disease. We do what we can with standard therapy, but we base our therapies on statistics and large randomized studies, which tell us very little about any one woman, her body, and her cancer. There is no right or wrong way to treat breast cancer. There is only your way. Whatever happens to you is 100% yours, regardless of the purported statistics. Putting together your own personal prescription for treatment and healing will ultimately be the best approach for you. This magnificent collection of chapters will help you with that journey.

CHAPTER TWO

Building Bridges from Conventional to Alternative Medicine

Debu Tripathy, M.D.

DEBU TRIPATHY, M.D., is a medical oncologist whose practice and research are dedicated to breast cancer. He has been the principal investigator on numerous clinical trials assessing newer chemotherapeutic and biological oncogene-targeting treatments. As part of a collaborative team with practitioners of herbal therapy, epidemiologists, and behavioral scientists, he has begun to design clinical studies to evaluate herbal therapy approaches for various indications in breast cancer. He has been granted an Investigational New Drug License (IND) by the Food and Drug Administration, the first of its kind, to study an herbal formula for its ability to reduce side effects of adjuvant chemotherapy for breast cancer. He has been awarded a grant from the State of California to obtain regulatory approval and has recently completed a clinical trial to assess Tibetan herbal formulae as sole therapy for metastatic cancer. Other studies include a clinical trial testing a Chinese herb for late-stage breast cancer and a randomized trial assessing an herbal therapy to treat menopausal symptoms in women with a history of breast cancer. Parallel laboratory studies are ongoing to determine which herbal extracts can inhibit breast-cancer cell growth and whether or not specific compounds in these herbs can be isolated and characterized. These multidisciplinary projects are early initiatives that will further our understanding of herbal and other alternative medicines in breast cancer using modern laboratory and clinical research tools.

You may hear people refer to acupuncture, herbal therapies, nutritional supplements, megavitamins, meditation, yoga, tai chi, and certain strict diets as complementary and alternative medicine. Some people make the distinction that alternative medicine includes therapies that are used as *substitutes* for conventional medicine, whereas complementary medicine involves the practice of using nonconventional therapies *in combination* with Western medical care. The emerging field of integrative medicine attempts to integrate the best therapies from both Western medicine and nonconventional practices, based on scientific evidence, to achieve optimal clinical outcomes concerned with both the disease process and the patient's quality of life.

But what exactly is alternative medicine, and why does it make some physicians so uncomfortable?

We may describe it simply as a treatment or approach not generally accepted by mainstream medicine, which has elements that are not always based on commonly accepted physiology, and for which clinical outcomes are not well documented.

Of course, there are many things on which a wide range of healers and health care providers agree. For example, most practitioners, alternative and mainstream alike, recognize the health benefits of a balanced, low-fat diet with weekly physical activity, and would recommend this lifestyle to their patients. It is unfortunate, then, that a chasm has grown between strong believers in alternative medicine and those in the conventional medical field. The alternative side is often accused of quackery, lack of rigorous science, and a rejection of proven, effective medicine. Conversely, the conventional medical field has been viewed as cold and nonhumanistic, with a failure to view the patient as a whole, while being overly reliant on technology.

Only recently have the two schools begun to work together toward a synthesis of medicine that seeks to expand our knowledge and combine the most useful aspects of each into an integrative approach. In this chapter, I will outline some of the background and concepts with which I think we can achieve this synthesis in the field of breast cancer, which, to date, has been on the leading edge of this movement.

A Movement toward Individualized Care

Early in my exposure to science, I was impressed by precision. I appreciated physics as perfectly predictable and pure. My academic comfort zones were subjects of a numerical and rational nature, whose questions could be answered with irrefutable exactness. I initially believed that biology was equally ordered and that it was just a matter of time before we mastered the complex biochemistry and physiology that made up the human body.

But my vision of order did not last long. It was rapidly overturned when I entered medical school and began to see the randomness and chaos that often accompany acute or severe illness. I discovered that many symptoms and syndromes did not fit neatly into a given classification of disease as described in my textbooks, nor did the recommended treatments result in the expected outcome in many patients. In a sense, I began to understand why a more mystical and artistic approach to medicine could complement the cold scientific knowledge and clinical textbooks. Over time, this realization provided a comfortable transition for me to start a research program in alternative medicine in parallel with my other studies of conventional treatments for breast cancer.

I still lapse into trying to cleanly categorize everything into discrete variables. When I view a chest X ray, I tend to have a checklist for every possible anomaly that could be present as well as an explanation for its cause. And I continue to be intrigued by the notion of using computerized databases of molecular and clinical information to help bring knowledge out of the seeming disarray that is typical of a large clinical practice such as ours at the University of California, San Francisco Breast Care Center. Is there a relationship between taking the birth control pill and the type of genes expressed in a breast cancer that arises years later? Much of the research in our Breast Oncology Program seeks to understand breast cancer at both the general and the individual level through the study of specific genes and proteins of a tumor as well as normal tissue. Nevertheless, I have come to accept that the elegant assembly of intricate biological processes is too complex relative to our limited knowledge for us to appreciate the basis of cancer in the same way a watchmaker would understand every gear and lock movement of an antique timepiece. The elements of cancer will act on a given person in highly unique ways, both at the cellular level and within the whole body. Therein lies the unpredictability that one must expect in the diagnosis and treatment of breast cancer—or, for that matter, any illness.

We are only beginning to assemble this information as we bank patients' tumor tissue to embark on this gargantuan task. As with many other cancer centers and laboratories around the world, there is a fresh and enthusiastic initiative to use new technology that allows us to analyze thousands of genes and proteins at a time. If we gather this information and use sophisticated statistical methods and computer-intense analysis, we might, over time, apply this new skill to predict how someone's breast cancer might evolve, and what treatments (conventional, biological, and alternative) might be the most effective. It is paradoxical that this high-tech movement in Western medicine to individualize cancer diagnosis and treatment comes hundreds and in some cases thousands of years after the establishment of many forms of traditional medicine that have relied on a highly customized and individualized approach.

Our Breast Care Center at UCSF has been involved in the development of a new therapy for breast cancer that illustrates both the triumphs and the shortcomings of modern cancer therapeutics. Herceptin is a recently approved drug that was specifically designed to interfere with the functional consequence of a genetic abnormality seen in about one quarter of breast cancer cases. This genetic abnormality is the amplification, or excess copies (in comparison to the usual two copies of every gene), of a gene termed HER2/*neu*. When Dr. Dennis Slamon at UCLA first noted that amplification of HER2/*neu* seemed to result in a more aggressive form of breast cancer, he, along with scientists at Genentech, a biotechnology company, developed and tested Herceptin, an antibody against the HER2/*neu* protein. We, along with other clinical investigators, conducted trials in patients with advanced breast cancer and noted that it was not always easy to even know which patients had tumors that made HER2/*neu*, since the test to measure this protein was not perfect and sometimes led to confusing results.

We also observed a tremendous difference among patients in their responses to Herceptin. Some had spectacular shrinkage of their tumors and improvements in their symptoms, and others seemed to have no benefit at all. While they all had the same genetic change in their tumor and received the same treatment targeting this change, it is clear that other factors affected their outcome. We still do not know how to determine who will be helped by Herceptin. Clinical trials have shown that on the average, patients live longer when Herceptin is added to chemotherapy, and this represents a first for a biological agent in a common type of advanced cancer. Still, it is sobering that a "magic bullet" approach does not have a more profound impact. This experience also serves as an important lesson about the uniqueness of the human body in health and illness. Specific diagnostic and treatment strategies are not likely to be effective in a complex disease such as breast cancer unless they are properly tailored to each individual.

Are the Alternative and Conventional Models of Medicine Really Different?

Pure science is blind to language or cultural distinction. The results of a particular experiment, when the experiment is repeated, should be comparable whether it is performed at the University of Iowa or the Polytechnic Institute of Pakistan. In fact, this type of reproducibility is one of the requirements of credible science.

On the other hand, the actual practice of medicine is no more immune to cultural mixing than is food, music, art, or religion. And if medicine is truly an amalgam of culture and science, it is quite plausible that many different medical traditions may be grounded in the same basic truths about biology. Hence, while diagnostic criteria and treatments may be radically different among conventional and alternative forms of medicine, the underlying pathophysiology and treatment strategies may be comparable. For example, traditional Chinese medicine and some other forms of Oriental medicine define illness as an imbalance or a disturbance that is based on many components, including symptoms, medical history, and other factors that may seem unrelated to an individual's illness such as qi stagnation, yin deficiency, or dampness. Therapies like herbal medicine and acupuncture are designed to "achieve center," in part by manipulating the body's own life force, or qi, to achieve harmony and health.

While this type of terminology may be foreign to many American physicians, we can easily make analogies in modern medicine. For example, pneumonia may be suspected when a patient has disturbed lung function (cough, chest pain, and shortness of breath) and evidence of infection such as fever and chills. Of course, in today's practice, this is usually confirmed with a chest X ray and bacterial cultures. Antibiotic therapy rids the body of the causative bacteria but also relies on the patient's immune system for complete recovery. This involves numerous biochemical and cellular processes that eventually return the system back to normal. Physiologically, this centering effect, or homeostasis, is akin to the resumption of harmony and balance sought by Oriental medicine. Think of the analogy of the blind men encountering an elephant: the one who falls into the broad and sturdy side of the elephant thinks it is a wall, the one who touches the tusk believes he has found a spear, the blind man who finds the swinging tail believes it is a rope, and the one who touches a leg thinks it is a tree. Each describes a totally different object based on what he perceives from his particular vantage point. Similarly, classifications of traditional Chinese medicine may very well parallel Western categories of disease. It may be only our incomplete understanding of physiology that prevents us from making straightforward comparisons to prove this theory.

Our research group at the UCSF Carol Franc Buck Breast Care Center has chosen traditional Chinese medicine as a model for interdisciplinary research in breast cancer because of its long tradition, the availability of standardized texts, its relative consistency in practice patterns, and the rigorous process of licensure and training required in many states, including California. Today, the profession has grown to include over ten thousand acupuncturists in this country, licensed to practice in thirty-eight different states.

Breast cancer is a prime field in which to begin to research and synthesize Western and Oriental medicine, not only because our knowledge is limited, but because breast cancer patients as a group have shown a great openness to alternative medicine.

Historically, Western approaches to breast cancer research have been founded on a series of randomized controlled trials. With this strategy, a large number of consenting patients are assigned by chance to one of two treatment groups that differ only by the drug or intervention being tested. This has allowed us to estimate the effects of the therapy rather precisely. One problem, however, is that the benefit of most treatments for common diseases is expressed as a statistical probability based on large population studies. For example, it has been shown that the antiestrogen agent tamoxifen can lower the risk of recurrence of early-stage breast cancer after surgery by about one half when the tumor is positive for estrogen receptors, indicating it will respond to hormonal therapy. Those odds were determined by large clinical trials in which half of the women were assigned to receive tamoxifen after surgery and the other half received a placebo (inactive pill). In these trials, twice as many women taking the placebo had a recurrence; so we have now concluded that tamoxifen is effective and lowers the risk of recurrence by approximately 50%. Double-blind, placebo-controlled clinical trials have been the gold standard in medicine because they allow us to make such precise judgments about effectiveness. However, these types of studies do not allow us to delve into individual differences based on the patient's personal characteristics or the uniqueness of her tumor cells, which are known to carry highly distinct genetic and biochemical changes. One could envision that some women are lowering their risk by much more than half, while others are getting no benefit at all, even though the overall average is a 50% reduction. So when a woman is told to take tamoxifen to lower her risk for recurrence, this can hardly be seen as a cure, even though tamoxifen does end up saving lives on a large scale.

This illustrates one of the problems of modern medicine, which treats a given disease as a monolithic entity and generally does not tailor therapy to the specific characteristics of an individual and her illness. While researchers have made a concerted effort to understand the unique genetic elements of the cancer cells arising from different women, we are far from being able to use this information to customize treatment. We are therefore practicing in a probabilistic realm, where most treatments have a given chance of working, but no guarantees can be made in an individual case. It may not be only chance or randomness that determines the outcome. There may be additional as-yet-unknown biological factors that could help us sharpen the prediction. Nevertheless, one can never fully predict whether or not a treatment will work, even though in some cases its effectiveness may approach 99% (very rarely is this the case in any cancer treatment). On the other hand, alternative approaches tend to take a more deterministic viewpoint: the many cues of the mind and body can provide the basis for a customized approach.

Research in Alternative Medicine:
A Starting Point

Our research program in traditional Chinese medicine has multiple strategies that address both the practice and philosophy of herbal medicine as well as the principles of scientific discovery and proof. We are certain to make mistakes, and we can only hope to learn from them in order to make every clinical trial and experiment more valuable and instructive than the one preceding it.

One of our starting points is the use of herbs or herbal formulas that have historically been used in a consistent fashion for a particular situation. Our first clinical trial was designed to alleviate the side effects of a specific chemotherapy regimen (adriamycin and cytoxan) that is commonly used after surgery for early-stage breast cancer. We decided to use a fixed combination of twenty-one herbs without individualization, and we are currently testing this combination via a randomized placebo-controlled double-blind study. This means that half of the patients are assigned by chance to take a placebo, or inactive powder that looks and smells like herbs, while the other half receive the active combination of twenty-one herbs. The herbs are taken three times a day as a powder dissolved in warm water, beginning 10 days before the first chemotherapy treatment. During this time, we can identify any side effects that may be due to the herbs. Neither the patient nor any of the physicians or nurses knows whether the active formula or a placebo has been assigned. Chemotherapy and the usual medications typically given for nausea, low white blood cell counts, and other side effects are administered in a very regimented way, just as they would normally be given in the office. Careful observations are taken at specified times: patients indicate on a questionnaire, using a scale of one to five, their degree of nausea, vomiting, and other side effects. We also record other measurements such as the white blood cell count and the amount of standard antinausea medication the patients need each day. About one month after all the chemotherapy has been completed, the study is over and the patient can then find out whether she was taking placebo or herbs.

The main purpose of this study is to make sure the therapy is safe and that side effects on the kidneys and liver, and other symptoms, are carefully measured. Since chemotherapy can also cause these types of side effects, we had to use a randomized placebo-controlled design rather than let everyone receive the experimental herbs. This study will enroll only sixty patients, so it will not be large enough for us to reliably know whether the herbs can reduce the side effects of chemotherapy. We might get a hint of this if the effect is large—for example, if the intensity of nausea or fatigue is cut in half. As with any study, we must plan and then execute a very detailed statistical analysis of the information before we can make any firm conclusions about safety and effectiveness. Likewise, we will need to apply this same approach to some of the other interesting studies we are doing with patients participating in this trial. For example, since certain herbs in the regimen are designed to stimulate the immune system, we will look at their effects on patients' immune function. We must interpret these findings carefully, however, because even if we show that the immune function of patients using the herbal regimen is strengthened, this does not necessarily mean that they will be at a lower risk of the cancer returning. No immunological strategy has been clearly and unequivocally shown to accomplish this, although some individual studies have hinted at it (see chapter 10).

How Should the Patient and the Oncologist Deal with Alternative Medicine?

If you are ready to explore complementary therapies with your doctor, you may find it difficult to discuss the subject. Many conventional physicians are reluctant to accept alternative medicine or recommendations from practitioners in the field. I think this elitist attitude stems, at least in part, from the very regimented and protracted training period that physicians go through. I remember vividly the sense of power I felt after finishing medical school, when I put on the white coat (which I have long since shed). Even for a novice intern, it was rather intoxicating. And speaking to patients reinforced that authority in a way that listening to them, or simply observing, never could. It was easy to reject any ideas that did not emanate from the hallowed halls of the School of Medicine. After all, how could those hard years of medical school have taught us anything but the divine truth?

During my residency, one of my patients brought a faith healer from the hills of North Carolina into her room. Gloria had leukemia, which had relapsed, and no further medical therapy was planned because of her dismal prognosis. I left the room thinking that prayer might help her and her family spiritually, but I was surprised to return and find Gloria feeling relieved of her nausea and headache, which had incapacitated her for the previous few weeks. She went home in a few days and ultimately succumbed, but I felt humbled that an incomprehensible method had helped Gloria in her last few days. Could she have possibly suffered even less had we encouraged the family to seek such help sooner?

Physicians (and other professionals, for that matter) mature after school, and as they become more removed from their formal education they broaden their knowledge from experience and other sources such as reading scientific literature and attending conventions. Therefore, if they have never observed any benefit from unconventional medicine or been exposed to it in journals or medical meetings, it is not surprising that they will be skeptical. In fact, they may consider it quackery and deception. Many of my colleagues express the need to protect patients from falling prey in moments of desperation. In a field that is only beginning to develop a scientific and research base, there is a catch-22 situation. How can influential clinicians and scientists endorse and carry out studies that will promote the understanding of those alternative treatments, when they and most of their colleagues view the entire field as unscientific?

How should you communicate with your mainstream physician about the sensitive issue of care obtained outside the system? Perhaps the most important factor here is the actual reason you are seeking this care. I tend to be much more proactive in discussing these matters when I understand what my patient is trying to achieve. Whether it is relief of symptoms or the desire to boost the immune system, I can at least provide my opinion about what I think is likely or possible with alternative treatments. Not being an expert in any of them, I cannot prioritize for my patients which methods may be most suitable, but my openness to even discuss the topic puts me on their team and not in opposition.

I would recommend that patients broach the subject with their doctors by seeking an opinion about a very specific situation. For example:

"Will this herb help avoid neuropathy (nerve injury) if I'm going to take a chemotherapy drug that is known to cause it?" The answer might help you reach your own conclusions. "There could be a chance the herbs will interact with other medications you are already taking" may be a useful answer if you are not willing to take any risk with drug interactions. However, an answer such as "There's no way that an herbal medication could do that" would leave you wondering if there was any harm in at least trying the herb. At the current time, there is not enough information and very little education regarding most forms of alternative and complementary medicine, so a physician's comments may reflect a lack of knowledge or, in some cases, a personal bias. However, your doctor may have enough personal experience to give you a more reliable response, for example: "Several of my patients did experience pain improvement with acupuncture after not responding well to different drugs," or "I read a recent report showing that the herb you are taking could affect the blood-thinning drug you are also taking."

Some physicians may feel that both their care and their control are being undermined by outside advice. Sometimes this sentiment might be justified—for example, if a patient were being urged to forgo an obvious and urgent treatment such as antibiotics for a life-threatening infection, or some form of curative surgery for cancer. At other times, the doctor's resistance may reflect some degree of arrogance and ignorance. If you encounter this, you must ask yourself if your desire to pursue the treatment in question (based on others' recommendations or any experience you might have had) is strong enough to encourage you to press your doctor further on the matter or even to find a different physician. Some doctors find it more comfortable to accept that their patient is using alternative medicine if they are not asked to participate in this treatment or discuss any details or opinions. In fact, most of the time, conventional and alternative medical care are not coordinated. While this is not an optimal situation, it may be better than abandoning one arm of your medical care when you find that both are valuable. If you are seeking a new physician or medical group, some cancer centers now offer alternative/complementary care options. However, in some cases, these centers are set up for marketing reasons and may not really deliver the types of care you're searching for, such as an experienced herbalist or acupuncturist. These facilities may not necessarily coordinate your care or provide education to conventional physicians about alternative approaches (or, for that matter, the physicians at such a center may not even be supportive of the integrated care initiative). When interviewing a new physician, you must decide what priority you place on such complementary care and express yourself accordingly.

I cannot offer my patients expertise in anything but conventional oncologic care, since I do not have the training or experience outside this area. This is the case for most practicing oncologists. But I can offer myself as genuinely interested in learning and researching other types of treatment. From a practical standpoint, this may mean presenting patients with the option to participate in one of our research studies. I also support coordinating care with practitioners of alternative medicine outside our center, and I provide whatever advice I can, based on the medical literature. However, in most cases, there is simply no right or wrong answer. In addition to working with outside alternative medicine practitioners, as part of our comprehensive approach to treating patients at the UCSF Breast Care Center, we offer services by licensed acupuncturists, art therapists, tai chi instructors, and a host of talented therapists in our joint psychosocial program. For patients seeking alternative and complementary approaches, I recommend the following:

1. Look for a practitioner who has extensive experience in breast cancer.
2. Ask for a clear description of why the proposed regimen would work, based on biological principles, and why this particular plan is being recommended for you.
3. Determine the range of benefits you might see and how likely you are to enjoy those benefits. Give the information a reality check by comparing it with other available therapies. For example, a greater than 50% chance of complete long-term remission in advanced breast cancer is almost unheard of; if it did exist and was documented, it would certainly have been reported in the news and medical journals.
4. Have a frank discussion about side effects, the frequency of these side effects, and possible interactions with other drugs.

What forms of alternative medicine would I myself be willing to recommend, based on the current state of knowledge in the field? The one approach that has the best backing of clinical trial data is the use of acupuncture for symptoms, particularly nausea and pain. Since there are many effective medications for these symptoms, acupuncture should be used in conjunction with these drugs unless the drugs are clearly ineffective or cause significant side effects. Moreover, acupuncture treatments must be given at regular intervals for best effect, and as with many forms of alternative medicine, the experience of the practitioner may affect the results. Another practice that I think is very useful, at least in improving one's outlook and psychological state, is the use of group or meditative therapies. This is clearly an area where one size does not fit all. Some individuals may feel more comfortable sharing experiences and insights with a small group, whereas others might prefer a more solitary practice of reflectiveness, perhaps coupled with yoga, music, or art. The field of psychoneuroimmunology is dedicated to studying whether these avenues can actually have a physiological impact against cancer that could improve medical outcomes. Some preliminary studies have shown that different forms of meditation and group interaction can have a favorable effect on the immune system, but clear effects against cancer and improvements in longevity have not been proven. While we await definitive studies, I think that mind-body techniques, at the very least, can help us more effectively cope and adapt to illness and stress.

The usefulness of dietary supplements, vitamins, antioxidants, and herbal therapies is less certain. Many of these agents can affect breast cancer cell growth in the laboratory, or have beneficial effects on one's immune system or hormone levels in the blood. Some small studies even show a decrease in breast cancer risk or breast cancer recurrence risk, but many other contradictory studies do not show such effects. More controlled clinical studies that are large enough to give us reliable answers are desperately needed. In a controlled study, there is a comparison group that does not receive the treatment in question; ideally, this assignment is made randomly, perhaps by computer or by flipping a coin. The control group receives a placebo (inert substance), but neither the investigator nor the patients know who has been assigned to which group. (This is referred to as a double-blind study.) This process eliminates bias, or factors outside the treatment itself, that might affect the results, such as a psychological boost from realizing that you are receiving a new and exciting therapy. In the absence of studies done this way, I therefore do not make firm recommendations about dietary treatments, herbal remedies, or nutritional/vitamin supplements. However, I do think that many common-sense approaches can be helpful, like eating low on the food chain (mostly fruit, grain, and vegetables) with lots of green leafy vegetables, which are rich in vitamins, and considering standard doses of vitamins if one's diet may be deficient. This may be useful not only against breast cancer but also against heart disease and other common maladies.

I personally have the greatest difficulties with alternative approaches that spurn some of the known and accepted standards for cancer care, such as surgery for early-stage operable cancer. I am equally apprehensive about belief systems that are contrary to known physiological principles, or those based on science and theory that have no historical or experimental foundation. Regardless of how passionately the belief is espoused, we need some form of proof to establish credibility. However, I also recognize the need to maintain a fully open mind to forms of healing that are very foreign or that diverge from what I see as established scientific principles. I hope we will all eventually be able to speak the same language in understanding what is required to openly embrace a particular approach.

Even though I am a coeditor of this book, there are bound to be points of view in it with which I disagree but which I feel should be aired. Obviously, all practitioners should share a commitment to open discourse and dialogue in pursuit of the truth. But there is always disagreement over the details of how and when the proof is sufficient.

Most practicing oncologists are aware of the common use of alternative medicine among their patients. Most do not feel qualified or interested in documenting the details of these regimens and are open to their use as long as it does not interfere with their treatment plan. I believe that oncologists should go the extra step—not only to document the nature of the therapies being used, but to understand the motivating factors and rationale behind these decisions and record any discernible positive or negative effects from these therapies. This is a tall order to fill in the modern-day era of fifteen-minute follow-up visits and a medical system that does nothing to promote adequate time for inter-action between physicians and their patients. However, this attitude needs to go beyond physicians and must include the office staff, insur-ance companies, and those who formulate health care policy. The entire cancer care field must become more attuned to the unmet needs and questions patients have—many of which deal with the field of alternative medicine. Once we understand the patterns of use, we can at least begin to prioritize which alternative therapies should be investi-gated first. Furthermore, regular gathering of patient information may even lead to some amount of evidence for or against the effectiveness of some approaches when numerous patients' records are formally analyzed. For all these reasons, I encourage oncologists to ask and record what their patients are using or considering.

I commend all the authors of this book for sharing their wisdom, art, and practice and for their willingness to put forth views that are bold and sometimes controversial. Counseling and treating individuals with breast cancer are complicated, and our arsenal to fight off the disease is far from complete. We encourage you to view our collection of chapters as a guide. Take from it what feels right to you, and use it for discussion with your caregivers, family, and friends. Over time, many of the fields covered in this book will converge, diverge, and evolve with conven-tional medicine. Let us hope that creative forces, open minds, and sci-entific objectivity will carry the day.

CHAPTER THREE

Choices in Healing

Michael Lerner, Ph.D.

MICHAEL LERNER, PH.D., is president and co-founder of Commonweal, a
health and environmental research institute in Bolinas, California, and of
Smith Farm Center for the Healing Arts in Washington, D.C. He is the
author of *Choices in Healing: Integrating the Best of Conventional and
Complementary Approaches to Cancer* (MIT Press) and co-founder of the
Commonweal and Smith Farm Cancer Help Programs, week-long
residential support programs for people with cancer.

The Fighter Pilot

This is a story about how one man was able to use a diagnosis of cancer to
heal his life. Edward, the father of a dear friend of mine from college, was
a fighter pilot in World War II, flying off an aircraft carrier in the Pacific.
He was very fortunate to come home alive. He married the widow of
another fighter pilot who had lost his life in Europe. He worked and
raised a family, but without much joy in his life for many years. Then one
day my friend called to say that her father had been diagnosed with a very
life-threatening abdominal cancer. He was not expected to live long at
all. My friend asked me to call him.

Edward and I became friends. I helped him find a gifted masseur, a
healer, and a practitioner of traditional Chinese medicine. I also helped
him find an oncologist he liked and a hospital that he preferred over the
first one he had been in. To the amazement of his family, Edward
changed dramatically. He improved his diet, he stopped smoking, and
he stopped drinking. He developed, in fact, a sense of joy and vitality
about life that far exceeded anything he had experienced for decades.

One day I asked Edward the question that I have often found useful in helping people with cancer toward real healing.

"If you didn't have cancer right now," I said, "and could do anything you wanted at all, what would you do?" Edward scarcely hesitated. "I'd start to fly again," he said.

"What is stopping you?" I asked.

"There's some dumb regulation in this state that if you have a cancer diagnosis you can't get a pilot's license again."

"Is there any way around that?"

Edward thought for a long time. "You know," he finally said, "I've often watched those glider pilots and thought that could be really fun to do." He paused. "I suppose," he said quietly, "that I could learn to glide."

Edward researched gliding. He discovered that one of the best gliding schools around was in the northern California desert. I live on the California coast, just north of San Francisco. One night while I was sitting at home, there was a knock on the door. I opened the door, and there were Edward and an equally weather-beaten old friend—another old fighter pilot, it turned out—completely unannounced, sheepish as sixteen-year-olds on a forbidden spree, asking for a place to bunk down for the night before they headed out to the gliding school in the desert.

Edward stopped by to see me again on his way back from gliding school. He had an advanced certificate as a glider pilot and a bright gleam in his eye. The best moment, he told me, was when he rode a thermal up to six thousand feet. He saw the snow-capped mountains off to one side. The desert stretched below him. He saw a shadow above him and looked up. There was a bald eagle. The eagle began to fly alongside him. In absolute silence, they soared side by side. The eagle looked him directly in the eye.

It has been many years now since Edward received the cancer diagnosis that was expected to claim his life within a relatively short time. He has had other health crises to deal with, but the cancer diagnosis and his response to it transformed his life for many years.

Edward's story is not unusual among people I have known who have been able to make creative use of a cancer diagnosis. One psychologist put it simply. A cancer diagnosis, he said, is often an excellent treatment for neurosis. That is, a life-threatening disease often helps us to radically shift away from self-defeating psychic patterns in the fight for life. My colleague Julia Rowland, a respected psycho-oncologist, says that if you ask women with breast cancer what the diagnosis has meant in their lives, you often hear a recital of a range of positive life changes that—if you did not know the cause was the diagnosis of a life-threatening disease—you would ascribe to a powerful positive event.

But many people experience nothing positive about a cancer diagnosis, and among them are people who were living more or less self-realized lives before the diagnosis. In a sense, we could say that they had no neurotic or self-defeating life patterns that the diagnosis helped them break out of. Yet, others who were already living self-realized lives are able to use the cancer diagnosis to explore new realms of self-actualization.

It is virtually impossible to generalize, except to say that if you are fortunate, a cancer diagnosis can be a teachable moment in your life. That moment can be a time when, if you are able to open up to the possibilities, the creative powers within you are uniquely ready to come to the surface to assist you in facing both the tremendous challenges and the possibilities of living through this very difficult experience.

Five Provinces of Choice in Cancer

I believe that when you are diagnosed with breast cancer—or indeed any other serious illness—five great provinces of choice open up before you, whether you are aware of them or not. And I believe that developing a conscious awareness of these provinces of choice, whether you are presently ill or not, can change your life for the better.

These five provinces are

Choices in healing
Choices in conventional therapies
Choices in complementary or alternative therapies
Choices in dealing with pain, grief, and suffering
Choices in facing death and dying

Indeed, every human being, in the course of a lifetime, implicitly makes choices in these five provinces of healing. But the sad truth is that most people never recognize that they are making these choices. They are never given the opportunity to consider how much difference making these choices consciously, with as much wisdom as they can summon up, can make, both for them and for those they care about.

Exploring these five provinces of choices in healing, and making these choices as consciously and skillfully as possible, is what I seek to help people with cancer do. This chapter focuses on the first of these five areas: choices in healing itself.

In a sense, you may encounter all five of these provinces of choice at each stage in the development of cancer or any other illness: at diagnosis, in choosing and undergoing conventional therapies, in choosing and using complementary therapies, in living with the hope that you have been cured and the disease will not recur, in facing recurrence if you have to live through that experience, in making new treatment choices and undergoing additional treatments, in living in remission with the hope that the remission will last as long as possible, in experiencing progression of the disease, in living with the hope that the progress of the disease will be as slow as possible or that new treatments will be developed while you are alive or that some alternative therapy might extend your life, and in facing the prospect of dying.

Even at diagnosis, for example, and even if the probability of cure is high, the prospect that this disease might be mortal surfaces in your consciousness. Thus, from the start of the illness, you may psychically be facing the inner encounter with death and dying, even though the objective probability that you will face death sooner than others your age may be very low. Even at diagnosis you may be grieving—grieving the loss of well-being and the uncertainties about the future you now face.

I regard each of these provinces of choice—in healing, in conventional therapies, in complementary therapies, in pain and suffering, and in death and dying—as chapters in a great book. In my imagination, this great book about choices in healing exists partially within us and partially outside of us. The parts of this great book that lie within us, and are unique to each of us, contain the wisdom that enables us to select what we need. The parts of the great book that we can find outside us include everything from the latest scientific studies of mainstream cancer treatments, to the complementary cancer therapies that make the most sense to us, to the greatest wisdom teachings of all traditions about life on the edge, to how to receive the love and support of our families and friends.

Because each of these five provinces of choice is in fact a chapter in a great inner/outer book, it is very important that you know you do not have to read all of these chapters at once. It is simply useful to know that they are there, and that you can turn to them when you are ready, and that they contain a wealth of wisdom that can transform the experience of cancer or any other disease. Skillful healing choices may help you to maximize the chances that you will achieve a cure—or extend life as much as possible.

Choices in Healing

Choices in healing provide the master key to each of these five provinces of choice. That is, a deep understanding of choices in healing provides guidance not only to choices in healing your life but to choices in conventional therapies, complementary therapies, pain control, and dying.

Here are some critical basic dimensions of choices in healing.

To begin with, *healing is fundamentally distinct from curing*. There are three ways in which the word *cure* is used in cancer. One definition of a cancer cure is a bit of statistical sophistry. You are sometimes said to be cured of cancer if you live five years without any sign of recurrence of the disease. That is not a real cure. That is five-year survival.

The second use of the word *cure* is the one that matters for you. You are by definition cured of a disease if you have been treated, the disease disappears, and you live as long as you would have lived if you never had the disease. That is a cure. An individual cure of this kind can in theory be achieved with conventional treatments, or complementary treatments, or some combination of both—or even with no treatments at all—as long as the disease disappears and you live as long as you would have lived if you had never had cancer.

The third use of the word *cure* in cancer goes beyond the individual, and it is also very important to you. A specific treatment for a specific type of cancer is said to be a cure for that cancer if, in some substantial proportion of cases, the treatment means that the cancer never returns. If a conventional cancer treatment exists that is curative for any form of cancer, I always strongly encourage patients to use it, and use it promptly, because, as we will see later, *there are no known systematically curative treatments for cancer among the complementary therapies*. That is to say, there are certainly many individual cases in which people have achieved cures using some combination of conventional and complementary therapies, and even occasionally cases in which people have used complementary therapies only. But to date there are no known systematically curative treatments of any kind of cancer among the complementary cancer therapies, while there are systematically curative treatments of some breast cancers (at least for the early stage) among conventional cancer therapies. Because life is so deeply precious, and because conventional therapies are the only current treatments known to have a scientifically demonstrated track record of systematically curing some cancers, a curative treatment should always start with conventional cancer therapies.

Healing is fundamentally distinct from cure, but it is also deeply connected to achieving a cure. Healing comes from within ourselves. It is the process by which we become whole again. It can take place physically, as when a bone knits together or a wound heals. It can take place emotionally, as when we overcome old or recent emotional wounds. Healing can take place mentally, as when we are able to replace destructive or outgrown ways of seeing ourselves and the world with wiser and more useful ways of understanding life. And healing can take place spiritually—if that word has meaning for you—as when we evolve in some meaningful way in relation to whatever guides us in life, to whatever we hold sacred. (I need to say, parenthetically, that I am in no way attached to whether the word *spiritual* is meaningful to you or not. Some of the most spiritual people I know have no use for the concept. We will talk about this more later.)

Since healing can take place at all these different levels—physical, emotional, mental, and spiritual—that also means that *healing can take place both in living and in dying.* Some of the most powerful healing experiences I have ever witnessed have taken place in people who were losing ground to a difficult disease, or who were actually dying.

This distinction between curing and healing is not some flaky idea of New Age healers. Rather, it is a distinction recognized throughout the best of the medical literature. Therefore, healing is fundamental to what we will explore together, since *healing is fundamentally our province,* not the province of the physician or health care professional. The physician may support or retard the healing process in us, but healing can truly come only from within.

Healing, therefore, is what we bring to the table in the confrontation with disease. And because each of us is an absolutely unique person, *healing at the physical, emotional, mental, and spiritual levels will be different for each of us.* This simple fact has profound implications: we must each find our own absolutely unique way to heal.

In the medical literature, this distinction between curing and healing leads to a set of fundamental distinctions that we ignore at our peril. We can say that *biomedical treatment is concerned with curing the disease and alleviating pain, while biopsychosocial medicine (or mind-body medicine) is concerned not only with curing the disease and alleviating pain but also with healing the illness and alleviating suffering.*

Thus, just as curing and healing are different but overlapping concepts, so are disease and illness, and pain and suffering. Curing, disease, and pain—the province of biomedicine—are all closer to the biomedical facts of the situation. Healing, illness, and suffering—the province of biopsychosocial medicine or mind-body medicine—are all closer to the human experience of these facts.

Imagine fifty women with precisely the same stage and grade of breast cancer. They all have the same disease, by definition. How many illnesses do they have? *The fifty women all have the same disease, but each has her own unique illness.* That is because each woman has her own completely unique way of experiencing the disease. This is essential to understand if you are to benefit deeply from this book. All fifty women might be treated in a similar way biomedically to cure the disease, but each should be treated differently, and treat herself differently, to heal the fifty different illnesses.

In fact, breast cancer is a particularly useful example of this distinction, because there are many different legitimate approaches to biomedical treatment of the same diagnosis in these fifty women. When there are important alternatives in biomedical curative treatment as well as in healing, as there often are, then part of healing the illness involves deep choices in biomedical treatment as well as in healing approaches to the illness.

It is vital to healing to pause here, for a moment, and truly let the significance of these simple truths sink in. For what you actually experience with a diagnosis of breast cancer, or any other life-threatening disease, is not the disease itself but the illness: your own experience of the disease. *And whether or not you are able to change the course of breast cancer, you can unquestionably alter the human experience of the illness.*

Moreover, everything that research has taught us about mind-body health suggests that in many instances, *the work that we do to transform the experience of the illness may also have an effect on the course of the disease.* This is because mind-body medicine has demonstrated that for many health conditions, there are—or may be—vital feedback loops between how we feel about our health and what course our disease takes.

Thus, working on healing as well as curing can be considered a win-win proposition. Healing work can help you go through the experience of this illness in the best way you can. And healing work may, in some cases, have effects on the disease process that may help you prevent recurrence or extend your life as well.

Healing with Imagery, Creativity, and Meaning

Let us assume we have concluded that work on healing is not just some flaky New Age concept but really merits our serious attention. How do you work on healing, really? I have suggested that each of our paths to healing is unique. But there are some pointers that may be helpful.

I have come to think of healing, particularly at the psychological and spiritual level, as closely related to three other concepts: *imagery, creativity,* and *meaning.* I want to say something about each.

The Uses of Imagery

Imagery, in the words of Rachel Naomi Remen, is the language of the unconscious. It goes beyond simple visual imagery, such as "Pac-man" healthy cells gobbling up diseased cancer cells. Many people with cancer try some stereotyped visual imagery and, discovering they cannot do it, decide that they are "no good" at imagery.

My friend and colleague, Martin Rossman, M.D., one of the best teachers of the uses of imagery in healing, taught me to ask people with cancer who have decided they are "no good" at imagery this simple question:

"If you think you are no good at imagery, tell me: *do you know how to worry?*"

If you know how to worry, Rossman points out, then you are by definition good at imagery. And most of us know how to worry. So the only question is, do you want to restrict your powerful skills at imagery to worrying, or do you want to explore other dimensions of the ways in which the unbounded forces of our unconscious communicate with us as well?

The truth is that imagery can come in many forms. Imagery not only can be visual—in fact, a majority of people are not primarily visual in imagery—but also can reach us through sound, touch, taste, smell, or simply a sense of knowing or intuition. Imagery can come to us in dreams, in writing, in art, in silence, in sudden moments of clarity, in the gradual dawning of realizations, and in almost every other possible way.

The Value of Creative Work

The story of my friend Edward, the fighter pilot, is a good example of someone who found, in gliding, an outlet for his lost creativity and zest for life.

The healing process can be seen in part as the search for reconnection with the creative healing force within us, for recovering our relationship with that creative fire.

It is important to consider the value of creative work in healing with cancer because so many of us, as adults, have come to forget or even to fear the creative force in our lives and to believe that we are not creative people. This is very clear in the Commonweal Cancer Help Program, where we routinely find that, of all the activities the program offers, there are two that participants routinely fear.

One is the sandtray, a Jungian technique developed originally for psychotherapeutic use with children too young to verbalize what is troubling them. A sandtray is a large rectangular wooden box, perhaps 20 inches wide and 30 inches long, with sides about 4 inches high, containing an inch or so of white sand. On shelves in the Commonweal sandtray room are hundreds of little toys and objects. The sandtray therapist—at Commonweal this is Marion Weber or Irene Gallwey—invites you to select any of the objects that attract you and place them in the tray. When you have placed as many objects as you wish in the sandtray, and it feels complete, Marion or Irene will invite you to reflect on what you have created and to say whatever you choose about it.

For many people, the sandtray naturally reveals a story, and it is often a story that they did not know they were going to tell in advance. These sandtray stories are often important healing stories. The truth is that facing a life-threatening illness often brings forth powerful unconscious processes that are unusually close to the surface and unusually ready for us to access, if only we know how. The sandtray is one way—one form of imagery, if you will—to access this deep unconscious creative force that "wants" to communicate with us.

The Greeks knew this. Greek healers knew that life-threatening illness often brings unconscious wisdom about how to heal very close to the surface, seeking only a setting where it can be released. The great Aesculapian temples of healing were places where patients came with the express purpose of awaiting a dream that would point out their path of healing. It is no trivial point that we need these Aesculapian temples ourselves, as much as we need hospitals. But we must invent our own Aesculapian temples, because our culture has forgotten the importance of dreams, of creative imagery, to our healing.

The other activity we can be assured that most people will fear during the Cancer Help Program is Poetry Night, when we write poems together. The idea of writing a poem is so petrifying to most Cancer Help Program participants that we even changed the name of the evening to Healing Language. It is petrifying for many people to imagine that they will be asked to engage in some kind of "creative writing," even when we explain that what we write that evening has nothing to do with meter and rhyme, but simply with listening to some of the words that others have written on previous retreats, meditating for a while, and then taking up pen and paper. When Rachel Naomi Remen brought poetry to the Cancer Help Program, she would offer a simple instruction after reading some poems and a brief time in silence: "Write something that is true."

Here are a few examples of poems from the Cancer Help Program.

One exceptional survivor of cancer, Erik Esselstyn, who outlived a dire diagnosis of pancreatic cancer, spoke for many of us in September 1988, when he wrote these lines:

Of courage and of love
I've learned anew
From breastless women.

Here is a poem that Susannah Abrams, who came to Commonweal in June 1992, wrote about her breast:

> My other breast is gone into the garbage pail,
> Cast aside, useless;
> Leaving my heart completely exposed.

Anthony Gallagher wrote a poem about an incurable cancer in June 1993:

INCURABLE

> This life is what
> I always wanted
>
> God's breath in the crows
> Cypress pretending to be wind
>
> Beer in the icebox
> Beans laughing on the stove
>
> My love ahead
> Her hands in her pockets
> Secrets in her hands
>
> And me
> In the rutted road
> Walking slowly home.
>
> But now it's just not enough.

And Ellen Mauck Lessy wrote this unforgettable poem about facing death with cancer:

SHROUD

> A word. With little power
> A word only: clichéd in silence
> and unknown in fact to all
> but orderlies and undertakers.
> The days of royal linen gone,
> supply rooms carry plastic squares.

Where is the celebration
of the life and body?

I'll come one day to wear
your mourning and my shroud,
but if you've loved me,
search the shelves at home.
You'll find a faded sheet
I've washed a hundred times
where we made love and slept,
the afghan knitted as a gift,
the old green spread that carried me
through college and the beach.
Bring something large enough
not for my body only;
more goes with me on this trip.
Wrap me in memory,
in remnants of life together,
not in that sterile white
made in the thousands for the everyman.
Let me be someone,
even in death;
send with me fragments
of people I have loved,
for I shall love them still.

Reading these poems, one can easily recognize how powerfully healing it can be to put into words some essential dimensions of the experience of the encounter with breast cancer. But going into the experience of Poetry Night, most people are as terrified of creative writing as they are of the sandtray. Now why is this? The answer, in both cases, is this: people have learned to fear that what they will produce will not be "good enough." They fear that they are not creative, that they will not produce a "good" sandtray or write a "good" poem.

With these culturally induced ways of dismissing and denigrating our own creativity, our birthright of access to the creative force within us may be shut off. Imagine yourself as a child, walking into a room with a sandbox and a lot of toys. Do you think the child would be afraid to play in the sand? The same is true of drawing or writing poems before our critical mind convinces us that we are no good at these activities.

We lose our outlets for our creative fire, and this loss is no small thing. Part of healing, therefore, may be reconnecting with this enormous power in ourselves.

Meaning and Survival

The third realm of inner work that I find deeply connected with healing is the exploration of meaning in our lives. You may know the book by Viktor Frankl, *Man's Search for Meaning*, which describes the essence of the relationship between healing and meaning. Frankl, a Jewish psychoanalyst, was a prisoner in Auschwitz during World War II. While trying to survive, and as a physician seeking to help other prisoners, he came to look closely at who managed to survive, both physically and psychologically, under these very extreme conditions.

Do you think it was the strongest who survived? Frankl found that those who survived were not the strongest, but rather those who had some *core of meaning* that made living worthwhile. As Nietzsche put it, "Those who have a why to live can bear most any how." This meaning differed from person to person. Eli Wiesel, a great Jewish writer who also lived through a harrowing experience in the Nazi concentration camps, reported the same thing that Frankl reported. It was the prisoners who had a deep core of meaning, of reason to live, who survived physically and psychologically. He and his father stayed alive, for example, trying to take care of each other. It was when his father died that Wiesel went through the worst of his camp experience.

For Wiesel, the core of meaning was not to abandon his father. For others, it was a deep belief in God. Frankl wrote that he watched men and women walk into the gas chambers "with a smile on their lips and a prayer in their hearts." Even when camp inmates simply could not survive physically, this core of inner meaning gave them a capacity to face death and unimaginable suffering from an interior place where there was something fundamental that the Nazis could not reach or destroy.

Larry LeShan, a great cancer psychotherapist who wrote the seminal books *You Can Fight for Your Life* and *Cancer as a Turning Point*, has reported that in his work with thousands of people with cancer, those who "do best" physically as well as psychologically are characteristically those who are able to use cancer as a turning point and who are able to find what LeShan has called "their own unique song." They have found their own unique core of meaning with which to face the experience of the disease.

Frankl puts it another way. There is what happens to us in life, and there is our response to what happens to us. We may or may not be able to change what happens to us, but we always have a degree of inner freedom in our *response* to what happens to us. The question of how aware and how skilled we become in exercising our freedom to choose our responses to the events of life is the fundamental question to which the great spiritual traditions are addressed. The spiritual traditions teach us the capacity to grow in wisdom and compassion so that we can respond, from the deepest place in ourselves, to whatever life brings us.

That capacity to choose wisely and compassionately, with a sense of our own uniqueness and our own destiny, is what making choices in healing is ultimately all about. To understand the nature of healing is to understand the greatest wisdom about how to live.

Sir Charles

I have learned as much about healing from friends with other illnesses as I have from friends with cancer. Charles Fox is one friend who has taught me as much about healing, while living with a difficult illness, as anyone I have met in my life. For his extraordinary services to life, I have internally "knighted" him, and I think of him as Sir Charles.

Born in England and raised in Kenya, Charles emigrated to California at age nineteen. He is a gifted novelist and lives in my town, a tiny coastal community of about two thousand souls. When I met Charles over twenty years ago, he was a dashing writer for *Car and Driver* magazine who liked to drive very fast cars. He had just been diagnosed with multiple sclerosis. He was beginning to walk with a cane.

Over the more than twenty years that I have known Charles, I have watched him go from walking with a cane to living as a quadriplegic, unable to move anything except his mouth and eyes. He has about 10% of his lung capacity left. He speaks with the aid of an amplifier.

Charles has been near death many times with his disease. A few years ago, he developed a sore on his buttocks from sitting in his wheelchair—a seemingly small event, but one that can be fatal for someone with minimal lung capacity and a weakened immune system.

Charles required surgery for the bedsore, which became infected. After surgery, he was confined to bed for three months so that his buttocks could heal. Without great care, the three months in bed might have led to other breaks in the skin. If the skin breakdowns had spread and the infection had continued, Charles would have died.

When I visit Charles, I never feel sorry for him. He has a vast repertoire of earthy stories, and an exquisite sense of timing and delivery when he tells these stories. We don't talk much about his illness when we see each other. We always watch the Super Bowl together. Sometimes we play chess.

During the twenty years I have known Charles, he has tried virtually every known alternative therapy for multiple sclerosis. He has used acupuncture, done bodywork with the late famous Israeli master Moishe Feldenkrais, eaten a variety of special diets, and practiced Buddhist meditation. He has kept careful track of the mainstream scientific literature on multiple sclerosis, waiting for a breakthrough and a cure.

Charles believes that all these therapies helped him for various periods of time and in various ways. The meditation, he says, has been especially useful—understandably, for someone who must perforce sit without moving.

What has helped Charles in healing most, without question, is love, which appeared most recently several years ago in the form of an extraordinary young Frenchwoman named Veronique. Vero is as small as Charles is large. They fell in love and married.

Watching Vero get Charles, whom I can barely move at all, out of bed and into his wheelchair in the morning, with the assistance of an ingeniously rigged pulley system, is for me nothing less than a small religious experience.

Charles and Vero's house is a crossroads of friends who drop in to read to him, sit with him, or take him on expeditions. He and Vero travel quite frequently, on a financial shoestring. They have lived in Mexico, France, and Spain over the past few years, both because they like the adventure and because costs are often lower there.

In the twenty years I have known Charles, never once have I heard him complain about what is happening to his body. As I sat with him during this last period of recovery from his wheelchair wound, while he lay in bed with a raging fever, I asked him how he did it.

He was lying on his back, staring up at the skylight a carpenter friend had just installed so that he could see the sky while confined to bed.

"In a way, the disease has been a gift," he said.

"In what way?"

"It stripped life down to its essentials," he said. "At a certain point, one tires of trying all these things to recover. One just wants to enjoy life for what it is. To live."

He paused.

"The Arabs have a saying," he said. "You have to ride a fast camel. Stay ahead of the news."

That is not a story about cancer. It is a story about living impeccably with something much more difficult than most cancers.

It is a story about a man who tried every possible active approach to healing, and for whom *not trying to recover physically* was itself, in its own time, the greatest healing. Or perhaps I should say the second greatest healing. The greatest healing for Sir Charles and all of us who are privileged to know him is his friendship and his love.

Two Useful Oversimplifications

In this chapter, I have taken refuge in two useful oversimplifications of the complex realities of healing for the sake of clarity. It is time to undo these oversimplifications, which have outlived their usefulness.

First, I have focused primarily on the psychological and spiritual dimensions of healing and their impact both on quality of life and potentially on prevention of recurrence and life extension as well. In fact, of course, there are many physical approaches to healing, such as diet and exercise, progressive deep relaxation and massage, yoga or qigong or other psychophysiological disciplines. The point here is that these physical approaches to healing are as deeply connected to enhancing psychological and spiritual well-being as they are to physical healing, just as psychological and spiritual healing can have profound physical effects on healing.

Second, I also oversimplified in suggesting that curative treatments primarily come from outside us, whereas healing comes primarily from within. This is true as far as it goes, but the deeper truth is that curative treatments may also depend to a large but unknowable extent on the regenerative forces for healing, both physical and psychospiritual, inside us. Any oncologist will tell you that some highly curative treatments inexplicably fail for some patients, while other rarely curative treatments inexplicably help some patients achieve total cures. In conventional therapies, a great deal of research on quality of life in cancer connects both psychological well-being and physical well-being to life extension with a wide range of cancers and cancer treatments. So healing, as it affects quality of life both physically and psychospiritually, appears in ways we do not yet understand. Sometimes healing is associated with life extension and prevention of recurrence—which is to say, curing.

It is also a great oversimplification to speak of healing as exclusively an inner province. We know from years of work in the Commonweal Cancer Help Program how powerfully healing can be stimulated by a supportive community of people who are going through a similar breast cancer experience and seeking to heal together. Healing can be powerfully assisted from without by physicians, friends, lovers, children, and sources of support that we may experience as fundamentally mysterious.

Healing, finally, is not an end, not a static state, not something to be achieved, after which we move on. Healing is a continuous evolutionary process within us, never ending, never complete. Healing is the journey itself. Healing is the purpose of life, the development of awareness, the deepening of wisdom and compassion, the use of will to ground insight in the acts of our lives. Healing literally means "movement toward wholeness." Wholeness encompasses both life and death, both losing and finding, both knowing and mystery.

CHAPTER FOUR

Chinese Medicine and Breast Cancer

Isaac Cohen, O.M.D., L.Ac.

ISAAC COHEN, O.M.D., L.Ac., is one of the leading authorities in the field of cancer treatment and traditional Chinese medicine. A pioneer in work designed to provide scientific translation of traditional medical concepts and therapies, he lectures internationally on the integration of TCM in cancer treatment. He was one of the founders of the complementary and alternative medicine program at the Carol Franc Buck Breast Care Center at the University of California, San Francisco and has established an ongoing relationship with the Chinese Society for the Integration of TCM and Western Medicine for the Prevention and Treatment of Cancer, Beijing, China. He has a doctorate in Oriental medicine from the Postgraduate Institute of Oriental Medicine in Hong Kong, has trained with the most renowned cancer specialists in China, and has studied extensively there. He spearheaded clinical and laboratory research to assess the efficacy of herbal therapies and has worked closely with University of California, San Francisco research scientists to discover mechanistic explanations for the clinical application of natural products.

> *Rain falls on the just and unjust alike.*
>
> —CHINESE PROVERB*

A few years ago, a woman in her early fifties came to see me, pathology report in hand. A mammogram had already revealed a 1-centimeter lump in her breast, a palpable lymph node under her armpit, and a fine needle biopsy had confirmed a diagnosis of infiltrating ductal carcinoma—in other words, breast cancer. She had done extensive reading and discussed things with her physicians, who confirmed that she had time—meaning one month—to explore her alternatives before resorting to

---

*The same idea appears in the New Testament in Matthew 5:45: "He causes his sun to rise on the evil and the good, and sends rain on the righteous and the unrighteous."

surgery. Intrigued by the possibilities of Chinese medicine, she asked whether I could treat her tumor with a noninvasive method.

Given the small size of the tumor, and the fact that there was little lymph node involvement and no evidence of metastasis, I agreed that it would be safe to delay conventional treatment methods for a few weeks and try herbal therapy and acupuncture. I did, however, explain to her that early intervention with Western medicine was the ideal route to achieve optimal results. Despite this advice from both her surgeon and me, she decided to try Chinese herbal medicine alone. I saw her monthly to evaluate her progress and make any necessary changes to her herbal prescription. After three months, in my opinion, her condition was the same. Since it wasn't good news but also wasn't bad news, my patient decided to continue. After an additional two months of treatment, we couldn't find the lymph node that was previously palpable under her armpit. The surgeon, however, thought that the tumor in her breast had increased in size. I was not sure that this was in fact the case but thought perhaps I was biased. With concern that the tumor had grown in size, both the surgeon and I strongly encouraged our patient to undergo surgery to remove the mass.

After the surgery, she was found to have no cancerous cells in her lymph nodes and no invasive ductal carcinoma. Her tumor had retreated to a small ductal carcinoma in situ (DCIS), which means that there are cancerous cells but they are contained within the walls of the duct. The change in diagnosis from invasive cancer to DCIS indicated there was a lower probability that the mass would ever develop into invasive breast cancer or spread to a distant location.

The fate of our patient had changed dramatically.

About Traditional Chinese Medicine

While there are hundreds of anecdotal case reports of breast cancer cures after the use of traditional Chinese medicine (TCM) as a sole therapy, there is not enough scientific evidence to justify the use of Chinese medicine to replace any of the current Western medical treatments: surgery, radiation, chemotherapy, and hormonal therapy.[1-3] There is no doubt, however, that Chinese medicine is useful in all stages of the disease to augment the benefits of conventional treatments, to prevent recurrence and metastasis in early stages of breast cancer, and to promote health, improve quality of life, and prolong life in advanced stages.[4-16] TCM is an altogether different form of medicine, with its own unique ways of describing human physiology and pathology. It has over a million practitioners worldwide.

In this chapter, we will look at how TCM treatments are currently being used in an integrated setting along with Western methods to treat women with breast cancer. Later on, we'll explore some of the history and principles of this ancient tradition.

History of Breast Cancer in Traditional Chinese Medicine

The development of a written medical system in China started sometime in the third or fourth century B.C., and reached a high degree of sophistication about 250 B.C. with the publication of the *Yellow Emperor's Classic of Internal Medicine*.[17-20] This canon describes the processes that affect life and health and suggests treatment principles, with some specific acupuncture and herbal prescriptions. Chinese medicine has had many developments since that time. As a medical system, Chinese medicine exists as a continuous living tradition that has served and still serves a large part of the world's population.[21]

The first government-sponsored medical university was formed in A.D. 453 by Qin Chengzu, the physician to the Southern and Northern dynasties. In the year 624, at the beginning of the T'ang dynasty, a very large medical school—for the first time with departments, faculties, and clearly defined curriculum—was established. The school even had eighteen hectares (about seven and a quarter acres) of herb gardens to help develop medical-agriculture specialists.[22]

The book *The Rites of the Zhou Dynasty* (1100–400 B.C.) mentions physicians specializing in the treatment of "swellings and ulcerations" or "necrosis and ulcerations." Those terms persist to this day to denote the study and treatment of tumors both benign and malignant.[23]

Early Chinese medical texts described different types of breast tumors and discussed their clinical appearance, physiological origin, and severity.[24-26] Over a hundred names were recorded for tumors in early medical literature. Most of them signify what we would regard as early cancerous conditions. The most common term for breast cancer was "breast rock."[27] In the *Yellow Emperor's Classic of Internal Medicine* we find the first clinical description of breast cancer. The prognosis was thought to be about ten years after diagnosis, and the process of metastasis and death was detailed.[28]

Other than locations, tumors were classified according to their physical appearance (obstinate jaundice, callous lips, flower blossom lesions), the sensation under the physician's fingers (rock, walnut, movable/immovable), recurring symptoms the tumors may cause (loss of luster, food regurgitation, distention).[29] Physicians based their clinical assessments on their analysis of the patient's history, breast examination, pulse palpation, and observation of the tongue as well as the skin of the inner corner of the eye.

Causes of Breast Cancer: The TCM View

Breast cancer in TCM is thought to be the product of a long accumulation of seemingly insignificant factors, which exert their effects for many years and slowly erode the body's ability to nurture, protect, and regulate itself. These effects may include environmental pollutants, climatic exposure, history of infectious diseases, availability of food (quantity), nutrient level in food (quality), dietary habits, mental and emotional attitudes, balance between work and rest, sexual life, inherited physiological makeup, and water balance and metabolism.

In TCM, breast cancer may result from the interaction of these factors over a long period of time. Each individual woman will have a different path to the initiation, formation, and development of her breast cancer. Each woman will also manifest the disease in a different way. TCM believes not only in a multitude of possible causes but also that breast cancer behaves uniquely in each woman.[30-36]

The Chinese outlined and detailed a complex picture of the body consisting of tissues, organs, and blood vessels as well as a grid of network communication systems called meridians that intersect and interact with all other tissues and organs. The meridians and blood vessels were believed to supply all the nutrients that command and control the body to achieve continuous balance and harmony. The highly essential "stuff" that runs in the network vessels—and you'll see in a minute why I call it stuff—is called qi (pronounced "chee").[37-39] The Chinese accepted that although qi flows in a very precise lawful order, there may also be chaos caused by the complexity of life's conditions, which constantly change over time. They likened life to the movement of clouds and river water: you can identify it, but you can't make it stop moving and changing.

In Chinese medicine, two parallel systems are viewed in tandem. One is the picture of the perfect: an ultimate state of things and being, a picture of heavenly balance and harmony. The other is a description of the lawful deviation from the perfect. Since many factors are at play, the Chinese described those deviations in terms of patterns or syndromes. The more you probe into the pattern, the more accurately you can describe its details and dynamics.

Basic TCM Treatments

Herbal Medicine

Herbal medicine is the primary mode of treatment for breast cancer in TCM. There are specific herbs for all the various manifestations of the disease and the side effects of mainstream treatments, and they can be used in conjunction with all other treatments.

Herbs are prescribed to address the specific complex of issues presented by each patient. Traditionally, herbal remedies are prescribed in combinations to work in synergy and to relieve one another's side effects. Usually, the formulas include five to twenty-five herbs, in varying doses.

Many practitioners provide herbs directly to their patients. In my practice, I write out prescriptions to be filled at a Chinese pharmacy, just as you'd take your physician's prescription to a standard pharmacy. (A list of herbal pharmacies is provided at the end of the chapter.)

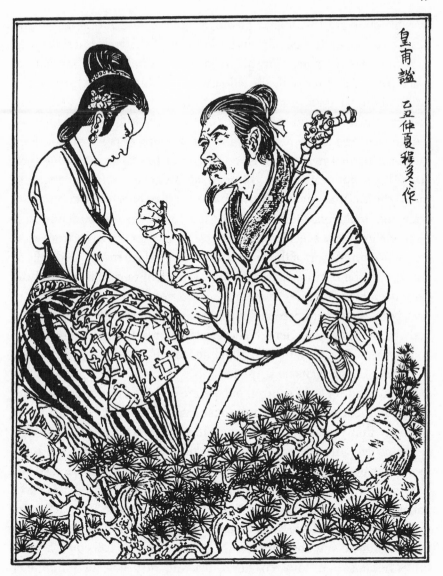

皇甫謐

乙丑仲夏程多之作

FIGURE 4.1. Huangfu Mi, author of *A Classic of Acupuncture and Moxibustion*, first published in A.D. 282, inserting an acupuncture needle.

Acupuncture

Acupuncture involves inserting fine needles in specific points on the skin in order to regulate the functioning of the body. (Acupressure, a form of massage of these same points, with no needles involved, is another possible strategy.) In Chinese medicine we believe that qi (energy) and blood circulate in the body through a network of channels (meridians) in a specific orderly fashion. The qi enters and exits individual meridians at exact times. You can needle the shin at a point called Stomach-36 to subdue abdominal pain. You can treat a headache by needling a point between the thumb and index finger on the Large Intestine meridian, or reduce nausea and vomiting by merely pressing a point on the Pericardium channel near the wrist on the inner (palm) aspect of the forearm. This is not hearsay or a cultural bias. Much scientific evidence and many clinical trials have confirmed the curative effects of acupuncture point manipulation. Modern science has found that acupuncture needling elicits many specific physiological responses, ranging from pain control to stimulation of the bone marrow to produce more blood cells or changes in the hormonal milieu. The concept of qi circulation and the existence of meridians is frequently questioned by contemporary scientists, but it is currently accepted that needling, at the very least, affects the body by provoking a variety of chemicals that reside in our central nervous system. These chemicals, called neurotransmitters, affect the body as a whole, changing its response to various ailments. This mechanism is well explained for pain control, but we are still far from understanding why acupuncture needling causes those internal changes.

In my first years of practice, even though I was a practitioner who made his living from practicing acupuncture, I was often surprised at the fact that patients reported a positive effect when points were needled at a distance from the complaint. I can't forget one of my first breast cancer patients, who initially came for treatment of intractable low back pain. She was "stuck"—she couldn't straighten up or bend forward. There was no comfortable way for her to even get a treatment. I needled a point under her nose and "tortured" her by twisting the needle for a minute or two. To her surprise and mine, her pain diminished dramatically, and she became more mobile. She is still my friend after more than ten years.

Many people are put off by the idea of acupuncture because they're afraid of needles or because the concept seems so strange to them. Actually, acupuncture can be administered with minimal pain, and most people find it very relaxing. In fact, most everyone falls asleep or "spaces out" during the treatment. The needles that we use are solid, unlike IV needles, which are hollow. The needle is usually inserted into

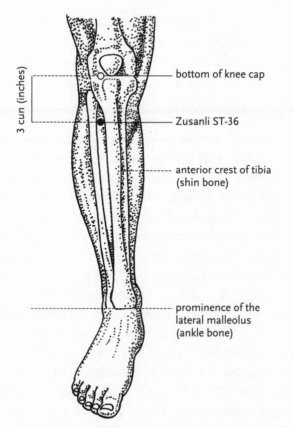

3 cun (inches)

bottom of knee cap

Zusanli ST-36

anterior crest of tibia
(shin bone)

prominence of the
lateral malleolus
(ankle bone)

FIGURE 4.2. Zusanli, Stomach-36 (ST-36) for the treatment and prevention of abdominal pain. Reprinted with permission from Deadman P, Al-Khafaji M, Baker K. *A Manual of Acupuncture.* Journal of Chinese Medical Publications, East Sussex, England. ISBN 0-9510546-7-8.

a muscle or into a space between a tendon and the muscular structure, so there is rarely bleeding when the needle is removed. Acupuncturists use sterile disposable needles.

Qigong

Qigong (literally, energy cultivation) encompasses a multitude of exercises and routines of gentle, rhythmical movements and self-massage aimed at controlling the breath, calming the mind, improving health and mental alertness, and preventing and treating disease.[40] (The more familiar tai chi is actually one type of qigong.)

Qigong has been practiced for centuries, and it is said to ward off evil as well as maintain good health. Research over the past thirty years supports this idea. There is good evidence that qigong can regulate heart function and blood pressure, enhance circulation and improve wound healing in people with diabetes, improve bowel function, eliminate harmful bacteria, reduce heartburn, help heal gastric and duodenal ulcers, and relieve chronic constipation. Qigong also increases the levels of endorphins and other chemicals associated with pain control and immunity. In clinical studies, qigong improved breathing and lung capacity.[41]

Research from China attests to the immune-boosting effect of the exercises. In a study of people with various types of advanced cancer at a Beijing hospital, about three quarters of the subjects received chemotherapy and did qigong, and the rest got chemotherapy alone. The drugs and dosages were similar, though not identical, in all cases. The qigong group practiced two hours a day for an average of three months.

The qigong group had significantly better results in normalized liver function and red blood cell profile, which translates to better supply of oxygen and energy in the body, phagocytosis activity (destruction of bacteria and other foreign particles), feeling of regained strength (82% vs. 10%), improved appetite (63% vs. 10%), and regularity of bowel movements.[42]

Many other studies have come up with similar results. I recommend qigong exercises to help women with breast cancer through chemotherapy and radiation, as well as to improve their health. Although qigong is best studied under the guidance of an experienced practitioner, there are many manuals and videotapes that teach some of the exercises.

Where East Meets West

The highest form of goodness is like water.
It knows how to benefit all things without striving with them.[43]

In modern Chinese cancer treatment, the prevailing attitude is to combine new and old, Western and Chinese, scientific and experiential.[44]

Most cancer patients in China today will use the treatments prescribed by Western-trained oncologists, surgeons, or radiologists as well as treatments by a TCM physician.

In China, there has been a trend in recent years to integrate conventional care with TCM treatment in an attempt to further optimize treatment outcomes; minimize the side effects of surgery, radiation, and chemotherapy; increase immune function; and extend the life span. As a doctor of Oriental medicine specializing in breast cancer, I typically work with the recommendations of my patients' mainstream physicians to coordinate a program of care that draws from both Western and Eastern traditions. Ideally, this integrated approach provides patients with more effective, personalized care—and certainly more options—than either school of medicine by itself.

Chinese medicine offers practitioners a comprehensive system of medical principles to apply in the treatment of breast cancer. This form of treatment is known as Fu-Zheng therapy, or "support the normal qi." (We'll discuss qi in more detail later.) The goals of the treatment include the following:

- Reducing tumor load
- Preventing the initiation, formation, and development of cancer
- Increasing the function and activity of the immune system
- Enhancing the regulating function of the endocrine (hormonal) system
- Enhancing and protecting the structure and function of the organs
- Strengthening the digestion and absorption of nutrients and improving metabolism
- Protecting the bone marrow and the generation of new blood cells
- Increasing the effectiveness of surgery, radiation, chemotherapy, and hormonal therapy
- Preventing, ameliorating, and controlling adverse side effects and diseases caused by cancer and cancer therapy
- Reducing the cellular resistance to chemotherapy and hormonal therapy[45,46]

In practical terms, the management of breast cancer will include surgery with herbal intervention beforehand to build strength and resistance.

Acupuncture can be used to help patients cope with the anxiety and tension surrounding breast surgery. This is followed by a postoperative herbal regimen and acupuncture to support recovery and prevent scarring, lymphedema (arm swelling), and pain. During chemotherapy, herbs and acupuncture alleviate side effects like nausea and vomiting and prevent toxicities like inhibition of bone marrow and damage to the heart. During radiation, herbs are prescribed to prevent fatigue and radiation burns and to enhance the effect of the treatment. For women with hormone receptor–positive tumors, we prescribe herbs and acupuncture to reduce the menopausal side effects and prevent certain toxicities like blood clotting. Even when the primary goal is to alleviate the discomforts and pain of conventional Western treatments, TCM will also be used to enhance the immune system, regulate the rest of the endocrine system, and provide dietary and lifestyle suggestions to promote better general health and ultimately improve the outcome.

Chinese medicine approaches disease by broadly inquiring into the patient's history to assess how the complex array of conditions he or she lives with corresponds to the current illness. TCM doctors look deeply into the patient's physical and psychological state. We consider environmental influences, bodily functions, eating habits, digestion, and much more; then we tailor the therapy to the individual's needs. In the treatment of breast cancer, this approach takes into consideration how the mind-body as a whole can aid in restoring many functions that are implicated in the formation, development, and metastasis of the cancer.

In TCM, we design each patient's treatment to work in accord with whatever stage she is in, whether it be right after diagnosis, before and after surgery, or in conjunction with radiation or the various types of chemotherapy. TCM will choose a treatment that works in synergy with the treatment prescribed by the patient's Western doctor.

The individual nature of TCM treatment makes it difficult to issue broad recommendations and simple medicines that fit all. This customized approach also presents a challenge for researchers who seek to measure the effects of TCM treatments. It is hard to conduct a clinical trial for one woman. Also, to restrict the treatment to a single regimen for everyone would limit the practitioner's independence and ability to choose the best option for each patient.

Each Woman Is Her Own Clinical Trial

One afternoon several years ago, an older woman came to see me in my office. At that time, Chinese medicine was much less popular than it is now, and it was much less accepted as a treatment for serious illness like cancer. This woman, who was in her early seventies, struck me as a very unlikely candidate to seek out Chinese medicine, especially with such a young practitioner as myself.

I learned that she had extensive lung metastasis from breast cancer that had been diagnosed a year earlier. Chemotherapy and radiation had helped temporarily, but each time the tumors came back even more aggressively. One of her friends, who had lived in Japan for many years after World War II, suggested that she try Oriental medicine as a last resort. This friend once had a terrible case of bronchitis that failed to respond to antibiotics, so her Japanese physician recommended herbal medicine. I could see my patient, who was a very proper lady, trying hard to hide her skepticism as she told me that her friend's bronchitis had disappeared soon after she started drinking a very vile-tasting herbal decoction. "Do you prescribe this sort of medicine?" she asked, with an effort to disguise her doubt as she pronounced the word *medicine*. Before I could answer, she said, "Well, you know my situation is quite different in nature. My doctor told me I have no longer than three months to live. So I thought I should try something as unharmful as herbal medicine." Again the word *medicine* came with difficulty.

I replied that we would try to make her feel as comfortable as possible and suggested that we treat her symptoms of weakness and painful breathing, while also trying to strengthen her appetite and restore her bone marrow from the chemotherapy damage. I emphasized that we should expect no miracle, but she seemed quite determined to try. I'm sure she did not want to die.

Fast forward three years. My patient was feeling very well. She frequently reported to me that she was able to outwalk most of her friends. Every time she told me this, she seemed genuinely surprised. Her tumors seemed to go through periods of small growth and long arrests, although they never shrank at all. One afternoon she came to tell me she had just visited her oncologist—the same one who had once given her three months to live. She announced that she was sorry, but she was going to stop the treatment with me. For the first time, she had mentioned to her physician that she was taking Chinese herbs. He became outraged. "There is no scientific evidence to support this form of quackery," he told her. Anyhow, there hadn't been any regression in her tumors; on the contrary, the tumors had grown. She said that although I seemed like a nice honest young man, she did not want to be involved in any quackery and needed to maintain a good relationship with her physician. That was the last I heard from her.

My experience with her raised many questions in my mind. In cancer therapy, we continually need to ask questions. What do we expect should be the result of a specific treatment? What constitutes a cure? How do we measure success and failure? For the oncologist, tumor regression was clearly the only measurement that counted. The patient's extended life and surprising energy were not enough to "prove" that Chinese medicine had any value whatsoever.

From my perspective as a TCM practitioner, each patient comes to me with a new story, only part of which resembles other stories. Whatever we may have learned from scientific investigations, large clinical trials, and specific clinical observations only constitutes information to enrich us for the next encounter with you, the new patient. I will bring all my knowledge to aid in tailoring the best treatment for you; yet, you will be your own prospective clinical trial. Your own experience is the only one that matters for you.

Surgery and Chinese Medicine

Surgery is still the best treatment for early breast cancer, and almost all women diagnosed with the disease will undergo it.[47-51] Therapeutic and reconstructive surgeries bring on a variety of unwelcome conditions that can be relieved with TCM, including pain, anesthesia-induced nausea, short-term diminished mobility, bruising, and fatigue. In my experience, one or two acupuncture sessions and an herbal formula a week before surgery can address several of these issues. We also use TCM to accelerate wound healing, increase peripheral blood circulation to aid the supply of nutrients and blood cells to the wounded area, aid nerve regeneration, reduce scarring, enhance the immune system, and pre-vent lymphedema—the swelling of the arm that can occur after the lym-phatic vessels have been severed by surgery.

Before surgery, certain herbs may complicate the job of the anesthesi-ologist and should be used with caution. These include ginseng root *(ren shen)*, Rehmannia *(shu di huang)*, salvia root *(dan shen)*, and ligusticum root *(chuan xiong)*, which thin the blood;[52-57] Atractylodis root *(bai zhu)* and *Carthamus* flower *(hong hua)*, which lower coagulation time and platelet aggregation function;[58-61] peony root *(bai shao yao)* and Millettia *(ji xue teng)*, which dilate peripheral blood vessels;[62-65] ephedra *(ma huang)*, which stimulates the sympathetic nervous system;[66-70] and citrus peel *(chen pi)* and *Lindera* root *(wu yao)*, which may elevate the blood pressure.[71-74]

The most important issue at this time is the fear and anxiety that arise after the diagnosis and the critical decisions you must make that will affect the rest of your life. What is the best treatment option? Should I have a lumpectomy or mastectomy? Should I have my lymph nodes excised, or should I ask for only sentinel lymph node excision?* How will I look after surgery? Should I have reconstructive surgery? What are the risks of an implant? What are the long-term side effects of reconstruction with abdominal tissue? Unfortunately, this chapter can't even try to address all these questions. But if you're grappling with them, I hope you'll take advantage of every resource available to help you make the right decisions: your health care providers, your support group, online communities, and the books listed in the Resources sec-tion at the end of this book.

Recovery from Anesthesia

Many women have nausea and constipation right after surgery. Acupunc-ture is extremely effective for these conditions, but unfortunately, most acupuncturists in the United States still don't have hospital privileges. It

---

*A sentinel lymph node excision is less invasive than an axillary dissection, since only the first lymph node to drain the site where the breast tumor is located will be removed. Sentinel lymph nodes are identified after blue dye and radioactive trac-ers are injected at the site of the tumor and then subsequently appear at the first lymph node that drains the cancer.

is sometimes very frustrating to know that our patients have suffered longer than necessary and received relatively ineffective treatments.

For self-acupressure, see the discussion of chemotherapy-induced nausea and vomiting later in this chapter. For postoperative constipation, in my experience one or two treatments on the same day get the gut going. You can complement the acupuncture with some herbs that stimulate bowel motility like rhubarb rhizome *(da huang)* and *Coptidis* root *(huang lian)*.[75-77]

Pain

Acupuncture and herbs have been used for centuries for pain management. Numerous modern studies detail the effects of both treatments and describe how they work.

The origin of most therapies we use today for surgical pain is in the medical literature for the treatment of war injuries. With so many wars throughout their history, the Chinese developed sophisticated methods to treat wounds inflicted by weapons. The treatments consisted of acupuncture, internal potions, and external ointments, salves, and liniments.[78]

Postoperative pain originates from severed nerve endings, swelling and inflammation, and bruising. Initially we use internal agents, since topical herbs may increase the risk of infection at the area of the incision. Herbs that help wounds heal and stimulate platelet aggregation are used, like *Astragalus* root *(huang qi)*.[79] Herbs that inhibit granulation (one phase of wound healing), like *Morindae* root *(ba ji tian)*,[80] should be avoided.

Bruising

Treatment of bruising should start only after the wound has somewhat granulated, which is usually about one week after surgery. Herbs that increase microcirculation, like ligusticum root *(chuan xiong)*, salvia root *(dan shen)*, *Carthamus* flower *(hong hua)*, and *persica* seed *(tao ren)*, are often used for this purpose.[81,82]

Fatigue

The fatigue experienced after surgery is caused partly by the anesthetic drugs. I think women often experience fatigue because pain and anxiety keep them awake. Addressing those problems helps eliminate the fatigue, so we try to help the patient relax her mind and body and get a good night's sleep. A commonly used herb for this is Zizyphus seed *(suan zao ren)*.[83,84]

Many studies in animals and humans show that both acupuncture and herbs can enhance strength and energy, lower recovery time after exertion, and reduce fatigue.[85,86] After surgery we mainly use tonics for qi and blood, like *Codonopsis* root *(dang shen)*, *Astragalus* root *(huang qi)*, and Lycium fruit *(gou qi zi)*.[87–89] All these herbs reduce fatigue, enhance immunity, and—in fruit flies, anyway—prolong life.[90]

Mobility

Qigong exercises are highly recommended to increase mobility and prevent lymphedema. Qigong movements are gentle in nature; the only weight they use is the weight of the person's own arm. The muscle relaxation inherent in the exercise prevents inflammation and the microtearing that leads to scarring, increases inflammation, and increases the risk of lymphedema.

Prevention of Excessive Scarring

Most scarring occurs within four weeks of surgery, but it does not end until more than eighteen months afterward. Although most women undergoing breast-conserving surgery will undergo breast irradiation to prevent local recurrence, same-breast recurrence often occurs at the scar area. Excessive scarring makes it more difficult to detect a tumor on mammograms.[91–93]

In TCM, we start work one month after surgery to prevent excessive scarring, which might increase the risk of lymphedema. A commonly used herb for this purpose is *Curcuma* rhizome *(jiang huang)*, which increases the reabsorption of fiber.[94] We use a messy poultice made with a combination of a few herbs, applying it one hour a day for forty-five days. The main ingredients of this poultice are *Galla rhei* Chinesis *(wu bei zi)* and *Solanum lyratum (shu yang quan)*.[95]

Chemotherapy and Chinese Medicine

Most women diagnosed with all stages of breast cancer are now offered chemotherapy to prevent recurrence[96-98] and eliminate any residual microscopic colonies of cancer cells that weren't reached by the surgery.[99-101] Chemotherapy is a systematic approach to killing the multiplying cancer cells.

For the past twenty years, such treatments have been shown to reduce the risk of recurrence significantly,[102-104] so much so that even with the risks and discomforts of chemotherapy, we recommend it to almost everybody. In some cases when large tumors are diagnosed, we apply chemotherapy to reduce the tumor size so we can do breast-conserving surgery.[105,106]

The most common regimens used in early breast cancer adjuvant chemotherapy are doxorubicin (Adriamycin) with cyclophosphomide (cytoxan), usually abbreviated as AC chemotherapy; cytoxan, methotraxate, and 5-fluorouracil (5-FU), usually abbreviated as CMF; and paclitaxel (Taxol) or docetaxel (Taxotere).

We often use Chinese medicine to complement chemotherapy. The herbal prescription usually includes several components that work together to bring about these effects:[107-116]

- Reduce side effects such as nausea and vomiting, fatigue, insomnia, and pain
- Reduce possible toxicities that might occur as a result of the chemotherapy, such as bone marrow inhibition, immune suppression, cardiac toxicity, and hepatic toxicity
- Enhance the benefits of the chemotherapy, e.g., lowering drug resistance and increasing peripheral blood flow, through the use of herbs that have a synergistic and/or additive effect
- Modulate the immune system, prevent immune suppression, protect the organs and glands involved in the production of immune cells

I can tell many, many stories about how taking herbs and receiving acupuncture help with the management of side effects and toxicities of chemotherapy. Since for most women it is the first (and hopefully last) time they are forced to undergo such treatment, they can only compare themselves to other women who did not include herbs as part of their treatment approach. Many of our patients report feeling that they're doing much better than other patients they see at cancer centers and in support groups who are not receiving complementary care with TCM. We have many reports of trials from China that show the usefulness of herbal therapy during chemotherapy.

Several studies that looked at the combination of TCM and Western therapies in early-stage breast cancer show that the five-year survival rate is greater when the combined approach is used. One study[117] showed that in 134 women with Stage II–III breast cancer who were receiving surgery, chemotherapy, and herbs, the five-year survival was 88.8%. In another study, 62 patients with Stage II–III breast cancer were divided into equal groups receiving standard surgery, radiation, and chemotherapy with or without herbs. The patients who took herbs used them for the whole duration of the observation. The five-year survival was 93% in the herb group compared with 32% in the other group. In another study[118] of 216 women with all stages of breast cancer who received integrated treatment, the five-year survival rate was 78.7%. These studies suggest that the combined approach is superior to conventional treatment alone.

One must say in advance that more research is needed to define the exact interactions of herbs and standard treatments and to quantify the results desired. At the University of California, San Francisco, Dr. Debu Tripathy, Dr. Mary Tagliaferri, and I, with the help of other scientists and clinicians, are trying to address those issues both in clinical trials and in laboratory analysis. During a visit to the Beijing Cancer Hospital at Beijing Medical University, our team was impressed that although Chinese women are usually diagnosed with breast cancer at a later stage than their Western counterparts (due to the lack of proper early screening policies and a social taboo that inhibits women from disclosing to their physicians that they have breast lumps) their five-year survival rate was higher than expected.

Nausea and Vomiting

Chemotherapy-induced nausea and vomiting continue to be among the most severe and distressing side effects endured by cancer patients. In chemotherapy regimens used for early-stage breast cancer, 30% to 40% of patients still experience nausea and vomiting within one week of receiving chemotherapy, even with the use of newer antinausea drugs.[119-122] In some cases, these side effects make a difference in the choices made by patients and physicians, and they can also lead them to discontinue the chemotherapy or reduce the dose.

A substantial amount of scientific literature supports the efficacy of both acupressure and acupuncture to treat chemotherapy-induced nausea and vomiting. In 1997, the strength of the scientific evidence for this application led a twelve-member National Institutes of Health consensus panel on acupuncture to conclude that "needle acupuncture treatment is effective for postoperative and chemotherapy-induced nausea and vomiting."[123]

Much of the scientific literature regarding acupuncture for nausea and vomiting has been published by J.W. Dundee and his colleagues at the Queen's University of Belfast.[124-130] In his studies, Dundee has evaluated the role of the most widely used acupuncture point for nausea and vomiting, Pericardium-6 (P-6), which is located between two tendons on the arm. Dundee's initial comparative studies examined the antiemetic effect of P-6 in 105 patients who had a history of nausea and vomiting during a previous round of chemotherapy. This study reported a 63% antiemetic benefit from the acupuncture. The findings from a smaller study provide evidence that the beneficial effects were limited to the specific acupuncture point, P-6, and were not felt when a "dummy" or "sham" acupuncture point was used. Subsequent well-controlled studies have similarly shown that acupressure or acupuncture applied to P-6 provides a treatment benefit in 60% to 70% of patients, compared with a 30% treatment benefit with sham acupressure or sham acupuncture, implying that point location is an important determinant.[131]

Acupuncture stimulation releases neuropeptides (proteins secreted by the nervous system) that stimulate the release of hormones and trigger changes in the autonomic nervous system and thus every tissue in

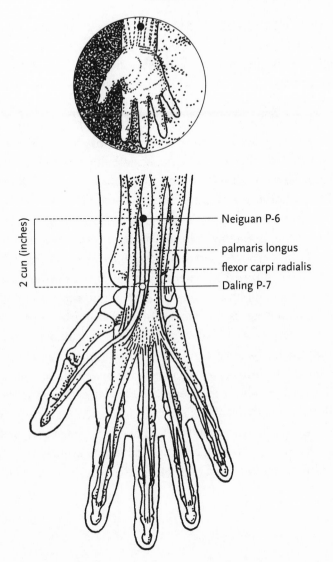

2 cun (inches)

Neiguan P-6

palmaris longus

flexor carpi radialis

Daling P-7

FIGURE 4.3. Neiguan, Pericardium-6 (P-6) for prevention and treatment of nausea and vomiting. Reprinted with permission from Deadman P, Al-Khafaji M, Baker K. *A Manual of Acupuncture.* Journal of Chinese Medicine Publications, East Sussex, England. ISBN 0-9510546-7-8.

the body. Neuropeptides are read by circulating cells, which respond with other internal biochemical secretions that complete the feedback cycle to the brain. It is through these neurotransmitters that acupuncture exerts its effects in the body.[132–134] Though we don't have specific knowledge of exactly how it controls nausea and vomiting, we have significant clinical proof that it works.

Stories like Angela's are the most convincing. Angela is a high-powered professional woman who came to us after her second cycle of AC chemotherapy, feeling horrible. The standard and nonstandard antinausea medications didn't seem to help her: when they stopped the vomiting, they led in turn to severe constipation, which increased her abdominal discomfort and nauseated her again for days. Frustrated, and determined to continue the course of chemotherapy, she decided to try herbs—something she never would have considered had not her surgeon and oncologist suggested the idea. While I can't say the herbs and acupuncture eliminated her symptoms entirely, by her own report they reduced her discomfort by about 80%. Being very pragmatic, she continued with herbal therapy and acupuncture throughout Taxol, her second kind of chemotherapy, and during radiation. She is currently taking herbs that work with tamoxifen.

Studies comparing herbal formulas with antinausea drugs have shown that the herbs are less effective for that purpose than the drugs, yet have fewer side effects.[135] We often give patients a low dose of antinausea herbs throughout the treatment, which reduces the amount of conventional antinausea drugs they need to take. We recommend that patients use the conventional drugs as needed. I advise my patients to drink fresh ginger tea regularly throughout chemotherapy, because ginger inhibits chemotherapy-induced nausea in both animals and humans.[136,137]

Constipation and Diarrhea

Constipation and diarrhea can result from chemotherapy[138–140] and can also be a side effect of the antinausea medications.[141,142] It's very important to drink loads of water, which also helps the bowels. Drinking the water slightly warmer than room temperature can minimize nausea during the first few days after chemotherapy. Of course, you should eat some fiber from both fruits and vegetables to help with your bowels. In Chinese medicine, we believe that cooked vegetables are easier on your gut and provide you with more nutrition when you are weak. The main herbs used during chemotherapy are shown in Table 4-1.[143,144]

TABLE 4-1. Herbs Used during Chemotherapy

CONSTIPATION	DIARRHEA
Trichosanthis fruit—*gua lou*	*Coptidis* root—*huang lian*
Rhubarb rhizome—*da huang*	*Fraxinus* bark—*qin pi*
Cistanches herb—*rou cong rong*	Magnolia bark—*huo po*

Fatigue

Many herbal regimens increase activity level and reduce recovery time after exertion in animals, and many herbal formulas reduce fatigue in people who are elderly or chronically ill.[145–152]

I usually urge women to slow down, ease their load, and not feel bad about needing more rest and time out when they're in treatment for breast cancer. Nancy wouldn't hear of it. She wanted to continue working full time in her executive position throughout her treatment (adriamycin/cytoxan chemotherapy, followed by Taxol, followed by radiation). She had two reasons for this. First, she wanted to keep herself occupied and not get dragged down by the treatment. Her second reason was the best I've heard: she didn't want to waste her sick leave and vacation time. She would much rather be able to take a nice long vacation far away at the end of the treatment, so she could make a quicker recovery.

And so she did. Nancy sailed through the treatments with such ease that in no time at all her support group came and demanded to have exactly what she got. She used an herbal combination that addresses all the symptoms of each of the regimens. The herbs that specifically combat fatigue are *Astragalus* root *(huang qi)*, Lycium fruit *(gou qi zi)*, and American ginseng root *(xi yang shen)*. Nancy took her long vacation and started to strategize her work life in a way that supports what she wants from her life. Meanwhile, I learned another lesson in how we can't give everybody the same advice about what to do with their lives.

Hair Loss

Unfortunately, hair loss is one of the milestones of breast cancer. The shock of being exposed in this way can be very traumatic. I have tried many herbs that are reputed to promote hair growth, and formulas that were once given to empresses to prevent hair loss,[153] but with no success. The best I can report is that herbs may help you keep your hair a little longer into the chemotherapy treatment, but in my opinion, that is not good enough.

Insomnia

You can't sleep, so you are tired. You are tired, so you try stimulants like caffeine and sweets. When you use them, you can't sleep. You take sleep-inducing drugs, so you feel drowsy the next day. But you're afraid of becoming addicted, so you don't know what to do. You try chamomile tea and valerian root tea, you hear the pros and cons of taking melatonin, you drink a glass of hot milk or down a shot of liquor—what a vicious circle.

In TCM we have a long record of treating what we call deficiency-induced sleep disorders, for which we administer strengthening, invigorating herbs that induce relaxation and natural sleep.[154,155]

TABLE 4-2.   Herbs That Affect Sleep

HERBS FOR INSOMNIA	HERBS TO AVOID WITH INSOMNIA
Zyziphus seed—*suan zao ren*	Ephedra herb—*ma huang*
Schizandra fruit—*wu wei zi*	Processed aconite root—*fu zi*
Biota seed—*bai zi ren*	Ginseng root—*ren shen* (at night)
Oyster shell—*mu li*	Citrus aurantium—*zhi shi*
Polygoni multiflori stem—*ye jiao teng*	Lonicera flower—*jin yin hua*

Leukopenia

Cancer patients frequently experience leukopenia, or decreased white blood cell (WBC) counts, caused by chemotherapy-induced bone marrow suppression. Studies have suggested that acupuncture can help maintain and restore WBC counts.[156-158] In forty-eight patients with chronic leukopenia, acupuncture stimulation led to an increased WBC count in over 90% of the patients.[159] Markers of immune function were also elevated in comparison with pretreatment levels. Another study of 121 patients with leukopenia who were undergoing chemotherapy showed a significant increase in WBC counts after five days of daily acupuncture and moxibustion (the technique of burning an herb [*Artemisia annua* leaf] above the skin to stimulate the acupuncture point).[160] Again, the clinical effect of acupuncture was measured, but exactly by what physiological mechanism it exerts its effect is unknown.

Several herbs and herbal formulations can help recover the number of WBCs rather quickly. Those formulas are not as effective as some of the currently used injectable forms of Western medicine used for neutropenia or a low white cell count. A formula containing 30 grams of each of the following ingredients—Fr. Illici Veri *(da hui xiang)*, Sophorae Flavescentis *(ku shen)*, and Caulis Millettia *(ji xue teng)*—increases the WBC count for each day of use, stabilizing the count after five days of use.[161] The tree fungus Tremella *(bai mu er)* has also been used to increase WBC rapidly.[162]

Mouth Sores and Loss of Sense of Taste

Chemotherapy often results in mouth sores, as well as continued erosion of the taste buds on the tongue, causing the sense of taste to either diminish or become hypersensitive. I have developed a mouthwash from two herbs that seems to work rather rapidly for those conditions. It contains equal amounts of trigonela seed *(hu lu ba)* and evodia seed *(wu zhu yu)* used as a gargle.

Peripheral Neuropathy

Women with peripheral neuropathy experience pain, numbness, and tingling, mainly in their hands and feet, caused by damage to the nerve endings induced by some chemotherapy agents. Acupuncture has a positive effect on the regeneration of nerve tissue, as evidenced by improved nerve conduction in patients with peripheral neuropathy.[163,164] The potential to improve on peripheral neuropathy symptoms resulting from the use of Taxol remains unstudied. The herbs Gastrodia root *(tian ma)* and Eucommia bark *(du zhong)* show a nerve-regenerating effect in animals.[165]

Appetite Changes and Weight Gain

Almost all women gain weight as a result of chemotherapy.[166-168] I believe that during the treatment it is not advisable to try to lose weight. Yet, knowing that you will most probably gain weight should be an incentive to eat low-fat, nourishing foods.[169] Moutan bark *(mu dan pi)* safely reduces weight without stimulating the adrenal glands in obese mice.[170] (It also works very well with our patients.) Acupuncture also helps in weight reduction for women who exceed their standard body weight by over 20% and who exercise regularly.[171] It is important to not use over-the-counter diet drugs or herbal products, since most have ingredients that can increase the risk of stroke and heart damage.

Early Menopause

Most women who are premenopausal at the time of diagnosis will enter menopause after chemotherapy.[172,173] Most of the time the effect is permanent. There is still controversy about the benefit or risk of continued menstruation and the risk of recurrence.[174] For very young women, the inability to conceive can be a huge loss.

In my experience, normal menstruation can be restored in many cases very safely with herbal medicine. I usually advise patients against trying very hard and at all cost to get pregnant for at least two to three years after diagnosis. Several herbs that can stimulate ovarian function are not estrogenic, although once the ovaries are stimulated, circulating estrogens and progesterone may increase.[175-180] It is thought that a slight elevation in circulating estrogen is correlated with an increased risk of breast cancer. So, stimulating ovarian function may not be a good idea right away.

Loss of Cognitive Function

Many women experience "chemo-head" after the second treatment. Unlike nausea, it comes on slowly, affecting short-term memory and the ability to do simple things like adding numbers or finding the right words. Little everyday tasks become a challenge: you might pick up your keys, put on your coat, and forget where you're supposed to be going. The deficit is significant and may last for years.[181-183]

Many people have been using *Ginkgo biloba (bai guo ye)* extract to help prevent and treat "chemo-head." Though a very good herb for dementia, it has a strong antioxidant effect that inhibits the formation of one of the active metabolites of adriamycin in the laboratory[184] and therefore may inhibit its activity. Since we don't know how it might behave clinically, I don't recommend that patients use *Ginkgo* during adriamycin-based chemotherapies.

Herbs used in China in some clinical trials have improved cognitive function.[185,186] The main herbs that were studied in clinical trials, *Alpinia oxyphylla* fruit *(yi zhi)*, evodia fruit *(wu zhu yu)*, and salvia root *(dan shen)*, actually restored damaged brain cells in experimental models.[187,188]

Traditional Chinese Herbal Therapy Aimed at Enhancing Immune Function

Patients with cancer often have depressed immune function, which usually worsens as the disease progresses and is compounded by chemotherapy and radiotherapy. Chemotherapy for early-stage breast cancer leads to a transient drop in the response of lymphocytes,[189] the immune cells responsible for recognizing and attacking viruses and cancer cells. The complexity of the immune system is still not very well understood. In general, we believe that there are four important steps in cancer control by the immune system: identification, recognition, attack, and knowing when to stop. The first step is for cells to produce a substance that can be recognized as a specific feature in the abnormal cancer cell. This substance is called an antigen. Once the antigen circulates in the blood, B-lymphocytes recognize the antigen and produce an antibody to it. The antibodies bind to the antigen and trigger several immune functions. T helper cells also recognize antigens and in turn produce a family of substances called cytokines, which stimulate the attack or withdrawal of the immune system from the antigen producing cells. Cytolytic T-lymphocytes recognize the antigen and immediately kill the cells expressing this antigen. Other players in this

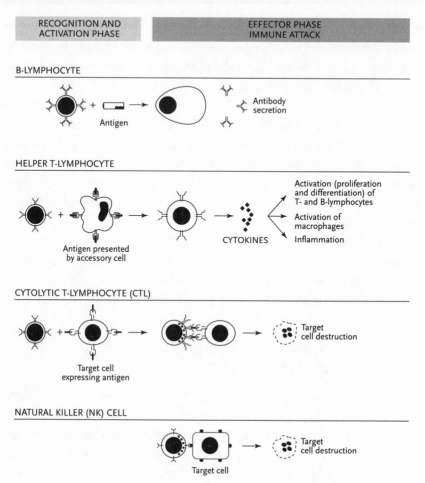

| RECOGNITION AND ACTIVATION PHASE | EFFECTOR PHASE IMMUNE ATTACK |

B-LYMPHOCYTE

Antigen

Antibody secretion

HELPER T-LYMPHOCYTE

Antigen presented by accessory cell

CYTOKINES

Activation (proliferation and differentiation) of T- and B-lymphocytes

Activation of macrophages

Inflammation

CYTOLYTIC T-LYMPHOCYTE (CTL)

Target cell expressing antigen

Target cell destruction

NATURAL KILLER (NK) CELL

Target cell

Target cell destruction

FIGURE 4.4. Lymphocytes. B-lymphocytes recognize antigens that are in the bloodstream and secrete antibodies. Helper T-lymphocytes recognize antigens that are on cell surfaces and secrete cytokines, which stimulate immunity and inflammation. Cytolytic T-lymphocytes recognize antigens on cell surfaces and destroy those cells. Natural killer cells use various receptors for recognition and then kill those cells.

complex response are the natural killer cells, which somehow don't need a full recognition of the antigen in order to kill those cells. The immune system needs to have a very specific way to empower itself to do any of its jobs. It isn't enough to have a big army with many soldiers. The soldiers have to be well trained, well equipped, and properly supplied. Most important, it has to know that there is a war, who the war is against, where the war is, and when to finish the war. For all these reasons, harnessing the immune system in the fight against cancer is very difficult. In one study, a correlation between lower immune function and subsequent risk of recurrence was seen.[190] An overview of trials of general immune stimulation for early-stage breast cancer did not show evidence that such stimulation improved the outcome.[191]

As stated above, one of the intended outcomes of Chinese herbal therapy is modulation of the immune system. In one study, patients with Stage III and IV stomach cancer receiving FAP (5-fluorouracil, epirubicin, and cisplatin) or FMP (5-fluorouracil, mitomycin C, and cisplatin) were randomly assigned to intravenous ginseng *(ren shen)* and ophiopogon *(mai men dong)* herb extract or placebo. A significant increase was observed in the ratio of CD4/CD8 cells, which are the subtypes of T-lymphocytes involved in specific immune attack, along with an increase in the overall T-cell count; all these indices dropped in the control group.[192] Several herbs have had different effects on immune cells and cytokine levels in laboratory, animal, and human studies, as shown in Table 4-3.[193–198] However, information on the influence of these therapies on recurrence and mortality in early-stage breast cancer remains unclear.

TABLE 4-3.

HERBAL AGENT	IMMUNE MODULATORY EFFECTS REPORTED*
Huang qi— Radix Astragali membranaceus	Increased CD4/CD8 ratio and phagocytic activity in patients with gastric cancer undergoing chemotherapy
	Stimulation of lymphocyte IL-2, IL-3, IL-6, TNFα, and IFN-γ
Dan shen—Salvia Miltorrhizae Radix Salviae Miltorrhizae	Increased T-lymphocyte production and function
Bai zhu—Rhizoma Atractylodis Macrocephalae	Increased phagocytosis, lymphocyte transformation, rosette formation, and serum IgG after chemotherapy

(continued)

TABLE 4.3. *(continued)*

HERBAL AGENT	IMMUNE MODULATORY EFFECTS REPORTED*
Fu ling—Sclerotium Poriae Cocos	Increased monocyte GM-CSF production Enhanced recovery of myelosuppression in mice after radiation Increased spontaneous rosette formation, lymphocyte transformation, and serum IgG
Gou qi zi—Fructus Lycii	Enhanced hematopoiesis, ameliorates lowering of number and function of T-lymphocytes, CTL, and NK cells in mice after cyclosphosphamide
Tian men dong—Tuber Asparagi Cochinchinensis	Enhanced humoral and cellular immunity
Wu zhu yu—Fructus Evodiae Rutaecarpae	Increased production of IL-1β, IL-6, TNFα, and GM-CSF in mononuclear cells in vitro
Xi yang shen—American ginseng Radix Panacis Quinquefolii	Increased TNF production, reversal of suppression of cytokine production in mice after cyclophosphamide Increased IL-2 and IFN-γ by murine splenic lymphocytes both in vitro and in vivo and IL-2 and IFN-γ production in mice after cyclophosphamide
Shu di huang—Radix Rehmanniae Glutinosae	Increased DNA and protein synthesis in lymphocytes, IL-2 production, T-lymphocyte proliferation, and NK and CTL activity in murine splenocytes Reduced immunosuppression effect in mice caused by cyclosphosphamide and steroids
Nu zhen zi—Fructus Ligustri Lucidi	Lessened leukopenia from chemotherapy or radiation
Liu zhi—Radix Salix	Improved regenerative capacity of bone marrow after chemotherapy

*In some cases, other herbs were included in combination therapy.[199]

TCM for Bone Marrow Inhibition

One aim of TCM is to restore blood production capability in the bone marrow. One herbal formula used to improve blood production is *shi quan da bu tang*, or All-Inclusive Great Tonifying Decoction, which was first introduced during the Han dynasty about two thousand years ago.

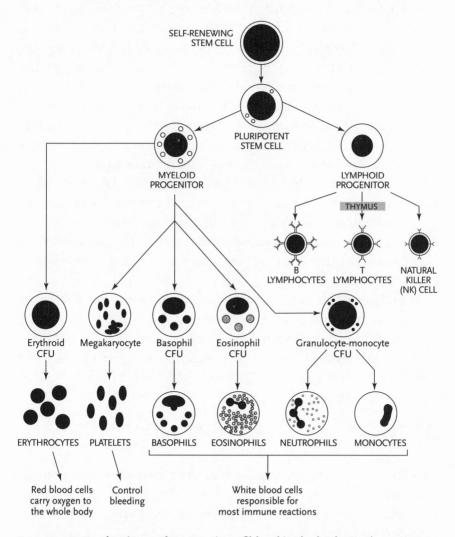

FIGURE 4.5. Production and maturation of blood in the body. Erythrocytes are red blood cells that carry oxygen to the whole body. Platelets help regulate and control bleeding. Basophils, eosinophils, neutrophils, and monocytes are white blood cells, which are responsible for most immune reactions.

This ancient formula contains ten herbs, some of which are commonly used TCM herbs and are familiar in the Western world. They include ginseng *(ren shen)*, *Astragalus (huang qi)*, licorice *(zhi gan cao)*, Chinese angelica *(dang gui)*, and cinnamon bark *(rou gui)*. Chinese researchers studied the effects of this formula to improve the WBC counts in 134 patients with cancer who had previously undergone chemotherapy and radiation therapy that resulted in low WBC counts. After treatment, 113 of the 134 patients had an increase in WBC levels to normal.[200] In a study of 58 patients with bone sarcoma undergoing chemotherapy with either cisplatin and dexamethasone (CD) or high-dose methotraxate and vincristine (MV), patients receiving standard care were randomly assigned to an herbal regimen or to observation alone. In the patients receiving herbal therapy, improvements in WBC and platelet counts were seen in the MV group, and there was less liver toxicity in the MV group. Patients receiving herbal therapy in both chemotherapy groups also showed significant improvement in post-therapy heart function (as measured by electrocardiography), less nausea and vomiting, and fewer skin rashes.[201]

Herbs from the berberidaceae family can increase white blood cells. Zedoaria root *(e zhu)* and cinnamon bark *(rou gui)* have been shown in humans and in animals to offset the bone marrow suppressive effect of chemotherapy.

Several herbs have bone marrow stimulatory (hematopoietic) effects, like Lycium fruit *(gou qi zi)*, Ligustrum fruit *(nu zhen zi)*, and ginseng root *(ren shen)*. The herbs Millettia *(ji xue teng)* and angelica root *(dang gui)* can also treat anemia by increasing the number of red blood cells.[202]

Radiation and Chinese Medicine

As with chemotherapy, during radiation therapy we try to achieve many aims with TCM intervention. Again, the idea is to keep the patient comfortable, minimize side effects, and try to enhance the effects of the radiation therapy.

In order to increase the cell-killing effect of radiation and control its local side effects, one needs to increase oxygenation to cells and promote peripheral blood flow.[203–207]

TABLE 4-4. Herbs Commonly Used during Radiation

ANTI-HYPOXIC EFFECT (INCREASE CELL OXYGENATION)	MICRO-CIRCULATION IMPROVING EFFECT	ANTIHISTAMINIC EFFECT,* ANTI-INFLAMMATORY EFFECT†	RADIATION SENSITIZING EFFECT
Codonopsis root—*dang shen*—Radix Codonopsitis Pilosulae	Ligusticum root—*chuan xiong*—Radix Ligustici Chuanxiong	Angelica root—*bai zhi*—Radix Angelicae Dahuncae	Ginseng root—*ren shen*—Radix Ginseng
Carthamus flower—*hong hua*—Flos Carthami Tinctorii	Salvia root—*dang shen*—Radix Codonopsitis Pilosulae	Gentiana root—*qin jiao*—Cortex Fraxini	Ganoderma lucidum—*ling zhi*
Lily bulb—*bai he*—Bulbus Lilii	Typha pollen—*pu huang*—Pollen Typhae	Lonicera flower—*jin yin hua*—Flos Lonicerae Japonicae	Ginseng and Longan formula—*gui pi tang*
Epimedium leaf—*yin yang huo*—Herba Epimedii	Leonuri herb—*yi mu cao*—Herba Leonuri Heterophylli	Scutelaria root—*huang qin*—Radix Scutellariae Baicalensis	Carthamus flower—*hong hua*—Flos Carthami Tinctorii

*Antihistaminic effect can reduce itching.
†Anti-inflammatory herbs can reduce swelling and redness in the breast and skin.

Two herbs can inhibit the effects of radiation. When given to animals, they increase their survival. They are Rehmannia root *(shu di huang)* and cinnamon bark *(rou gui)*.[208]

Fatigue

From the TCM perspective, radiation-induced fatigue is caused by an accumulation of heat toxin, causing dryness and therefore disturbing the yin fluids. (See the discussion of yin and yang later in this chapter.) This in turn causes what Chinese medicine calls "yin vacuity blazing fire." What those strange words feel like is that you are very tired but agitated at the same time. It becomes hard to fall asleep or stay asleep through the night. This usually does not start until the third week of radiation therapy. Weekly acupuncture treatment relaxes this sort of agitation, and comprehensive herbal therapy attempts to counter the damage to the fluids and the inflammation.

Burns and Skin Protection

I recommend that women undergoing radiation apply *Aloe vera* gel (fragrance-free) to the skin two or three times a day. If an itchy, red, rough sensation starts to develop on the skin, I give them an herbal ointment called *ching wan hung* to apply once or twice a day. I find it miraculous for mild to moderate radiation burns. The ingredients of the ointment are still kept secret by the manufacturer. Beware—it stains everything it touches, so if you use it, don't wear your favorite white blouse.

Scarring

Scarring from radiation is different from scarring caused by surgery. Since the radiation exposure covers a large area, the beams pass through and scatter to areas in the interior of the body, mainly the lungs and—if the cancer was in the left breast—to the heart. Though radiation technology has improved significantly in the past decade, preventing heart and lung fibrosis is important. Again, the herbs we use are those that increase microcirculation, decrease collagen activity, and promote the breakdown of scars.

Hormonal Therapy

Hot Flashes and Night Sweats

Menopausal symptoms are prevalent among breast cancer patients as a result of early menopause caused by chemotherapy, stopping hormone replacement therapy, or treatment with hormonal agents like tamoxifen. Hot flashes, night sweats, insomnia, dry skin, and vaginal dryness, as well as weakening of bones and increased risk of heart disease, are thought to be related to waning estrogen levels. Acupuncture has often been shown to help control menopausal symptoms in over 90%

of subjects.[209–211] The effectiveness of acupuncture appears to be lower if the symptoms have lasted for a longer time.

Susan, a seventy-year-old woman, came to see me before undergoing radiation therapy. She had many prior health problems, ranging from joint and muscle pain, digestive disorders, and nerve damage from injuries to severe menopausal symptoms that worsened when she stopped using hormone replacement therapy (HRT) after receiving a diagnosis of breast cancer. Susan warned me that she was very sensitive and that it took her weeks to adjust to new medications. She said that it was rare for her body to agree to new medications, including natural ones. Her reactions ranged from nausea and vomiting to neurological symptoms like numbness and tingling to severe constipation, diarrhea, acute stomach pain, and heartburn. She was terrified about what radiation would do to her and even more concerned about tamoxifen, since she had already experienced menopausal symptoms for twenty years even while using HRT.

Susan made it clear to me that she couldn't stop working. We started with what I thought was the appropriate herbal formula. At her next visit, she stated that she didn't feel she could tolerate the formula. She developed a rash on her arms and chest and was gassy and nauseated. After thorough interrogation, I suspected that she had a sensitivity to one of the herbs in a formula of twelve herbs. It takes some experience to determine what could be causing someone to react to a formula of many ingredients. Usually in TCM we do not often see side effects other than minor digestive discomfort or frequent urination. When we do, we change the treatment principle or modify the whole formulation. I omitted the suspected herb from the formula and, after a week of feeling well without the side effect, she began to trust me.

Susan did very well through radiation therapy, and her menopausal symptoms are mostly controlled with the herbs and acupuncture. Even five years later, after her course of tamoxifen, whenever she is out of herbs the menopausal symptoms return and become quite severe.

Decreased Libido

Many women experience diminished libido when taking tamoxifen.[212] I think many issues affect one's sexuality after a breast cancer diagnosis.

The breast is much more than a gland for milk production and distribution of nutrition to offspring. The visual aspect of the breast and breast sensation contribute to sexual play and pleasure. The physical and psychological assault to the breast after diagnosis is something we haven't addressed in the medical world.

You're also not likely to crave sex when you've been made so tired by the treatments for breast cancer. Many women become menopausal as a result of chemotherapy, or they have to stop HRT. The consequences are several mechanical difficulties with arousal and intercourse, like vaginal dryness and atrophy (shrinkage of the vagina). On top of that, tamoxifen does seem to lower one's sex drive. Giving estrogens is out of the question because of the theoretical risk of breast cancer recurrence.

Sexuality has occupied the minds of Chinese physicians for many centuries, and Chinese libraries are full of very detailed treatment strategies and technical manuals on the subject. TCM physicians are told that the question of sexuality is one of the ten essential questions for the diagnosis of any internal disorder. In TCM, we divide decreased libido into four aspects and treat them as necessary: (1) lack of mental desire, (2) lack of physical arousal, (3) mechanical inability, and (4) relationship problems. TCM has herbs for the first three problems—and for number four, we have advice. It isn't unusual for couples to go through difficult times after the diagnosis and treatment of breast cancer. The fear and anxiety for both partners can be enormous. Many significant others I've talked to don't know how to switch roles from caregiver back to lover. The best advice I have is this: don't let it go totally, talk about sex, and be patient with yourself and your lover. In TCM, sexual play is considered important for one's health and well-being. We believe that sex helps maintain healthy relationships between the mind and the vital organs.

Vaginal Dryness

There are internal and external potions for the treatment of vaginal dryness. The most common herb combinations are those that strengthen kidney essence and liver blood. With tamoxifen, some women have vaginal discharge in addition to dryness. There are many reports of successful treatment of noninfectious vaginal discharge with TCM.[213,214]

Osteoporosis

The loss of bone mass and the weakened functions of bone remodeling and repair are the cause of osteoporosis. As is usual with the body, a complex array of biological activities controls the formation and maintenance of the bones. Osteoporosis is a major health concern because of the risk of fractures that take a long time to heal, and the pain that results from the loss of gait and posture.[215–217] The single most important thing you can do is exercise. Get your heart, lungs, and muscles working. Place impact on your bones with movement, and your body will activate its own restorative capacity.

To date, we have two types of drugs to help prevent bone loss. We don't have drugs that build bones.[218] Several studies have detailed the effects of TCM in osteoporosis.[219–223] In TCM we use the herbs in Table 4-5.[224–226]

Cardiovascular Health

The most significant risk of tamoxifen therapy, though it is still a very small risk, is the formation of blood clots in the blood vessels.[227] Again, we use herbal agents that may reduce the risk of tamoxifen vascular toxicity.[228]

TABLE 4-5.   Herbs with Effects on Bone

Bone Calcification Promoting Effect	Promote Healing of Fractures	Possible Estrogen Receptor Modulating Effect	Researched Formulas
Psorala fruit— *bu gu zhi*— Fructus Psoraleae Corylifoliae	Deer horn— *lu rong*— Cornu Cervi Paruum	Psorala fruit— *bu gu zhi*— Fructus Psoraleae Corylifoliae	Modified Rehmannia Six—*liu wei di huang wan*
Drynaria root— *gu sui bu*— Rhizoma Drynariae	Sarcandra herb— *jiu jie feng*	Cypery tuber— *xiang fu*— Rhizoma Cyperi Rotundi	Kidney-nourishing and bone-strengthening pill

Endometrial Proliferation

The greatest concern among women who are prospects for taking tamoxifen for five years is the increased risk of uterine cancer.[229] Though one can't discount this risk, the incidence of uterine cancer attributable to tamoxifen is very low. Many herbs have been used for endometrial cancer and for regulation of the endometrium (uterine lining).[230,231] We use a low dosage of these herbs as a preventive measure for endometrial cancer.

Metastatic Disease

Unfortunately, we don't have a cure for breast cancer once it has spread to a distant area like the bones, lungs, liver, or brain. Chemotherapy, hormonal therapy, radiation, and other treatments now being explored

TABLE 4-6. Herbs with Cardiovascular Effects

Anti-thrombotic Effect	Cholesterol Reducing Effect	Lower Plasma Lipids Level	Coronary Vasodilation/ Flow Increasing Effect	Anti-atherosclerotic Effect
Chinese Angelicae Sinensis— *dang gui*	Radix Polygoni Multiflori— *he shou wu*	Radix Paeoniae Lactiflorae— *bai shao yao*	Citri Reticulatae— *chen pi*	Ginkgo bilobae— *bai gou ye*
Rhizoma Corydalis Yanhusuo— *yan hu suo*	Radix Platycodi Grandiflori— *jie geng*	Rhizoma Polygonati— *huang jing*	Radix Salviae Miltorrhizae— *dan shen*	Radix Polygoni Multiflori— *he shou wu*
Rhizoma Sparganii Stoloniferi— *san leng*	Radix Ginseng— *ren shen*	Semen Cassiae— *jue ming zi*	Fructus Trichosanthis— *gua lou*	Chinese Angelicae Sinensis— *dang gui*
Radix Ligustici Chuanxiong— *chuan xiong*	Cortex Lycii Radicis— *di gu pi*	Fructus Crataegi— *shan zha*	Rhizoma Gastrodiae Elatae— *tian ma*	Fructus Rosae Laerigatae— *jin ying zi*

do not yet show complete promise. They are used to relieve the symptoms caused by the cancer and, hopefully, to slow down its progression.

In seasonal rain
along a nameless river
fear too has no name.

—BUSON (1644–1694)

I believe that the combined use of TCM and conventional treatments slows down the progress of the disease, prolongs life, and improves the quality of life for women. Many anecdotal reports and some small observational studies show the benefit of using an integrated approach. One such study of thirty-two women with Stage IV breast cancer compared the effect of chemotherapy with a prepared emulsion of Coix seed *(yi yi ren)* to the effect of chemotherapy alone.[232] The herb-chemotherapy combination had a 66.7% effect, and 26.7% of patients experienced complete remission, whereas the chemotherapy alone had a 47.1% effect, and 11.8% of the patients experienced complete remission. In another small observational study of fourteen women with breast cancer that had advanced locally to the soft tissues and bones, CMF chemotherapy was combined with radiation therapy, tamoxifen, and herbal therapy. Twelve of the women survived after one year, seven after three years, and five after five years.[233] Another group of seventy-seven women with Stage III and IV breast cancer were given a glucose solution of Garcinia resin *(teng huang)* intravenously and orally. The effective rate was 76.6%, and 19.5% of the participants had a greater than 50% reduction in the tumor size.[234]

Four years ago a woman in her early thirties came to my office with a diagnosis of breast cancer that had metastasized to the bones. She had several spots along her spine and had just finished thirteen courses of various kinds of chemotherapy, resulting in many severe side effects, and she had been hospitalized with dangerous neutropenia (very low white blood cell count) on several occasions.

Sarah had had her first encounter with breast cancer seven years earlier during a pregnancy. She had a very small tumor and one positive axillary (armpit) lymph node. At that time, she received six cycles of chemotherapy and radiation. Approximately two years later, a new lesion, defined as premalignant, was detected in the same breast. She underwent a prophylactic dual mastectomy.

On the day of the one-year anniversary of her mastectomy, Sarah dreamed that she had a recurrence. She awoke from the dream to discover that she had a broken left rib. Several weeks later, after a scan, she was diagnosed with metastases to her bones. This was slightly less than three years from her original diagnosis of breast cancer.

Fifteen months before her initial diagnosis, right after her first child was born, Sarah noticed that her breast was abnormally lumpy. She had repeated clogging and infections in her right breast and felt unable to produce enough milk from it. She had a history of painful fibrocystic breasts and had actually received mammograms and ultrasound at the age of twenty-five for suspect lumps. But in general, Sarah was very athletic, active, and healthy. Her only notable health concern before having breast cancer was that her menstrual period was accompanied by severe pain and discomfort and the menstrual flow was irregular. After the first round of chemotherapy she became menopausal. That made her more comfortable, but she was concerned about her hormonal health.

Sarah came to my office six months after the last chemotherapy. At that time, she had been taking tamoxifen for four months, and she had just learned that her cancer had progressed slightly. There wasn't much I could offer her. I prescribed her some nasty-tasting herbs to help with both the control of cancer and her general weakness after chemotherapy. Throughout the forty-eight months she has been taking Chinese herbs, she has been feeling fairly well and is relatively symptom free. Her cancer has progressed slightly in one spot in her lower spine and has practically disappeared from many of the spots in her upper spine. Five months ago, after the progression, we decided to give Sarah chemotherapy in order to regain control of the cancer.

I believe that the combination of hormonal and herbal therapy along with the recent chemotherapy is helping to manage the disease. It isn't a smooth sail, but we are also not crashing on the rocks. Sarah's quality of life is dramatically better than it was before she began the herbal therapy, and the progress of her illness is much slower than anticipated.

My hope with Sarah is to slow down the progression of her breast cancer so that she lives with it as a chronic disease—a disease that needs monitoring and attention but doesn't inhibit her life. Sarah reminds me that she wants to witness my getting old!

To Promote Organ Health as Well as Fight Cancer

The colonization of breast cancer cells in a distant organ eventually causes that organ to fail in its normal functioning. The tumor physically and physiologically impairs the organ. I usually try to keep the organ as healthy as possible while trying to fight the cancer cells. The longer and healthier the function of the organ is maintained, the fewer symptoms women will feel. Also, in recent years it has been shown that some physiological bone abnormalities coincide with the invasion of breast cancer to the bones. I believe we will find such abnormalities to be the case in all organs to which breast cancer metastasizes.

Anticancer Herbs

Gina was diagnosed with breast cancer eight years ago. At the time of diagnosis she had two tumors of 7 centimeters each, which she found while examining her breast in the shower. She had a mastectomy, and eight of twenty-five lymph nodes were found to have metastatic breast cancer. Since Gina was in her early thirties, the most aggressive therapy was administered to her. She received three cycles of regular chemotherapy, followed by high-dose chemotherapy with stem cell replacement. After the high-dose chemotherapy, she had radiation to the chest wall and began taking tamoxifen soon afterward.

Approximately forty-two months ago, while still taking tamoxifen, she was diagnosed with metastatic breast cancer. She had multiple enlarged lymph nodes in both lungs, with a pleural effusion (fluid in the lungs), and tumors in the bones. She received ten months of chemotherapy with Taxol and Taxotere. Her oncologist thought that the chemotherapy had reached its maximum benefit, and though she still had lung and bone nodules, he proposed to take a short break from chemotherapy to allow her body to recover.

Gina was seeing an herbalist throughout her chemotherapy and felt that he was surely helping her maintain relatively good health with minimal side effects and toxicities. Unfortunately, he became very ill, and

Gina switched her care to me. We talked over the whole situation and decided to give herbal therapy a chance to work as a sole treatment for four months. For eleven months her condition was totally stable. Besides minor fatigue and occasional aches and discomforts—the kind that alarm anybody with a history of breast cancer—she felt well. After fourteen months, Gina felt her breathing become labored. Scanning revealed fluid in her lungs and some progression of her lung tumors. Gina started a clinical trial of a new experimental agent, and two months later the cancer had progressed. We immediately suggested chemotherapy, and after three months we found that it had progressed again. Gina has resumed taking herbs for the past four months, and her condition is again stable.

Gina has learned to have a remarkable relationship with her cancer. She anticipates it with some ease. Her case is a good reminder that cancer has its own life, which none of us knows or understands. We can't really tell anybody how that person's cancer will behave. We can speculate for large numbers of people; yet, we can say very little to an individual. When we look at the whole field of breast cancer, we can tell the story as we know it, but we can't tell a thing about one woman and her future.

Many herbs have been studied for their cytotoxic, or anticancer, activity. As a matter of fact, over 60% of chemotherapy agents are made from natural products.[235,236] The herbs mentioned in Table 4-7 have been tested in laboratory studies and in animals. These herbs can inhibit the growth of cancer cells or the formation of tumors in mice, or they can reduce the volume of tumors in tumor-bearing animals. The effectiveness varies among the herbs, and their modes of action are different. Clinically, we use one or more of these herbs when treating women with cancer. The dosages for active cancer are generally much higher than they are for general use, and they should be used with extreme caution.[237-244]

The herbs are divided according to their traditional categories. This is to show that we traditionally ascribe different modes of action to an herb even if it is used for a similar condition like breast cancer.

Acupuncture for Chronic Pain Caused by Cancer

The theoretical principles written two thousand years ago for treating pain with acupuncture still apply today. Scientific studies demonstrate

TABLE 4-7.   Herbs with Anticancer Activity

Tonics	Clear Heat Toxins	Clear Heated Phlegm	Blood Vitalizing Herbs	Softening Hard Mass Herbs
Radix Ginseng— *ren shen*	Herba Taraxaci— *pu gong ying*	Fructus Tricho-santhis— *gua lou*	Radix et Rhizoma Rhei— *da huang*	Pseudobulbus Shancigu— *shan ci gu*
Semen Coicis Lachyrma-jobi— *yi yi ren*	Spica Prunellae Vulgaris— *xia ku cao*	Folium Artemisia Argyi—*ai ye*	Semen Vaceariae Segetalis— *wang bu liu xing*	Herba Solani Nigri— *long kui*
Radicis Acantho-panacis Gracilistyli— *wu jia pi*	Herba Lobeliae Folium— *ban bian lian*	Folium Eriobotryae Japonicae— *pi pa ye*	Gummi Olibanum— *ru xiang*	Herba Sargassii— *hai zao*
Fructus Psoraleae Corylifoliae— *bu gu zhi*	Folium Hibiscus— *fu rong ye*	Bulbus alli sativi— *da suan*	Myrrha— *mo yao*	Concha Ostreae— *mu li*

that acupuncture relieves pain by stimulating nerve fibers that are embedded in the muscles, which then send impulses to the spinal cord and ultimately affect the midbrain and the pituitary gland. These three centers are activated and release neurotransmitters such as endorphins, enkephalines, and monoamines to block the "pain messages."[245] When needles are placed close to the site of pain, either on a specific acupuncture point or at the tender spot (a trigger point), all three centers are activated. In TCM practice, local and distal needling is applied to enhance the overall pain-relieving (analgesic) treatment.

Pain management with drugs can be effective when properly applied, but in many cases pain control is inadequate. Narcotics and other analgesics can cause constipation, nausea and vomiting, fatigue, and difficulty concentrating. On occasion, tolerance to pain medication can develop, which requires higher doses of narcotics and a risk of depression to the central nervous system, the heart, and the lungs as well as liver and kidney toxicities.[246,247]

There are many reports describing the use of acupuncture for pain control.[248-251] One large study of 286 patients with bone metastases reported significant pain relief in 74% of patients when acupuncture was attached to low-current electric stimulation. This was also associated with a much lower need for narcotic analgesics in the long term.[252] In a randomized study of 48 patients with stomach cancer who were receiving chemotherapy, the use of acupuncture was compared with conventional pain management with narcotics and anti-inflammatory agents. Drug therapy had better immediate (twelve-hour) pain control, but for long-term pain control (at two months), Chinese medicine delivered comparable results, without the side effects or risks associated with the drugs.[253] The body's natural pain-control mechanism is mediated by the release of opiate-like substances called plasma neurotransmitters. After two months, these substances had increased only in the acupuncture group. Other studies have reported that acupuncture can be safe and effective in relieving pain and the clinical course of shingles (herpes zoster)—a side effect experienced by patients undergoing chemotherapy.[254]

Prevention

Health maintenance and disease prevention are the ultimate goals of TCM. The following old story illustrates this well:

> A lord of ancient China once asked his physician, a member of a family of healers, which of them was the most skilled in the art. The physician, whose reputation was such that his name became synonymous with medical science in China, replied, "My eldest brother sees the spirit of sickness and removes it before it takes shape, so his name does not get out of the house. My elder brother cures sickness when it is still extremely minute, so his name does not get out of the neighborhood. As for me, I puncture veins, prescribe potions, and massage skin, so from time to time my name gets out and is heard among the lords."[255]

Prevention of breast cancer is probably very complex and difficult to achieve. In order to reduce some of the risk factors, we need intervention from the time we are in our mother's womb. Unfortunately, what we know about risk factors in breast cancer does not amount to very much. It isn't like lung cancer, where the connection with smoking is powerful and clear.

There are two aspects to prevention. The first has to do with maintaining a healthy lifestyle in light of what is known about risks related to diet, exercise, and other factors. This category encompasses all that we can do in our own lives, and includes minimizing exposure to environmental carcinogens and avoiding untoward medical interventions that can increase the risk of cancer. Education, action, and knowledge of our own bodies enable us to influence our destiny.

It's important to note here that many times, when we interact with medical care providers, we end up feeling that we have no control over the course of our life or our illness. At the other extreme, we may feel guilty, believing that we contributed to the illness. But to dwell too much on either of these ideas is self-defeating. I have many patients who ate organic food and low-fat diets, meditated, exercised, and did everything "right," yet still have to deal with breast cancer.

The second aspect of prevention requires addressing the biological mechanisms and medical conditions that we know contribute to the initiation, formation, development, and spread of breast cancer: conditions such as hyperplasia (an unusual increase in cells), breast density, and benign breast lumps like cystic breast or fibroadenomas. In China, many studies have shown that herbal intervention and acupuncture can diminish these factors very effectively.

Regulation of Possible Contributing Factors

Several biological conditions can be targeted with herbs in the interest of breast cancer prevention.

We believe that mutagenicity, the capacity of cells to change their fate and adapt to their local community of cells, is the first step in the possible development of cancer. The reason the breast is a problematic area is that breast cells have to undergo change and differentiation in response to the possibility of conception and lactation. Therefore, controlling differentiation and preventing mutations must be done without hindering the capacity of breast cells to differentiate and die normally.

Several herbs have an antimutagenic effect. They reduce or eliminate the capacity of a variety of chemical substances to change the fate of cells. Some of these herbs are peony root *(bai shao yao)*, Dictamni bark *(bai xian pi)*, and Fr. Psoralae *(bu gu zhi)*.[256]

Other herbs have a strong antioxidative effect. They prevent the effect of free radicals on the cells, thus lowering potential DNA damage. Some of these herbs are Lycium fruit *(gou qi zi)* and *Galla rhei* chinensis *(wu bei zi)*.[257]

Another group of herbs, like Atractylodes root *(bai zhu)* and Poria cocos *(fu ling)*, inhibit tumor promotion and might be used as chemopreventive agents. They were able to lower the effects of chemicals known to promote tumors in animals.[258]

Cinnamon bark *(rou gui)*, helps prevent the lethal effect of radiation exposure. It also inhibits its enzymatic activity that hastens the transfer and activation of regulatory proteins. This inhibition limits the triggering effect of oncogenes toward tumor formation.[259]

Many herbs have an antiviral effect. Women infected with Epstein-Barr virus are thought to be at an increased risk for breast cancer even if the virus may seem to be dormant in the body.[260]

All the above examples are suggestive of possible mechanisms and future exploration of herbal medicine in the prevention of breast cancer.

Breast Lumps

We can measure and treat breast hyperplasia (an unusual increase in cells) in order to reduce the incidence of breast cancer. From analysis of the data obtained from screening women, science arrived at some understanding that proliferative breast hyperplasia increases the risk of breast cancer by a factor of 1.9. That means that whereas right now 25 out of 1000 women will have breast cancer, if a woman has a diagnosis of breast hyperplasia her chance is multiplied by 1.9, so now it is 48 out of 1000. If there are any atypical cells, the risk increases to 5.3 times that in women with nonproliferative lesions. The risk of developing breast cancer from just having a palpable cyst is even higher, at 2.81.

The risk is higher for women younger than 45, at 5.94, and decreases significantly with age to 1.73 for women older than 53. The type of cyst does not matter, suggesting that treating any palpable cyst may reduce the risk of breast cancer.[261] If we can intervene and reduce the rate of proliferative breast hyperplasia and breast cysts, we believe it will reduce the incidence of breast cancer. Also, since we don't have a convincing model to assess which women with proliferative hyperplasia or breast cyst will be diagnosed with breast cancer, treating the proliferative disorder early might be a plausible way to reduce the risk.

There are many reports of effective treatments of breast disorders using TCM. I will summarize a few.

Five studies involved a total of 757 women aged 13 to 55 with a history of chronic fibrocystic breast disorder, defined by the presence of pain, cysts, and distinct lumps. They were treated for one to six months. Several herbal formulas were used in the trials, and the formulas varied according to TCM classification. The average total effect rate in all the studies, defined as complete resolution of lumps, pain, and cystic changes for at least three months, was 68.4% (518 women). If we include the women who had a partial effect, defined by marked improvement, the average effect of the herbal treatment was 89.4% (677 women).[262]

In a separate study, 120 women aged 20 to 62 (average age 41) with discrete breast lumps thought to be noncancerous were treated with Chinese herbs. The diagnosis was done by radiological assessment. The formulas were administered according to traditional Chinese symptom sign differentiation. The patients could use only the prescribed herbs during the trial. The herbs were given in capsules. Forty-six women (38.3%) had complete resolution of the lumps for at least three months. Fifty-six (46.6%) had greater than 50% reduction of the lumps. Twelve (10%) had less than 50% reduction, and 6 (5%) had no improvement. One treatment course was three months of herbal therapy. Of the women who had complete resolution of their lumps, 36 (30%) had complete resolution after one course (three months) and the 10 (8.7%) remaining had a complete resolution after six months. No notable negative side effects were experienced by the study participants.[263]

One has to remember again that the fantastic responses were for benign breast lumps, not cancerous lumps. The lumps were treated as a strategy to prevent breast cancer, not to treat breast cancer after it occurred.

In a clinical trial of 96 women with breast lumps, acupuncture and herbs in combination were effective in resolving the lumps and pain associated with fibrocystic syndrome. The women took *er xian tang* (Two Immortals decoction—just the name will make you feel better) and were prescribed acupuncture at various points on the Stomach, Liver Governing, and Conception vessels (see "The Meridian System" below for a discussion of the vessels in TCM). Of the 96 women, 58 (60.4%) were cured by the three-month follow-up point, and 17 (17.7%) were markedly improved. The total effect rate of the trial was therefore 78.1%. The selection of the acupuncture points was based on traditional theory and modern research. The authors noted that the analysis of patients' blood before and after the trial showed that the hormones associated with the hypothalamus-pituitary-ovarian axis—the hormones that are associated with normal menstrual cycle as well as with breast cancer—were normalized. In many experiments, modulation of estrogen, progesterone, and follicle-stimulating hormone was detected after the stimulation of acupuncture points.[264]

Breast Density

After age, the strongest predictor of breast cancer risk is breast density. On mammography, variations in the female breast depend on relative differences in the amounts of fat, connective tissue, and epithelial tissue, which makes up the lining of the ducts and lobules where breast cancer starts. Fat appears dark, whereas connective and epithelial tissues appear lighter or white. Women whose breasts appear dense (more white on the mammogram) in more than 50% of the total breast tissue area have a three- to fivefold increased risk of breast cancer compared with women who have less than 25% breast density.[265-269] This relationship is even stronger in women with a family history of breast cancer.[270] However, breast density remains one of the least recognized risk factors for breast cancer. Increased breast density is common among women diagnosed with breast cancer and occurs in 33% to 42% of all cases. By contrast, only 10% of patients have a family history of breast cancer. Because breast density is a significant risk factor, it raises the possibility that a decrease in breast density indicates reduced risk.

A study of 460 women with benign breast lumps and increased breast density who were treated with herbs reported a positive effect on the resolution of lumps and reduction of density. The women ranged in age from 19 to 58 (average age of 38.5); 79.6% were 28 to 45 years old and 20.4% were 46 to 58 years old. Of all those women, 206 had lumps and increased density in both breasts, 148 had symptoms on the left only, and 106 on the right only. All the patients were monitored for six months after the end of the treatment. The patients were classified into three syndrome groups and were given a single herbal formula. Of the 460 women, 108 (23.5%) showed complete response, defined as the complete disappearance of lumps and shadows with X-ray and infrared-ray assessments; 222 (48.3%) showed marked improvement (greater than 50% reduction); and 96 (20.9%) showed some improvement. I included the improvement group because it was defined as showing more than 50% reduction of density but less than 50% reduction of the mass.[271]

Unfortunately, none of the above data have been directly correlated to reduction of breast cancer risk. Long-term follow-up is very expensive, and the practical Chinese consider it unreasonable to waste efforts on looking at the connection between breast density and cancer risk, since we already know it is a risk. While the above trials were flawed, they suggest enough to warrant further investigation. Our group at UCSF hopes to open a randomized trial to assess breast density reduction in 2003.

Hormonal Regulation

Breast cancer risk factors include a woman's reproductive history, the time of her first full-term pregnancy, the number of pregnancies, her use of hormone therapies, and lactation. A woman's reproductive system is regulated and influenced by many hormones, like estrogen, progesterone, and follicle-stimulating hormone, that promote, control, and inhibit one another to provide the ability to ovulate, conceive, carry the baby to full term, and provide it with nutrition through lactation. Several theories have been suggested as to why estrogen and progesterone may increase the risk of breast cancer. We now know the story is very complicated and will require further research.

Normal breast development, normal reproductive function, and normal menopause are probably keys to maintaining good health in many ways but also to preventing breast cancer. TCM has a wide array of treatments that help regulate good reproductive life from its beginning until after menopause. Since the method in TCM is to view health and disease along one continuum, many treatments were designed to prevent hormonal disregulation. As an example, the treatment for menstrual pain involves not just painkillers but also herbs that regulate the whole hormonal milieu that is associated with it. Chinese physicians believe that maintaining balance and harmony wards off all diseases.

The use of what we now call phytoestrogens is very old. The herbs that affect estrogenic response are selected according to their clinical effect and the woman's age. We do not give a young girl the same herbs we give a postmenopausal woman, and we regulate the menses of a twenty-five-year-old and of a forty-five-year-old differently. The correct responses require different herbs.

We will need to further define scientifically the biological specificity and selectivity of these compounds. We will also have to further define their clinical application and quantify their effect on breast cancer prevention.

As you can see from this overview, TCM is being used today in many practical ways to relieve symptoms and promote better health and well-being before, during, and after breast cancer treatment.

It's fascinating to think that we can provide our patients with a better, more complete level of care by augmenting the latest medical science with a system that extends back thousands of years. While it would take volumes to give a full account of the history and principles of Chinese medicine, the following pages offer an introduction.

Basic Tenets of Traditional Chinese Medicine

Yin and Yang

The Chinese claimed that everything in the universe is composed of an interplay between two opposing principles: yin and yang. Yin signifies the feminine, motionless, cold, dark, water principle, and yang is the masculine, active, hot, light, fire principle. Regardless of the different values we (or society) might attach to any of these qualities, in the Chinese system one principle is not "better" than the other; rather, they are equally important and necessary. There is no yin without yang and no yang without yin. Everything in the universe has yin and yang. The sky is yang; the ocean is yin. Day is yang; night is yin. A cloudy day has more yin within the yang, and a sunny day is more yang within yang.

Yin and yang mutually oppose each other; interact with each other; promote, support, and build each other; and suppress each other. Yin and yang can overwhelm each other and control each other. This innate duality within the unity allows for all change and movement that occur in nature. Every thing and phenomenon has its essence of yin or yang and at the same time has its relative "yinness" or "yangness." When we encounter a patient, we apply the yin-yang principle to all the symptoms, signs, and functions. We also try to recognize the subtle interplay of yin and yang. Yin can transform to yang and vice versa. You can get a sunstroke that causes chills, and a frostbite that burns. In breast cancer, we need to determine whether the fast proliferation of cells originates from some overactive or underactive function of the body. For example, weak elimination, a yin symptom, could allow carcinogens to linger inside the body and affect the controlled proliferation of cells. Yet, once cells are proliferating, it is certainly an overactive yang symptom. We may even see aspects of inflammation near and around the

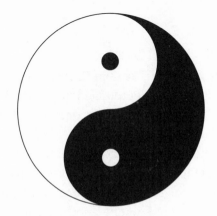

FIGURE 4.6. Yin/yang symbol.

tumor, which is a defense reaction: a yang phenomenon. Yet, the number of activated white blood cells available for the body to fight the cancer is low, which is a defense deficit: a yin aspect.

TABLE 4-8.   The Common Attributes of Yin and Yang

YIN	YANG
Moon	Sun
Dark	Light
Cold	Hot
Damp	Dry
Still	In motion
Feminine	Masculine
Relaxed	Aggressive
Heavy	Light
Substantial	Functional
Murky	Clear
Internal	External
Responsive	Active
Interior	Exterior
Downward	Upward
Inward	Outward

Five Phases Doctrine

Five Phases theory is another way the Chinese express systematic correspondence and reciprocal interdependency. Five different essential, basic processes or movements are represented by the symbols Wood, Fire, Earth, Metal, and Water.

All things and phenomena affect one another constantly according to determined sequence and timing. The relationships between and among the symbols in the Five Phases are to produce one another, control one another, and overcome one another. These lines summarize the sequential evolution of the phases and their relationships:

Wood produces/engenders fire
Fire produces/engenders ashes/earth
Earth produces/engenders minerals/metals
Out of water comes minerals/metal
Water produces/engenders wood.

Wood overcomes earth
Earth dams water
Water extinguishes fire
Fire melts metal
Metal cuts wood.

Whether or not these relationships are plausible in reality, the Five Phases system helps TCM physicians think very carefully about what causes disease. It requires them to look further and deeper into the mechanisms of any symptom or sign before they can make a diagnosis.

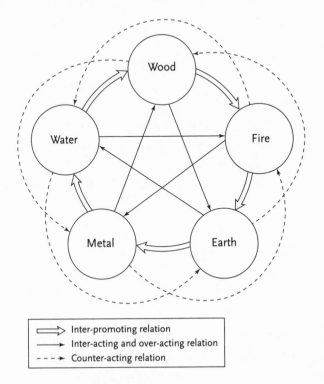

FIGURE 4.7. Five phases in Chinese medicine.

For example, abdominal bloating and distention can be a result of wood overacting on earth, or earth not being produced/engendered by fire, or earth overcoming water. In each instance earth is implicated; yet, the functions that are in discord are different. More than a final theory of categorization, the Five Phases are a useful method to teach us to look at various relationships at once and not just trust simple appearances.

TABLE 4-9. The Most Frequent Assignments to the Five Phases

	WOOD	FIRE	EARTH	METAL	WATER
Color	Blue/Green	Red	Yellow	White	Black
Climate	Wind	Hot	Damp	Dry	Cold
Season	Spring	Summer	Late summer	Autumn	Winter
Human sound	Shouting	Laughing	Singing	Weeping	Groaning
Emotion	Anger	Joy	Pensive-ness	Grief	Fear
Taste	Sour	Bitter .	Sweet	Pungent	Salty
Yin organ	Liver	Heart	Spleen	Lungs	Kidneys
Yang organ	Gall-bladder	Small intestine	Stomach	Large intestine	Bladder
Orifice	Eyes	Tongue	Mouth	Nose	Ears
Tissue	Tendons	Blood vessels	Flesh	Skin	Bones
Hollows	Axilla	Chin	Groin	Elbow crease	Knee crease
Fluids	Tears	Sweat	Drool	Snivel	Spittle
Reflection	Nails	Complexion	Lips	Body hair	Hair
Soul	Ethereal	Spirit	Ideation	Animal	Mind

Qi

Qi is a fundamental concept in Chinese philosophy, medicine, and life. Everything in the universe—organic and inorganic, static or mobile—has qi, is defined by its qi, and is composed of qi. However, in contrast to Western philosophy, it is not some primordial matter or mere energy, soul, or spirit. As my tai chi teacher, Master Chang, once said, you can describe qi, but real understanding can come only from one's inner experience.

So, what is qi? According to Master Chang, it is above all a real sensation that can be literally experienced. Qi is the innate vibration of each substance—the vibratory state of any thing, living or still, at any moment. It is therefore the matrix that connects energy with the matter upon which it is acting. Qi is like the glue or plasma that contains and adheres energy to matter. A famous Chinese riddle illustrates this. When a flag is moving on a ship's mast, is the flag moving? Is the wind moving? Is the air moving? Is our mind moving?

All movement in the body—voluntary, involuntary, willed, or psychophysical—is initiated and accompanied by qi. Walking, breathing, heartbeat, thinking, dreaming, growing, aging are governed by the movement of qi. Qi defends the body from the influence of environmental evils. Qi promotes the harmonious transformation of food, drink, and air into blood, qi, sweat, urine, and tears, and it regulates the innate rhythmic cycles of growth, maturation, and decay. Qi governs and maintains the body's substances and organs in their proper places: blood in the vessels, uterus and bladder in place, stomach and intestines from herniating. Qi is responsible for basal heat and the even distribution of warmth in the whole body.

Since qi is in constant movement, disharmonies of qi result from disrupted or irregular qi movement, which can take several forms:

- **Qi deficiency/vacuity:** Not enough qi can be generated for a specific function or for the body as a whole. The usual result is functional difficulty. General qi deficiency manifests clinically as lethargy, lack of desire to move physically, inability to concentrate. Most modern Chinese literature states that qi deficiency is at the root of breast cancer.

- **Collapsed qi:** The qi is so insufficient that it can no longer hold the substances or parts in their proper place, like a prolapsed uterus or rectum.

- **Stagnant qi:** The movement of qi is impaired, impeded, obstructed, or occluded. The smooth and orderly operation of the whole is then disturbed. Qi stagnation usually results in distention, pain, or tenderness.

■ **Rebellious/counterflow qi:** This is a particular form of stagnant qi in which qi is going in the wrong direction. Clinical symptoms of rebellious qi in the lungs result in cough, nausea, and vomiting. The specific type of counterflow qi has to be identified for treatment of nausea and vomiting to be successful.

Blood

In Chinese medicine, blood circulates in the blood vessels and through the meridians. It nourishes all the tissues and organs, maintaining the organs and tissues and preventing their decay. Blood also activates the sense organs.

Blood originates from the distilled essence of food, nutritive qi, and the "clear part of the breath. Qi is the commander of blood, and blood is the mother of qi."

There are two major blood disharmonies:

- **Blood deficiency/vacuity:** The signs are pale face, dizziness, and dry skin.
- **Blood stagnation or congealed blood:** Blood is not moving smoothly. The signs are sharp pain, cysts, and tumors.

In China, great significance has been given to blood stasis as a major contributing factor in chronic diseases and cancer. Many studies have detailed the relationship between blood viscosity, coagulation mechanisms, and cancer prognosis. It was found clinically that when they used herbs that invigorate and vitalize the blood, patients had less metastatic recurrence.

Essence

Essence, or jing, is the fluidlike substance that promotes reproduction and development.

The fusion of the parents' essences in conception forms one's prenatal essence. The prenatal essence determines one's growth patterns. Postnatal essence is derived from the purified parts of ingested food.

The function of essence is to initiate growth, development, and aging and to control the processes that are associated with the timely operation of specific functions. Foremost of these functions is the proper maturation and operation of the reproductive system. Essence and qi may be distinguished from each other by their speed: qi is more immediate, whereas essence is the slow controller of life's cycles.

Pathologic states of essence include congenital diseases, late or improper maturation, premature senility, and sexual and reproductive dysfunction. In breast cancer we sometimes consider essence disorders to be associated with improper hormonal function or incomplete breast development and differentiation, which are thought to be risk factors for breast cancer.

Spirit

When emotions have not yet emerged, that is called balance;
when they are active yet all in proportion, that is called
harmony.

—THE RECORD OF RITES, CA. EIGHTH CENTURY B.C.

Spirit, or shen, is the substance responsible for conscious activity in humans. In Chinese medicine, lack of spirit or overactive spirit will interact with qi, blood, and essence and will possibly result in physical changes and disharmony. The spirit is the mechanism that connects in the organism all the conscious, unconscious, and subconscious activities. This system commands voluntary movement, instinctual reactions, and the bowels.

The second function of the spirit is acquiring memory and activating memory, and the third function is intelligence. Understanding, reason, judgment, common sense, and critical thinking are all traits of the spirit. The relationship of mental faculties to the body and its activities will determine the balance, evolution, and development of the mind.

Very frequently, women state that their spirit is tired after the physical and emotional insult of breast cancer therapy. We now know that there is actually some damage to women's cognitive functions as a result of treatment. Some of the cognitive deficit is reversed when energy returns, and some of the deficit is more permanent. In Chinese medicine, we sometimes use herbs for calming the heart and nurturing the spirit to address or prevent the effects of treatment.

Body Fluids

Body fluids and their dynamics are very important with regard to breast cancer. They are sensitive to changes in the condition of qi, blood, and the organs as well as to emotional states and the weather. Qi, blood, and body fluid form the media through which the whole body communicates. In modern medicine, we now understand that proper water balance is crucial for maintaining health and longevity. We also recognize that some mucuslike substances are important regulators of cellular functions.

The Organs

Very early, the Chinese described only twelve main organs that were associated with the twelve main meridians. The organs are classified into a yin group and a yang group. The yin organs are the liver, heart, spleen, lungs, kidney, and pericardium. Their function is to produce, transform, regulate, direct, and store qi, blood, essence, and spirit. The yang organs are the gallbladder, small intestine, stomach, large intestine, urinary bladder, and triple burner, which is considered an organ although it has no physical entity. These organs receive, break down, transport, and excrete food and drink. Though most of the organs are named and anatomically located in the same way as in modern medicine, the functions ascribed to organs vary greatly from the functions attributed to them by modern science. The organ called the triple burner doesn't have a specific anatomical location even in Chinese medicine; it is purely a combination of related functional activities.

Six "curious" organs are also mentioned in the Chinese medical literature. They are the brain, uterus, marrow, bone, blood vessels, and gallbladder. The gallbladder is considered both a yang organ and a curious organ because it has the function of excreting bile as well as refining it.

Each of the twelve organs and six curious organs has its own unique functions. Many times those functions have nothing to do with what the physical organ does from a modern physiological point of view. For instance, it is thought in Chinese medicine that the heart stores and rules the spirit. Dysfunction of the heart's spirit or qi or blood can result in spirit disorders such as insomnia, forgetfulness, difficulties responding to the environment, and more severe conditions like hysteria, insanity, and psychosis.

The Meridian System

The body has twelve primary channels and eight extraordinary channels. Unlike blood vessels, the channels are an invisible network. They link the whole body from the depth of the marrow to the organs and all the other structures. The meridians are what unifies and harmonizes the smooth, correct flow of the fundamental substances. There is mounting scientific evidence that acupuncture can change many aspects of our physiology; yet, there is no direct evidence that the meridian system as described by the Chinese actually exists. The flow of qi in the channels constitutes the first concept of circulation and physiological rhythms in the history of medicine.

Each of the twelve main meridians is associated with an internal organ. The eight extraordinary meridians serve as reservoirs of qi, blood, and essence. Only two of the eight extraordinary vessels have pathways on the body's surface.

The breast body is governed by the Stomach meridian. The nipple is governed by the Liver channel. Through the breast, the Spleen and Pericardium meridians pass. The Gallbladder meridian runs through the outer aspect of the breasts. It also has a branch that connects with the Stomach channel near the collarbone and runs across the breast to connect to the Pericardium meridian. The Large Intestine Divergence channel follows the breast. The Heart channel intersects with the Lung channel at the breast. The Great Connecting vessel of the stomach issues from below the left breast. The Conception vessel and the Penetrating vessel spread through the breast.

Diet and Exercise

In TCM, the causes of disease are divided into three basic categories: internal causes, which stem from the emotions; external causes, which refer to climatic conditions; and the causes that are neither internal nor external. Of this latter category, diet is one of the most important.

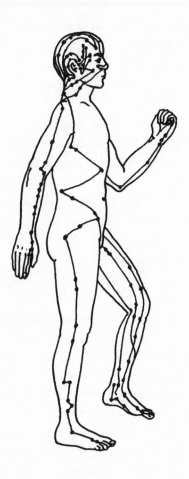

FIGURE 4.8. (a) The meridians (channels) of acupuncture (side view).

Chinese medicine evaluates food not only by what nutrients and chemicals it contains but also by how it is prepared and by the strength and health of an individual's digestive system, constitution, and specific lifestyle. Internal predispositions and medical conditions make certain foods harmful for certain people.

The ancients recognized that breast cancer evolves from high-fat, greasy, flavorful, high-energy (high caloric intake) diets and the prolonged consumption of alcohol. This is corroborated by modern science—minus the flavorful foods. The Chinese emphasis on flavor as well is interesting.

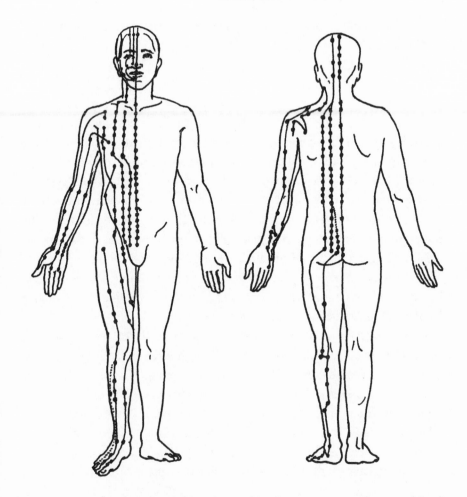

FIGURE 4.8. (b) The meridians (channels) of acupuncture (front and back view).

What makes things flavorful is present in minuscule quantities in our food. The flavor molecules are measured in parts per billion of a microgram. Yet, our desire for food is generated by those parts per billion molecules. Science is just catching up on how different odors can affect the regulation of the menstrual cycle and sexual response. The elucidation of the importance of taste may clarify its relationship to health and disease. In TCM, the desire for or large consumption of one taste—sweet, salty, or hot—over a long period of time affects specific physiological functions in the body and can result in disease.

In private conversations with some of the greatest cancer authorities in China, I asked them why they believe women in their country have significantly less breast cancer than women in the Western world. They noted that whereas this was true in the past, the rate of breast cancer is now rising in the major metropolitan areas, like Beijing and Shanghai. They believe that high-fat and high-calorie diets are an important factor. In addition, the Chinese are eating more fried food, which means a higher intake of rancid oils and free radicals that can promote carcinogenesis. The Chinese cancer specialists made an interesting observation. For the first time in China's history, almost everyone in the metropolitan areas has an abundance of food. This newly acquired sense of wealth draws many people to indulge in what they perceive as food for the wealthy. Since oil, animal products, frying, and condiments are expensive, using them regularly becomes an expression of one's freedom and luxury. And as China's dietary habits become more like those of the West, so does its risk of cancer.

Physical activity is another factor the Chinese have long considered essential to good health, and current Western science certainly supports this. Exercise decreases the risk of breast cancer, mainly in postmenopausal women. In younger girls, exercise reduces body mass and delays the onset of menstruation, thereby reducing risk. Physical activities seem to be related to many endocrine functions. According to Chinese medicine, physical activity should be done with moderation. Too much activity and exertion can damage the body and not allow it proper recovery time.

TCM and the Future

TCM intervention has a very long, very well documented history of use. The fact that your physician doesn't know this history and doesn't accept its premises does not mean that it doesn't exist or is meaningless. The application of TCM treatments is simple and inexpensive. We can easily use some of the recent developments in biology to study the molecular and genetic mechanisms of herbs.

The future of TCM in the treatment of breast cancer demands clearer investigation and documentation. Scientific studies will have to be conducted to evaluate all its benefits, effects, and risks. Research into TCM poses many problems from a conventional point of view, since TCM is an individualized form of treatment and therefore all results are considered anecdotal from a Western scientific standpoint. We need to develop new methods for assessing these individualized approaches. The new model should include assessments of toxicity and long-term effects other than tumor reduction and disease-free interval that are more in tune with our patients' experience.

On the prevention front, I think we should use molecular markers and early screening methods that detect risk factors, not just early disease. We should then develop totally nontoxic treatments for conditions like breast atypical hyperplasia, and monitor the outcomes for many years. We should start observations and education with the daughters and close family members of women who have been diagnosed with breast cancer, while treating them with nontoxic interventions.

We can and need to apply the TCM philosophy of dynamic whole to the interaction and intervention of breast cancer. The fact that we are all different hasn't yet been factored into our medical model. We try to regard everything as conforming to a single pattern, and therefore we lose the opportunity to investigate differences. New computer analysis will allow us to observe the effects of various changes in our physiology that, if followed carefully, can help us learn who benefits from what treatment, for how long, and why.

Until the day this very specific individualized information becomes available, I encourage you to benefit from the experience and knowledge of TCM as well as Western medicine. Again and again I have seen that the two together have a lot more to offer than either one alone. In modern medicine, we typically tell women that their only option is to replace one horrible thing with a mildly lesser horrible thing. I don't accept it, and I hope you will not either.

Resources

Practitioners of TCM

To find a practitioner of Chinese medicine, see Resources at the back of this book.

Qigong

For books, tapes, and videotape instruction about qigong, see Resources at the back of this book.

Herbal Pharmacies

SHEN NONG HERBS
1600 Shattuck Ave.
Berkeley, CA 94708
510-849-0290

SPRINGWIND HERBS
2325 Fourth St. #6
Berkeley, CA 94710
510-849-1820

MAYWAY CORP.
1338 Mandela Pkwy.
Oakland, CA 94607
800-262-9929

KPC PRODUCTS, INC.
16 Goddard Ave.
Irvine, CA, 92618
800-572-8188

GOLDEN FLOWER CHINESE HERBS
P.O. Box 781
Placitas, NM 87043
800-729-8509

SHEN HERBS
1385 Shattuck Ave.
Berkeley, CA 94709
877-922-4372

Recommended Reading

Cohen, Kenneth S. *The Way of Qigong: The Art and Science of Chinese Energy Healing.* New York: Ballantine Books, 1997. Wonderful explanations of the philosophy and practice of qigong; very well documented.

Ellis, Andrew, Nigel Wiseman, and Ken Boss. *Fundamentals of Chinese Acupuncture.* Brookline, Mass.: Paradigm Publications, 1988. A text of traditional acupuncture principles and techniques.

Filshie, Jacqueline, and Adrian White. *Medical Acupuncture: A Western Scientific Approach.* Edinburgh: Churchill Livingstone, 1998. Summarizes the current scientific literature and clinical applications of acupuncture.

Kaptchuk, Ted, O.M.D. *The Web That Has No Weaver: Understanding Chinese Medicine.* New York: Congdon and Weed, 1983. Excellent book for the basic concepts and tenets of Chinese medicine.

Lu, Henry C. *Chinese Natural Cures: Traditional Methods for Remedies and Preventions.* New York: Black Dog and Leventhal Publishers, 1994. Describes some of the dietary principles used in TCM.

Ni Maoshing, Ph.D. (trans.). *The Yellow Emperor's Classic of Medicine.* Boston: Shambhala, 1995. A translation of the earliest Chinese medical classic.

Pan Mingji. *Cancer Treatment with Fu Zheng Pei Ben Principle.* Fujian: Fujian Science and Technology Publishing House, 1992. Summarizes the experience of treating various cancers with integrated Western and Chinese medicine.

Reid, Daniel. *Chinese Herbal Medicine.* Boston: Shambhala, 1987. Good simple introduction to Chinese herbs.

Reid, Daniel. *The Complete Book of Chinese Health and Healing: Guarding the Three Treasures.* Boston: Shambhala, 1994. A good manual of Chinese medicine's philosophy and health recommendations, written in a very accessible language.

Shen Ziyin and Chen Zelin. *The Basis of Traditional Chinese Medicine.* Boston: Shambhala, 1996. A comprehensive survey of Chinese medicine and its treatment modalities, written by two eminent experts from China.

Shi Lanling and Shi Peiquan. *Experience in Treating Carcinoma with Traditional Chinese Medicine.* Shandong: Shandong Science and Technology Press, 1990. Summary of the authors' clinical cases of various cancers treated with Chinese medicine as sole therapy.

Stux, Gabriel, and Richard Hammerschlag. *Clinical Acupuncture: Scientific Basis.* Berlin: Springer, 2000. Summarizes the current advances in acupuncture research.

CHAPTER FIVE

Diet and Breast Cancer

Lawrence Kushi, Sc.D.

LAWRENCE KUSHI, Sc.D., graduated from Amherst College and the
Harvard School of Public Health. He is the Ella McCollum Vahlteich
Professor of Human Nutrition at Teachers College, Columbia University.
Dr. Kushi is an internationally recognized nutritional epidemiologist who
has published numerous research articles in the area of diet and cancer.
He has also been a member of various committees including the
American Cancer Society's 1996 Advisory Committee to revise guidelines
for nutrition and cancer prevention, the 1996 National Institutes of
Health Consensus Development Conference on Acupuncture, and the
American Cancer Society's 1999 committee to develop guidelines on
nutrition and physical activity for cancer patients, their caregivers, and
their families. Dr. Kushi is also the son of Michio and Aveline Kushi, the
foremost proponents of macrobiotics; the macrobiotic diet is one of the
most widely used alternative comprehensive dietary approaches to
cancer in use today.

There is no universal consensus about the relationship between diet
and breast cancer. Despite hundreds of studies, mainstream medicine
has yet to agree on a definitive set of dietary recommendations for
women, either before or after diagnosis. Nevertheless, evidence that
cancer results from both genetics and environment suggests that diet
and lifestyle may play a role not only in causing cancer but in preventing it as well—and possibly even treating it.

This chapter will focus primarily on the role of diet in breast cancer,
with an emphasis on macrobiotics. True, as the son of leading authorities on macrobiotics, I have a particularly personal connection to the
subject. But more to the point, macrobiotics is a major alternative
dietary approach to cancer, one of the few that is truly comprehensive.

I hope this discussion will help educate and empower the woman
with breast cancer to seek out her own path. Here is the story of one
who did.

My twin sister and I were born on September 27, 1952, in Easton, Pennsylvania. Our ancestry was Irish and Pennsylvania Dutch (German), and our food was typical postwar American fare: chicken, eggs, lots of dairy, some beef, ice cream, chocolate, cheese, sugar, cakes, refined white flour, canned or frozen vegetables. We ate almost no whole grains and never heard of mineral-rich sea vegetables. From an early age, I suffered from hypoglycemia (low blood sugar) and was overweight, because I craved sweets my whole life. I tried many diets in order to slim down. For example, one diet had me eating protein pills at every mealtime and consuming 48 eggs in a single week! At age thirty, I adopted a lacto-ovo-vegetarian diet, choosing not to kill animals anymore. But then my diet consisted mainly of cheese omelets, pizzas, ice cream, and chocolate. By this time I was working very hard on a Ph.D. and was staying up working all night at least twice a week. My weight peaked at about 170 pounds.

My background in mathematics and science, including a master's degree in high-energy physics, had led to employment in the newly emerging computer field. I had worked in the United States and Europe as a programmer, analyst, technical writer, and consultant. In the mid-1980s, I worked as a teaching assistant in the physics department of my fourth graduate school. I had become very disillusioned with Western science, because I had never met an advisor whose ideas made real sense to me. I was searching for something more meaningful.

In early July 1985, at age thirty-two, I developed what looked like mastitis, an infection of the breast. In two weeks, about one quarter of my left breast had become swollen and painful, hard under the skin from three o'clock to six o'clock, with red, hot edema of the skin over it. Also evident were the classic symptoms of the skin looking like orange peel (peau d'orange) and a ridge between normal skin and the furthest border of the inflammation. Antibiotic drugs had no effect, and neither mammogram nor ultrasound revealed anything conclusive. On July 22, a surgical biopsy confirmed inflammatory breast cancer. There was extensive tumor (a 6 × 6 cm mass) inside and outside the ducts, with severe chronic inflammation and extensive invasion to the lymph vessels. The skin had many spots where the cancer had spread. Fortunately, no lymph nodes could be felt under my armpit.

I began doing extensive Medline computer searches of all the relevant literature at the medical school at Yale University, where I was a graduate student in physics. All confirmed that practically no woman was alive two years after this diagnosis, despite mastectomy, chemotherapy, and/or radiation treatment. My kind but pessimistic oncologist told my husband that I probably had only two or three months to live, even with medical treatment. I was young for this ailment: the average patient was age fifty-two years at onset, and postmenopausal. All the medical literature I consulted said "etiology unknown" for this type of cancer. My oncologist suggested that it was genetic; yet, no one in my family had ever had breast cancer of any kind before. Therefore, he said, it must be a latent gene. This was not very satisfying for me.

The day after diagnosis, my oncologist started chemotherapy treatments for me once a month, for four months: cytoxan, adriamycin, and 5-fluorouracil (CAF) both intravenously and by mouth. The side effects included loss of hair within three weeks, nausea, early drug-induced menopause, heart palpitations, weakness, and extreme loss of white blood cells. The inflammatory skin component became better after one or two treatments, but the hardness of the diffuse tumor remained. By October, my white blood cell count was dangerously low for me to proceed with further chemotherapy. Even though I asked the hospital dietitian for a special diet to reduce my great weight, my medical doctors told me that during chemotherapy, I had to maintain my weight. They encouraged me to eat anything, especially high-protein foods, and recommended a high-calorie chocolate drink. I knew Western doctors had almost no training in nutrition, and no idea about food causing cancer. My intuition told me that the best course would be opposite to what the doctors recommended.

In September 1985, my twin sister had given me Dr. Anthony Sattilaro's book *Recalled by Life*, about a physician and chairman of Methodist Hospital in Philadelphia. Using a macrobiotic diet, he had recovered from prostate cancer that had metastasized to his bones. After he weaned himself from extensive medical treatments and switched from gourmet French food to simple fare of whole grains, vegetables, beans, and sea vegetables, medical tests declared him free of his cancer in less than one year. According to macrobiotics, cancer is caused primarily by a long-time imbalance in our diet and way of life. This made complete sense to me. It seemed that all my life I had known my diet was very wrong, and that I would become deathly ill at an early age. But I also felt intuitively that I would somehow recover, and lead a life totally different from that of my first thirty-three years.

At home, I immediately threw away all the cheese and chocolate in my kitchen and read every book I could find on macrobiotics, beginning with *The Cancer Prevention Diet* by Michio Kushi, with Alex Jack. I also started to take cooking classes from a local macrobiotic center in Middletown, Connecticut. Very carefully I studied the concepts of yin (expansion) and yang (contraction), the complementary opposite energies that make up all things.

I discovered that to recover from this extreme form of breast cancer, I needed to first eliminate the dairy food whose protein and fat primarily made up the mass of the tumor. Macrobiotics holds that dairy goes naturally to the milk-producing part of a woman's body, while sugar, oil, and other stimulants cause the tumor to spread like wildfire. I also had to stop the eggs, cheese, and baked flour products, which had stagnated in my pancreas and caused the chronic hypoglycemia that drove me to eat all those comforting sweets and dairy products. I began to see food and the body in terms of the Oriental concept of energy, which was easy with my physics background. If the energy of improper food could cause energy blocks or stagnations like tumors in the body, then proper food could also release these blocks and eliminate the symptoms of cancer. I was determined to let food be my medicine. I carefully avoided all sweets, oils, and excessive fat and protein, as well as all refined flour products, and I ate only foods recommended in the "Breast Cancer" chapter of Michio Kushi's *The Cancer Prevention Diet.*

I went for a second opinion at Tufts New England Medical Center and found a group that advocated only chemotherapy and radiation therapy, without surgery. My research indicated that at M. D. Anderson Cancer Center in Houston, radiation therapy twice daily for six weeks could help tumors of this type temporarily, so I asked my radiation oncologist to do this, until January 1986. He confessed that all medical treatments in this case were more art than science, but he would try his best. I found in seeking further opinions that there were as many recommendations as there were doctors, so I asked those whose opinions with which I agreed to write letters to my own doctors to direct treatments. In particular, I found a surgeon opposed to surgery, and in this way I convinced my own team of physicians not to do a mastectomy. I tolerated the radiation treatment well, especially because I balanced the very yin treatment with additional miso soup and sea vegetables once I started macrobiotics.

Finally, my oncologist was pressuring me into six months more of chemotherapy. I had decided that I would rather die than bear more torture from the drugs. On January 28, 1986, I met Michio and Aveline Kushi for my first consultation at a Way of Life seminar in Boston. Aveline kindly presented me with an autographed copy of her newly published *Complete Guide to Macrobiotic Cooking*, which I treated as my new Bible. Michio told me in his light and amusing, yet provocative, way that I would commit suicide if I ate one more piece of chocolate.

He recommended a version of the standard macrobiotic diet tailored for my condition, including four special home remedies to be prepared from household foods:

- Grated carrot and daikon radish to dissolve my excess body fat and help me lose weight.
- Sweet vegetable drink—a tea made from cooking onion, cabbage, carrots, and winter squash—to help clean the egg and cheese fat out of my pancreas, which had been causing my extreme hypoglycemia and chocolate binges.

- Ume-sho-kuzu—a Japanese salty and sour drink made from a thickening root starch, an alkalinizing pickled plum, and soy sauce—to strengthen my intestines and relieve the chronic constipation that is at the root of many upper body ailments.
- Barley and cabbage breast plaster—a paste made from cooked pearl barley (Job's tears) and raw green cabbage worn nightly for two months. This plaster was most effective: after just four or five days, I found that old hard breast calcifications I had had for many years were beginning to soften and dissolve.

As my disease was so far advanced, even Michio Kushi was cautious, and he gave me two programs to choose from: one based on diet alone, the other a combination of diet with additional chemotherapy. Although my husband preferred that I take more drugs, he supported my decision to use only macrobiotic food as my medicine, and he created a "nest" at home where I could just cook, make special remedies, take walks, sing happy songs, and sleep. He also kindly kept away anyone who brought my energy down, including my kind and well-meaning, but pushy, oncologist.

For the next two months I followed the healing diet that Michio had recommended. Every second of my time I spent trying to save my life, because if I did anything else, I felt I could easily lose my life. I never once doubted that I would recover. Macrobiotic philosophy enabled me to understand the energy that had caused the tumor to grow, and to create the energy of food that would cause it to be balanced and dissolve. I learned how food transmutes into blood, and what we eat becomes our body, mind, and spirit. With each new meal, I felt that my blood was being made into a cleansing solvent that could penetrate my remaining tumor and dissolve all the heavy dairy fat and protein of which it was composed. With my cleaner body and cleared mind, my intuition became sharper, and I could experience the power of the universe—heaven's and earth's forces—healing me directly.

At the end of March 1986, on Good Friday, I was awakened at about four A.M. by nearly uncontrollable diarrhea. I had read that the body sometimes "discharges" excess animal food in such strong ways, so I was not so concerned. But the next morning, to my happy surprise, I realized that the remaining hardness of my breast tumor was suddenly and miraculously gone! This was just two months after I had started a serious practice of macrobiotics under the guidance of Michio and Aveline Kushi. In the time that modern Western medicine had said that I would probably die, a traditional Eastern diet had helped save my life. I was so grateful.

I began and still continue to record what foods I eat daily, and to record the condition of my body each morning. This self-research has confirmed for me the cause-and-effect relationship between diet and health. For example, I found that the cosmetic use of small amounts of sesame oil on my face for six weeks in June 1986 seemed to bring back the redness on my breast. It appeared that the oil entered my bloodstream as if I had eaten it, and it was like throwing oil on a flame. Following Michio's advice, I stopped the oil treatment and again ate grated carrot and daikon. The inflammation disappeared with diarrhea after about five days. After this, I stayed very strict with my diet and lifestyle for more than two years. I widened my diet to include fruit, bread, and oil only when I was told it was safe by my counselor and then extended it to the standard macrobiotic diet, which I follow to this day.

My salvation, I think, lies in the following facts:

- The initial chemotherapy was yang to balance my extreme yin condition.
- I took only a modest amount of drugs to control the acute initial symptoms of inflammation, and then stopped.
- I carefully avoided all foods that resembled those that caused the tumor to grow, and I never cheated on my healing macrobiotic diet.
- I stopped my graduate studies and quit my consultant job to focus on just getting well.
- At all times I felt in control of both the Western and the Eastern treatments.
- Every day I spent cooking like a pharmacist to save my life.
- I had a supportive and loving family, who had blessed me with a strong constitution, changed to a macrobiotic diet with me, and even studied shiatsu to give me massages.

- I still had a little intuition left to know what was good for my recovery.
- I did not believe I would die just because the doctors said I would.
- I had a strong imperative to live and a Big Dream for my life.

About two years after recovering, I began to study formally at the Kushi Institute in Becket, Massachusetts. It seemed to me that with my newly found knowledge, I had to change my life to help others who were also unfortunate enough to have a diagnosis of cancer or other serious disease. I see very many people making the same mistakes with diet and way of life that caused me so much pain and suffering. I served as a coordinator of the Way to Health Program, a one-week seminar designed to help people, primarily cancer patients and their families, begin macrobiotics. Because of my science background, I was often called upon to coordinate medical research and teaching for the Kushi Institute. For the past several years, I have served as an assistant to Michio and Aveline Kushi at their home in Brookline, Massachusetts.

It is now fourteen years since I was diagnosed with cancer. I am returning to my old passion, high-energy and nuclear physics, but from the macrobiotic vantage point of alternative science. We are conducting experiments in low-energy nuclear transmutation, attempting to form heavier elements such as iron from lighter elements such as carbon and oxygen. We are also investigating natural, alternative methods of energy generation and storage, including directly harnessing cosmic energy received from heaven, and centripetal energy generated from earth. Just as cancer, heart disease, and other illnesses can be healed with peaceful, gentle means, it is our hope that someday unlimited sources of energy and scarce elements will become commonly available, and help heal the planet and promote peace in this world.

I am very, very grateful to be alive. I am grateful to my family for giving me life and eternal support. I am grateful to medical doctors for their original diagnosis and for controlling the inflammation at the beginning so the cancer did not spread. I am grateful to Michio and Aveline Kushi and other teachers for bringing the traditional wisdom of the unifying principles of nature to America, for teaching me the cause of my cancer, and for bringing foods and

recipes that helped save my life. And I am very grateful to the
patients and champions of alternative medicine who helped add
both quality and quantity to the precious years of my life.

—FORMER BREAST CANCER PATIENT

Although the above story is about inflammatory breast cancer, a relatively rare and aggressive form of the disease, the lessons it illustrates
are important. First, it indicates that dietary change can have important
and profound influences on health. Second, it reveals the relative lack of
knowledge and experience most conventional physicians have in this
area. Finally, it shows us the important role of intuition, belief, and a
willingness to take responsibility for one's actions in the quest for health
and recovery. This chapter will directly address the first of these points:
the role of diet in breast cancer. I hope it will provide knowledge to
health care professionals and empower women with breast cancer to
seek out their own path in the absence of definitive information.

Food, Nutrition, and Life

Cancer is a chronic disease that may be influenced at many stages of its
development by nutritional factors. The evidence that cancer is a result
of a genetic-environmental interaction suggests that diet and lifestyle
may play a role not only in causing cancer but in preventing it as well. It
has been known for centuries that cancer kills its victims by depleting
the body of essential nutrients. Cancer was described in many traditions
as causing consumption, or wasting. The depletion syndrome is caused
in part by the different metabolic activity created by the tumor and in
part by the body's defense strategy. Current studies of populations
around the globe show that different diets and lifestyles affect not only
the incidence of breast cancer but also the age of incidence and survival.

Many nutrients are now known to affect DNA replication and cell differentiation, two aspects of the cell's life that are abnormal in cancer. We
now know that we all come from a common ancestor and our genetic
basis is similar, regardless of where we come from on earth or how different we look. The differences we observe largely result from how we have

adapted to the climate and the geographical terrain, which in turn dictates what kinds of food and how much food we have. In different regions of the world, people eat differently. The variety of food, the amount of food, and the methods of food preparation and storage account for much of the difference that we see in the health status of different populations. The simple fact that we have a larger quantity and variety of food, which we are able to keep fresh, has dramatically increased our longevity and our health status during the past century. Yet, abundance and longevity come with a price. Since cancer mostly occurs later in life, we believe that high-calorie intake, high fat in the diet, and longer exposure to nutritional influences increase our risk of getting cancer.

In general, food and its nutrients give us the energy required for our daily activities. They also provide essential building blocks for the formation of our structure and growth and for the regulation of various bodily functions. We need to consume carbohydrates, proteins, fats, vitamins, minerals, and amino acids to maintain life. The question that we all have is: what are the proper quantity, proportion, and variety of each of the essential food elements? In the past few decades, a seemingly endless number of diets have been proposed for many purposes. Unfortunately, most of them focus not on health but on weight loss, and diet has become synonymous with weight control. Often, the diets in question do not account for an individual's health conditions or the energy demands dictated by lifestyle. Our food has changed so dramatically in the past century that we spend 90% of our food money on processed products.[1] We consume larger quantities of higher-fat food,[2] fewer fresh ingredients, and more foods flavored with artificial ingredients.[3] We eat out more often than in the past, which contributes to our problem with obesity.[4] Our food is fortified with different vitamins and minerals, which in specific cases can both detract from health and contribute to it.

The attempt to tailor a single diet that fits all breast cancer patients is unreasonable. We should also make a distinction between using food and nutrition for the maintenance of health and as medicine for the treatment of an illness. In relation to breast cancer, we might ask whether diet can be used by an individual to cure an existing disease, or prevent disease from occurring or recurring. If so, what is the proper diet, and how long should we follow it?

Diet and the Prevention of Breast Cancer

The role of diet and nutrition in the development of cancer has been a major focus of cancer research for many years. It is fair to characterize much of this work as focused on two main areas: (1) exploring and understanding how dietary factors may lead to the onset of cancer, and (2) examining dietary patterns, nutritional status, and related phenomena and comparing them with the patterns of cancer incidence and mortality.

The former types of studies have largely been laboratory based, involving tissue cultures or laboratory animals, while the latter have primarily been conducted in human populations using the tools of epidemiology and prospective clinical trials (wherein an intervention such as dietary manipulation is actually tested as an experiment). Ultimately, these studies, which include everything from cross-cultural comparisons to randomized clinical trials, provide the basis for determining whether there is a causal relation between a dietary factor and cancer incidence or prognosis. It is important to recognize that the most definitive evidence comes from controlled randomized trials of diet. To date, very few of these have been completed.

In the area of diet and breast cancer, literally hundreds of epidemiological studies have examined different aspects of food and nutrition and their relationship to breast cancer. The issue that has probably attracted the most attention over the years is dietary fat.[5] We can trace this interest to the strong geographical association between dietary fat intake and breast cancer incidence (or mortality), as illustrated in Figure 5.1.

In this figure, adapted from an analysis by Prentice et al. in 1988,[6] the availability of fat calories in the diet in twenty-one countries with good cancer registry data is strongly associated with breast cancer incidence. These and similar findings across other countries,[7] within countries,[8] or in comparison of migrants to one country with breast cancer rates in their country of origin,[9] indicate that there are strong environmental influences, most likely related to dietary patterns and to dietary fat intake, that may influence breast cancer incidence and mortality rates. In the laboratory, manipulating the dietary fat content of rats can dramatically affect the development of breast cancer. This also suggests that dietary fat and dietary patterns are important in breast cancer development.[10] But despite the intriguing geographical trends and suggestive data, no con-

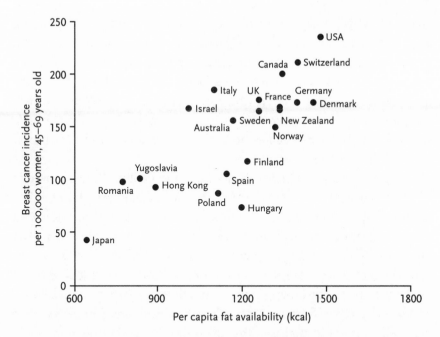

FIGURE 5.1. Rates of Breast Cancer in Different Countries Based on Fat Intake

nection has been established between dietary fat intake and the development of breast cancer when this idea is tested in very specific, controlled clinical trials. In fact, it is now generally accepted that dietary fat intake in adulthood probably has little or no influence on the development of breast cancer even when fat intake is very low (below 20% of energy).

The evidence suggesting that diet has no relationship to breast cancer has been growing since 1987, when the results of the first prospective cohort studies of dietary fat and breast cancer were published. These findings were probably best summarized in an article published in the *New England Journal of Medicine* in 1996.[11] In this article, Hunter and colleagues pooled the data from seven large prospective cohort studies of dietary fat and breast cancer that were conducted in various locations in the United States, Canada, the Netherlands, and Sweden. Overall, the analyses of these pooled data included 337,819 women and 4980 cases of breast cancer. Ultimately, there was no association between dietary fat and risk of breast cancer in any of the studies. Individually, two of the studies suggested a modest increased risk with increased fat intake.[12] This was true regardless of how the data were analyzed: whether as percent of energy from fat (number of calories), as grams of fat consumed, or in examination of subcategories of fat intake, such as by animal fat or vegetable fat intake (shown in Table 5-1). Even at very low fat intake levels, below 20% of calories, there was no association with lower risk of breast cancer. A subsequent article examined further whether there might be interactions of fat intake with other risk factors such as body size or age at menarche for breast cancer, but no evidence was found.

Despite the summarized findings from the Pooling Project, there is still a great deal of interest in the possible role of diet in breast cancer. For example, some prospective cohort studies have observed an increased risk of breast cancer associated with intake of red meat.[13,14] This was reported earlier in a large study in Japan, in which women who consumed red meat on a daily basis had more than twice the risk of developing breast cancer as women who consumed red meat only on occasion.[15] Additional analyses from the Iowa Women's Health Study have indicated that well-done meat increased the risk of breast cancer.[16] One theory is that this increased risk may be caused by a greater consumption of certain heterocyclic amines, which are produced when meat is cooked. These can become carcinogenic once they are metabolized in the body.[17]

TABLE 5-1. Relative Risk Estimates for the Association of Breast Cancer on Dietary Fat

DIETARY VARIABLE	CATEGORY OF INTAKE					
	1 (LOW)	2	3	4	5 (HIGH)	P TREND*
Total fat	1.0	1.01	1.12	1.07	1.05	0.21
Saturated fat	1.0	1.03	1.04	1.00	1.07	0.41
Monounsaturated fat	1.0	1.07	1.11	1.10	1.01	0.73
Polyunsaturated fat	1.0	1.07	1.03	1.06	1.07	0.32
Animal fat	1.0	0.96	0.96	0.92	0.99	0.70
Vegetable fat	1.0	1.04	1.02	1.05	1.08	0.19
Energy	1.0	1.01	1.13	1.04	1.11	0.15

*Probability value for the test for linear trend across the five categories of fat intake. From the Pooling Project of prospective cohort studies of diet and breast cancer, adapted from Hunter et al., 1996.[18]

It is possible that scientists have not yet been able to establish a connection between fat intake and breast cancer risk because of problems in the research methodology. For example, several of the studies conducted so far have not set out with the primary purpose of specifically evaluating the relationship of fat intake to breast cancer risk. Several of the studies we now rely on to assess the relationship between diet and breast cancer were designed with different objectives, and they yielded findings about dietary fat along the way. These tangential results may offer us only an incomplete or inaccurate picture of the situation. Another research problem stems from the difficulty in Western countries of identifying a substantial population of women who are truly on low-fat diets. Without enough qualified subjects, it is impossible to conduct studies on a scale large enough to produce definitive results. Finally, one of the most important factors in breast cancer risk may be diet during infancy, childhood, and early adolescence—but this information is difficult to capture accurately on questionnaires given to adults and therefore has not been subject to analysis. Nevertheless, if one is waiting for clinical evidence that it's worthwhile to minimize dietary fat, one need only think of coronary heart disease, where the connection is clear and undisputed. Whether or not fat is ever implicated as a breast cancer risk, there's no doubt that dietary fat, especially the saturated fats found in meat and dairy products, promote heart disease—which is, after all, the nation's leading killer. So there's no question that decreasing one's dietary fat intake is a positive step toward good health.

Hormonal and reproductive factors are closely associated with breast cancer risk, though the manner in which they may lead to breast cancer is unclear. However, early nutrition determines the rate of growth and development in women. Rapid growth leads to earlier age at onset of menstruation, which is a known risk for breast cancer.[19] Rapid growth and development are measured when increases in height and weight are compared across generations and societies. Two studies conducted in the United States did not find an association between dietary fat or total caloric intake and the onset of menstruation.[20] A third study conducted in Germany showed that high fat and total calorie intake, combined with a low level of physical activity, were associated with an earlier onset of menstruation. All three studies consistently reported that height, weight, and body fat composition were strongly associated with earlier age of menstruation; yet, only the German study reported on the level of physical activity. Higher consumption of proteins or lower consumption of dietary fiber was also correlated with earlier menstruation,[21] and girls who were vegetarian started menstruating at a later age.[22] It is important to note that the average age at onset of menstruation varies significantly between nations but not significantly within a group. In the United States, the average age is twelve or thirteen years, while in rural China the average age is seventeen or eighteen years—and in that area, the incidence of breast cancer is about fivefold lower. An interesting observation was made in Norway in relation to food consumption, age of menarche, and breast cancer risk. The women who were born between 1930 and 1932 and experienced the famine of World War II during the years of their anticipated onset of menstruation had a 13% lower risk for breast cancer.[23]

Trying to make sense out of all these data is not easy. Yet, we may be able to conclude that a diet high in fat and calories, which is also high in protein from red meat and is accompanied by low physical activity, increases the risk of cancer. That risk is higher for women who are tall and overweight, and if the onset of menstruation was earlier, the risk increases. Nevertheless, we have to remember that the risk we are talking about is still relatively small when compared with a risk such as lung cancer from cigarette smoking.

Like the information on high-fat and high-calorie food, high consumption of carbohydrates, in the form of starch, is associated with increased risk of breast cancer in some studies[24] but not in others.[25] At the other end of the carbohydrate spectrum, diets with high fiber content, mainly fruits and vegetables, may play a protective role in breast cancer.[26] More specifically, the risk is reduced if the fiber is from fruits, vegetables, and crude fiber but not from cereals.[27,28] Several reasons why fiber may protect from breast cancer have been suggested. One is that soluble fiber, found mostly in fruits and vegetables, lowers the reabsorption in the intestine of estrogen secreted by the liver.[29] Fiber is also thought to decrease the risk of breast cancer by reducing obesity and insulin sensitivity, both of which are associated not only with increased risk but also with poorer prognosis.[30]

More recently, there has also been growing interest in the role of folic acid and associated nutrients in relation to breast and other cancers. Of particular interest has been the possible role that inadequate folate, a B vitamin found in leafy vegetables, may play in carcinogenesis. There is increased risk of breast cancer with low folate intake in the presence of high alcohol consumption.[31-33] These findings suggest that vegetables and other foods high in folate may confer some protection against breast cancer. Other areas of growing interest in relation to breast cancer include the possible role of soy and other foods containing phytoestrogens, as well as the relatively high carotenoid and antioxidant content of many fruits and vegetables. These areas are covered elsewhere in this book, and much of this epidemiological literature was summarized recently in a large monograph from the American Institute for Cancer Research and the World Cancer Research Fund on Diet, Nutrition, and the Prevention of Cancer.[34] Their findings are given in Table 5-2.

TABLE 5-2. Judgments by the American Institute for Cancer Research/ World Cancer Research Fund Panel on Diet, Nutrition, and the Prevention of Cancer Regarding the Likelihood That Various Dietary Constituents or Related Factors Modify the Risk of Breast Cancer

STRENGTH OF EVIDENCE*	DECREASES RISK	NO RELATIONSHIP	INCREASES RISK
Convincing		Coffee	Rapid growth Greater adult height
Probable	Vegetables and fruits	Cholesterol	High body mass† Adult weight gain Alcohol
Possible	Physical activity Dietary fiber Carotenoids	Monounsaturated fat Polyunsaturated fat Retinol Vitamin E Poultry Black tea	Total fat Saturated/animal fat Meat

(continued)

TABLE 5-2.   *(continued)*

STRENGTH OF EVIDENCE*	DECREASES RISK	No RELATIONSHIP	INCREASES RISK
Insufficient	Vitamin C Isoflavones and lignans Fish		Animal protein DDT residues

*See AICR[35] for specific definitions of these terms as used by the panel.
†For postmenopausal breast cancer.
Adapted from AICR, 1997.[36]

Diet and Prognosis (Outcome) After a Diagnosis of Breast Cancer

Although substantial epidemiological research has been done on diet and the risk of breast cancer, surprisingly few studies have examined the relationship of diet to breast cancer prognosis and survival. Indeed, few studies have examined the broad spectrum of complementary and alternative therapies as factors in recurrence or survival from breast cancer.[37] In the area of diet, this is unfortunate, given the belief that dietary factors play a major role in breast cancer.[38,39] All reported studies were retrospective, that is, they were not clinical trials in which diet was actually prescribed ahead of time and tested as an experiment, with careful analysis of the resulting risk of breast cancer recurrence.

The relative scarcity of studies on diet and breast cancer prognosis is particularly striking, since the mechanisms that may explain how diet relates to cancer risk may also teach us something about the role of diet in treating the disease. Some dietary factors act to prevent cancer by biological mechanisms. For instance, cruciferous vegetables may alter the metabolism of carcinogens. Folate (one of the B vitamins) affects the expression of DNA. Soluble fiber may decrease factors that influence cell proliferation and thereby inhibit the growth of an invasive cancer. As a specific example, genistein, an isoflavone that is found in high concentration in soy foods, has been demonstrated to reduce the formation of new blood vessels,[40] among other physiological roles.

Because tumors need a blood supply in order to grow, we may hypothe-size that diets high in soy may inhibit tumor progression. (For further discussion, see chapter 6.)

Thus, very little scientific information directly addresses the question whether dietary change after diagnosis is helpful to women with breast cancer. For example, to date, only fourteen studies have examined whether dietary fat intake may be a prognostic factor for women with breast cancer. While these have design limitations that demand cautious interpretation, several of them suggest that higher dietary fat intake may compromise survival. These fourteen studies are summarized in Table 5-3. Eight of them reported results connecting an increased risk of mor-tality after breast cancer diagnosis with increased fat intake.[41-48] For ex-ample, in one of these studies, among 471 women diagnosed with breast cancer, post-diagnosis consumption of red meat was associated with a 30% increased risk of recurrence, or a relative risk of 1.30.[49]

Those results, specifically related to dietary fat intake, are also summa-rized in Figure 5-2, which presents the relative risks of mortality after breast cancer, comparing high fat intake with low fat intake. The majority of studies consistently find that higher fat intake is associated with a poorer prognosis. For example, if the relative risk is 1.21, then there is a 21% increased risk of mortality after a diagnosis of breast cancer in a woman with higher fat intake than in one with lower fat intake. A relative risk of 3.17 indicates that the risk of dying of breast cancer with a high-fat diet compared with a low-fat diet is 217% greater. As noted in Figure 5.2, eight of the eleven studies found that high fat intake was associated with an increased risk of mortality after a diagnosis of breast cancer.

Only a few of the studies were explicitly designed to address whether dietary habits after diagnosis affect outcome. Among the three studies (noted by the asterisks in Figure 5.2) that collected information on what women were eating after they were diagnosed with breast cancer,[50-52] only one had information on dietary habits both before and after diagno-sis. Thus, only one study could address the question whether dietary change after diagnosis may influence prognosis. In this study, dietary habits after diagnosis were not collected at a consistent point in time because the primary purpose of collecting dietary data was to address questions concerning the cause of disease, rather than disease outcome. Two of the other studies with post-diagnosis information reported

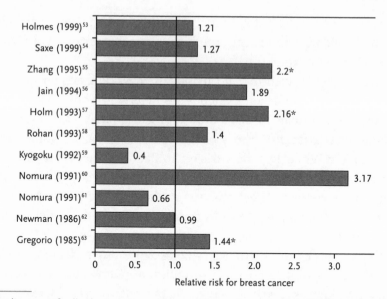

*Studies specifically designed to address whether dietary habits after a breast cancer diagnosis affect mortality.

FIGURE 5.2.   Dietary Fat and Risk of Death after Breast Cancer.

findings consistent with a poorer survival with higher fat intake.[64,65] As noted in Table 5-3 and Figure 5.2, the relative consistency of the findings from these studies, despite these design flaws, do suggest that dietary change should be examined in the context of breast cancer prognosis.

One important dietary habit that has been linked to both incidence of breast cancer and breast cancer prognosis is alcohol consumption. The greater the amount of alcohol a woman drinks, the stronger her risk of getting breast cancer or of having a recurrence.[66–69] Also, heavier drinkers tend to be diagnosed with later-stage breast cancer, which may explain the role of alcohol in the spread of breast cancer.[70] Drinking three glasses of alcohol or more per day is associated with a 40% to 70% increased risk of breast cancer, in comparison with nondrinkers.[71,72]

Clinical Trials of Diet and Breast Cancer Prognosis

At least two ongoing large randomized trials are examining the effects of low-fat diet on the recurrence of and survival from breast cancer. Survival of breast cancer patients after surgery was consistently greater in

Japan, where fat intake is low, than in the United States, where fat intake is substantially higher, regardless of stage at diagnosis.[73-76] Even factors like tumor grade and lymph node involvement could not explain the differences in outcome between the patients in Japan and those in the United States.[77] This difference in survival rates illustrates why large-scale dietary intervention trials are important. These observations are supported by animal studies in which fat intake, especially linoleic acid, directly stimulates breast cancer metastasis.[78-82]

One of the two ongoing large-scale studies is the Women's Healthy Eating and Living (WHEL) Study, based at the University of California at San Diego, which was inspired by the use of alternative dietary therapies for cancer.[83-85] This study uses a predominantly vegetarian diet that promotes the use of juicing, in the belief that the women will be able to ingest large amounts of the various phytochemicals (plant nutrients) that may be important in cancer prevention and treatment without having to take pills as supplements. A second study based at the American Health Foundation, the Women's Intervention Nutrition Study, will focus on the effects of low-fat diets.[86] As of this date, recruitment in this study is complete, and the women will be monitored for a few more years before the study is complete.

These randomized clinical trials are important tests of specific dietary interventions that we have reason to believe may favorably influence breast cancer recurrence or survival. The scientific rationale for these studies is based largely on other studies suggesting that a diet high in fruits and vegetables and low in animal foods decreases the risk of cancer.[87] This type of diet forms the basis for cancer-prevention guidelines as promoted by organizations such as the American Cancer Society[88] and the American Institute for Cancer Research.[89]

Complementary or Alternative Dietary Approaches for Breast Cancer

Although mainstream nutritional science recommends a diet high in vegetables, fruits, and whole grains for cancer prevention, no such recommendations are yet part of the treatment of breast cancer. Interestingly, the major alternative dietary approaches to cancer have generally

TABLE 5-3.   Epidemiologic Studies of Diet and Breast Cancer Recurrence or Survival

Reference	No. of cases	No. of outcomes	Follow-up (years)
Gregorio (1985)[90]	676 206 local 312 regional 158 distant		15–23
Newman (1986)[91]	300		5–7
Ewertz (1991)[92]	1,744		
Nomura (1991)[93]	182 Japanese 161 Caucasians		7–12
Kyogoku (1992)[94]	212	47 breast cancer deaths	9–13
Rohan (1993)[95]	412	112 breast cancer deaths	5.5
Holm (1993)[96]	149 ER+	30 recurrences	4
Ingram (1994)[97]	103	21 breast cancer deaths	6
Jain (1994)[98]	678 Canadians	76 breast cancer deaths	7–12
Zhang (1995)[99]	698		0–6
Jain (1997)[100]	676		
Hébert (1998)[101]	471	109 recurrences	7–9

Diet Period	Diet Variable	Relative Risk (95% CI)
Before diagnosis	Total fat (per 1,000 g/mo)	1.14
	Total fat (per 1,000 g/mo)	0.93
	Total fat (per 1,000 g/mo)	1.16
	Total fat (per 1,000 g/mo)	1.44 (p<0.01)
After diagnosis	Total fat	0.99
	Total fat	No association
Before diagnosis	Total fat	0.66 (0.25, 1.76)
Before diagnosis	Total fat	3.17 (1.17, 8.55)
Before diagnosis	Total protein (hi vs lo 4th)	1.4 (0.5, 3.9)
	Total fat	0.4 (0.1, 1.3)
	Animal fat	1.3 (0.4, 4.1)
	Vegetable fat	0.5 (0.2, 1.7)
Before diagnosis	Total fat (hi vs lo 5th)	1.40 (0.66, 2.96)
After diagnosis	Total fat (% E)*	1.08 (1.00, 1.16)
	Saturated fat	Increased risk
Before diagnosis	β-carotene	Decreased risk
	Fruit	Decreased risk
	Total vegetables & fruit	Decreased risk
Before diagnosis	Total fat (% E)	1.89 (0.96, 3.70)
	Saturated fat (% E)	2.32 (1.22, 4.40)
	β-carotene (IU)	0.48 (0.23, 0.99)
	Vitamin C (mg)	0.43 (0.21, 0.86)
Before diagnosis	Total fat (% E) (hi vs lo 3rd)	2.2 (1.0, 4.7)
	Saturated fat (% E)	1.7 (0.8, 3.5)
	Monounsaturated fat (% E)	1.8 (0.9, 3.8)
	Polyunsaturated fat (% E)	1.3 (0.6, 2.6)
Before diagnosis	Total fat	Increased risk
After diagnosis	Red meat (times/day)	1.30 (1.03, 1.64)
	Butter, magarine, lard	1.12 (0.66, 1.89)
	Beer (drinks/day)	1.41 (1.02, 1.97)

(continued)

TABLE 5-3.   *(continued)*

Reference	No. of cases	No. of outcomes	Follow-up (years)
Hébert (1998)[102] *(cont.)*		73 breast cancer deaths	7–9
	222 premenopause	? recurrences	7–9
		? breast cancer deaths	7–9
Saxe (1999)[103]	149	28 recurrences	5–7
		26 deaths	5–7
Holmes (1999)[104]	1982	378 deaths	4–14

*% E = percentage of total energy from total fat

Diet Period	Diet Variable	Relative Risk (95% CI)
After diagnosis	Red meat (times/day)	1.43 (0.74, 2.79)
	Butter, margarine, lard	1.16 (0.86, 1.58)
	Beer (drinks/day)	1.58 (1.00, 2.78)
After diagnosis	Red meat (times/day)	1.93 (0.89, 4.15)
	Butter, margarine, lard	1.67 (1.17, 2.39)
	Beer (drinks/day)	1.58 (1.15, 2.17)
After diagnosis	Red meat (times/day)	2.60 (0.96, 7.03)
	Butter, margarine, lard	1.03 (0.61, 1.76)
	Beer (drinks/day)	2.33 (1.35, 4.00)
Before diagnosis	Total fat (10% E)	1.42 (0.82, 2.46)
	Saturated fat (20 g)	1.89 (0.47, 7.59)
	Monounsaturated fat (15 g)	2.33 (0.76, 7.11)
	Bread & cereal (7 servings)	0.55 (0.33, 0.93)
Before diagnosis	Total fat (10% E)	1.27 (0.71, 2.27)
	Saturated fat (20 g)	1.45 (0.32, 6.62)
	Monounsaturated fat (15 g)	1.77 (0.53, 5.87)
	Bread & cereal (7 servings)	0.87 (0.58, 1.29)
After diagnosis	*92 dietary variables examined; selected findings comparing high with low intake include*	
	Vitamin A	0.78 (0.58, 1.06)
	Alcohol	0.92 (0.66, 1.27)
	Dietary fiber	0.69 (0.50, 0.97)
	Lutein & zeaxanthin	0.87 (0.62, 1.21)
	Calcium	0.66 (0.48, 0.91)
	Protein	0.65 (0.47, 0.88)
	Omega-3 fatty acids	0.77 (0.56, 1.07)
	18:2 *trans* fatty acid	1.45 (1.06, 1.99)
	Poultry	0.70 (0.50, 0.97)
	Dairy	0.72 (0.52, 1.00)
	Fish	0.80 (0.60, 1.07)
	Vegetables	0.81 (0.59, 1.11)

advocated a near-vegetarian diet that embodies the spirit of mainstream dietary guidelines for cancer prevention.

As outlined in several sources (see *Choices in Healing: Integrating the Best of Conventional and Complementary Approaches to Cancer* by Michael Lerner[105]; a publication by the Office of Alternative Medicine entitled *Alternative Medicine: Expanding Medical Horizons;*[106] or the Office of Technology Assessment's publication *Unconventional Cancer Treatments*),[107] two of the major comprehensive dietary approaches to cancer are the Gerson diet and the macrobiotic diet. The phrase *comprehensive dietary approach* distinguishes these diets from other nutritional programs that require patients to ingest a specific food or supplement rather than making a major change in their diet. A comprehensive approach includes not only eating different foods but changing one's eating habits and methods of food preparation. It does not preclude the use of specific supplements but emphasizes the importance of fundamental dietary change.

The Gerson Therapy

A fundamental aspect of Gerson therapy is a vegetarian diet. Other important recommendations for cancer include the use of juices, similar to the intervention under study in the WHEL trial. Indeed, the WHEL trial dietary intervention was inspired in part by the Gerson therapy.

The main theory underlying the Gerson approach to cancer is the idea that "the body must be detoxified—activated with ionized minerals, natural food so that the essential organs can function. For healing the body brings about a kind of inflammation. That is a tremendous transformative reaction. This renders the body hypersensitive or allergic to the highest degree against abnormal or strange substances (including bacilli, cancer cells, scars, etc.)."[108] Also related to detoxification, Gerson therapy advocates extremely restricted fat intake and moderate protein restriction (part of the rationale for a vegetarian diet), as well as limited sodium and potassium supplementation. Vitamin C supplementation is also usually recommended. Other aspects of the Gerson approach to cancer include coffee enemas and the administration of pancreatic enzymes, calf's liver extracts, and thyroid supplementation with iodine. While the literature that supports some of these specific recommendations is spotty at best (see Lerner for a full review),[109] the dietary change that is one of its fundamental aspects can be supported in part by a generous interpretation of the scientific literature. Objective scientific information specifically supporting the Gerson approach to cancer management, more specifically to the management of breast cancer, is not yet available, although breast cancer is one of the cancers described as being helped by this approach to cancer.

Macrobiotics

Macrobiotics is described in substantial detail here both because of its popularity as a comprehensive dietary approach to cancer and because of the familiarity of the author with macrobiotics.

Broadly, the word *macrobiotics* has been used to describe a philosophy, a cultural movement, and an eating pattern. The word *macrobiotic* was used by the eighteenth-century German physician Hufeland to describe a program for good health and prolonging life.[110] It was used more recently by British sinologist Joseph Needham to describe the philosophy underlying much of the Chinese view of science and medicine.[111] However, in recent decades macrobiotics has come to be thought of in the context of cancer through the work of the Japanese philosopher George Ohsawa and his students, one in particular: my father, Michio Kushi.[112]

The vast majority of people who would describe themselves as following a macrobiotic lifestyle probably have not been diagnosed with cancer or other serious illnesses. Therefore, it is a misperception that macrobiotics is strictly a diet for the treatment of disease. Michio Kushi, the most well-known authority on macrobiotics in the world, has authored books describing the philosophical bases of macrobiotics as well as his own motivations for devoting his life to macrobiotics.[113,114] His dedication to macrobiotics came out of his studies in political science and a search for solutions for world peace. He wrote, "I realized that it was essential to recover genuine food, largely of natural, organic quality, and make it available to every family at reasonable cost. Only then could consciousness be transformed and world peace achieved."[115] Kushi described his use of the word *macrobiotics*:

> I adopted "macrobiotics" in its original meaning, as the universal way of health and longevity which encompasses the largest possible view not only of diet but also of all dimensions of human life, natural order, and cosmic evolution. Macrobiotics embraces behavior, thought, breathing, exercise, relationships, customs, cultures, ideas, and consciousness, as well as individual and collective lifestyles found throughout the world.
>
> In this sense, macrobiotics is not simply or mainly a diet. Macrobiotics is the universal way of life with which humanity has developed biologically, psychologically, and spiritually and with which we will maintain our health, freedom, and happiness. Macrobiotics includes a dietary approach but its purpose is to ensure the survival of the human race and its further evolution on this planet. In macrobiotics—the natural intuitive wisdom of East and West, North and South—I found the Medicine for Humanity that I had been seeking.

Despite the broad view of macrobiotics presented by these excerpts, macrobiotics has come to be known largely as a dietary approach to cancer. This is evidenced in part by the Office of Technology Assessment's publication *Unconventional Cancer Treatments,* in which macrobiotic diets are listed along with the Gerson treatment and Kelley regimens as a common dietary approach for the treatment of cancer.[116] In addition, the American Cancer Society periodically announces that macrobiotic diets are on its list of unproven methods of cancer management.

The East West Foundation, founded by Michio Kushi as a nonprofit organization for the promotion of macrobiotics, sponsored conferences on diet and cancer as early as 1974. The recognition of macrobiotics as an alternative measure for cancer prevention was spurred by the publication in 1979 of a book by Jean and Mary Alice Kohler, *Healing Miracles from Macrobiotics: A Diet for All Diseases.*[117] Jean Kohler was a professor of music at Ball State University who had been diagnosed in 1973 with pancreatic cancer and had been given a poor prognosis. He discovered and turned to macrobiotics, and the cancer went into remission; his experiences with macrobiotics are detailed in this book.

However, the major impetus behind the reputation of macrobiotics as an alternative cancer treatment came from the 1982 publication of *Recalled by Life: The Story of My Recovery from Cancer,* by Anthony Sattilaro and Thomas Monte.[118] The book described the experiences of Anthony Sattilaro, who was diagnosed with metastatic prostate cancer at the age of forty-nine in 1977. What made Sattilaro's case of particular interest was that he was an anesthesiologist and head of a hospital in Philadelphia. Despite his medical training, he turned to macrobiotics as an alternative approach to his cancer and credits it, among other factors, with sending his cancer into remission. His personal story became the basis not just of his book but also of articles in the *Saturday Evening Post, Life* magazine, and other periodicals. This exposure created a great deal of public interest in macrobiotics in the context of cancer therapy.

On the heels of Dr. Sattilaro's book came the publication in 1983 of Michio Kushi and Alex Jack's *The Cancer Prevention Diet*[119] (published in a revised edition in 1994), which, despite its name, was devoted largely to macrobiotics in the treatment of cancer. The book also detailed the philosophical bases behind macrobiotics. As the most prominent spokesperson for macrobiotics, Michio Kushi provided in this book the best overview of the macrobiotic approach to cancer, of which diet is the centerpiece. While dietary guidelines are individually modified depending on the specific cancer and other aspects, there is a "standard macrobiotic diet" that forms the basis for dietary recommendations for cancer.

Macrobiotic Dietary Guidelines

The standard macrobiotic diet provides a framework that is modified depending on one's age, sex, level of activity, personal needs, and environment. In the context of cancer therapy, individuals are encouraged to work with a qualified macrobiotics counselor. For specific cancers, these recommendations may be further modified. The Kushi Institute, founded by Michio Kushi and located in Becket, Massachusetts, began a certification program for counselors approximately fifteen years ago.

The standard macrobiotic diet can be broadly described as one that emphasizes whole plant foods. It is therefore a high–complex carbohydrate, low-fat, predominantly vegetarian diet. To the extent possible, foods to be consumed should be organically grown. The diet consists of the following types of foods:[120,121]

- 50% to 60% whole cereal grains. These include brown rice, barley, millet, oats, wheat, corn, rye, buckwheat, and other less common grains.
- 25% to 30% vegetables, preferably locally grown. This may include small amounts of raw or pickled vegetables.
- 5% to 10% soups, or about two bowls per day, preferably made with sea vegetables such as wakame or kombu and other vegetables, and seasoned with miso or tamari soy sauce.
- 5% to 10% beans of various types, such as azuki, chickpeas, or lentils; bean products such as tofu, tempeh, or natto; and sea vegetables, cooked with the beans or as separate dishes.
- Occasional foods to be consumed a few times per week or less often include white-meat fish, fruits, seeds, and nuts.

Foods that are generally avoided in a standard macrobiotic diet include meat and poultry, animal fats including lard and butter, eggs, dairy products, refined sugars, and foods containing artificial sweeteners or other chemical additives. In the context of cancer, these restrictions may be absolute for a period of time until recovery. The stories of both Professor Kohler[122] and Dr. Sattilaro,[123] as well as that of the breast cancer patient which began this chapter, detail an initial period during which all animal foods and fruit were avoided, followed subsequently by periods during which these foods were reintroduced into their diets.

Biomedical Literature Related to Macrobiotics and Cancer

Although no dietary surveys have been conducted of people with cancer who are following a macrobiotic diet, there have been some surveys of people following a macrobiotic lifestyle. A survey of fifty adults following a macrobiotic diet conducted by Brown and Bergan[124] and analyzed by Kushi et al.[125] demonstrated that fat intake averaged 23% of total calories, saturated fat intake averaged 9%, and carbohydrate intake 65%. Reflecting the extremely low animal food consumption in this study, dietary cholesterol intake averaged 73 mg/day. These values contrast markedly with the United States averages of approximately 37% of calories from fat and 14% from saturated fat.[126]

The dietary pattern outlined in the standard macrobiotic diet is consistent with recommendations for cancer prevention from the American Cancer Society and the AICR/WCRF.[127] While neither of these reports specifically mentions macrobiotics or macrobiotic diets, the practice of macrobiotics appears to represent one possible way that patients may apply those recommendations. Indeed, on the basis of those recommendations and other research, it is reasonable to propose that the standard macrobiotic diet carries substantially lower cancer risk than the standard United States diet. Several studies have demonstrated consistently that people following a macrobiotic diet are at lower risk of cardiovascular disease than people in the general population because of their substantially lower blood cholesterol levels,[128–132] lower blood pressure,[133,134] and higher plasma levels of antioxidants relative to cholesterol.[135] These findings are perhaps not unexpected, given the low-fat, low–saturated fat, and high–whole grain dietary pattern of the standard macrobiotic diet. The studies may be relevant to the breast cancer patient, as some studies suggest that higher blood cholesterol levels are an indicator of poorer prognosis from breast cancer.[136]

In addition to the general macronutrient differences between a standard macrobiotic diet and the standard American diet, certain foods that are part of the daily standard macrobiotic diet have possible anticancer effects. For example, in a cohort study of 265,000 people in Japan, miso soup consumption appeared to have an inverse association with the risk of breast cancer.[137] Several case-control studies suggest an inverse association of tofu and other soy products with risk of breast cancer[138] (the role of soy products in breast cancer is covered elsewhere in this book). Miso has been observed to inhibit the formation of mammary tumors[139] and has also been proposed to have antioxidant properties.[140] It has also been suggested that sea vegetables, perhaps through their high concentration of alginic acid, a type of dietary fiber, may decrease the risk of breast cancer.[141,142] Beans and bean products, especially those derived from soybeans such as miso, tofu, and tempeh, also appear to contain other compounds, such as protease inhibitors[143] and the phytoestrogenic isoflavonoids mentioned earlier, that may play a role in cancer prevention.[144]

Other Aspects of the Macrobiotic Approach to Cancer

In addition to the central role of diet, macrobiotics often recommends other methods to facilitate recovery from cancer. These take the form of external applications, including body scrubs with hot, wet towels, and compresses or plasters, such as those made with pearl barley and leafy greens that are recommended for softer breast tumors. Some of these were described by the patient whose case history introduces this chapter. A hot body scrub may be recommended twice daily in the morning and evening to help activate circulation, promote clear and clean skin, discharge fat accumulated under the skin, and open skin pores to promote smooth and regular elimination of any excess fat and toxins.

A plaster made from pearl barley (Job's tears) and leafy greens for softer breast tumors is prepared as follows: Pressure-cook pearl barley as you would brown rice. Mash to a paste in a suribachi (mortar and pestle). Finely chop an equal amount of large leafy green vegetables (e.g., Chinese cabbage, collards, bok choy, green cabbage) and mash together with the barley in the suribachi. Grate ginger (about 3% to 4% total volume of plaster) and mix thoroughly. Add enough volume of white unbleached flour to make a paste. Spread the paste about one-half to one inch thick on a cotton cloth. Apply a warm wet towel to the breast area first to heat it up and stimulate blood circulation. Then apply the plaster directly to the breast tumor area. Wrap and bind it with a bolt of cotton cheesecloth and safety pins, and cover with a cotton towel. Apply for three hours or overnight. Repeat daily until the tumor softens and dissolves. A similar plaster, prepared from brown rice and miso, is recommended for harder breast tumors.

Additional "way of life" recommendations for general good health are listed here. Some of them may be emphasized in the context of the macrobiotic approach to cancer.

- Use pots and pans made of stainless steel, ceramics, or cast iron, rather than aluminum.

- Cook with gas or wood, not electricity, and never with microwaves.
- Minimize baking in the oven.
- Eat regularly in a relaxed manner, two to three meals per day as desired.
- Late-night eating or snacking is not recommended. It is best not to eat for the three hours before sleeping.
- Each meal should be centered on grains: 50% or more.
- Variety in the selection and preparation of various kinds of dishes is very important. A strict diet does not mean a narrow or monotonous diet.
- Walk outside in fresh air for half an hour or longer every day.
- Exercise or sports are also beneficial, but not to the point of exhaustion.
- Wear only 100% cotton clothing next to the skin; outer garments may be of other materials.
- Use 100% cotton bedsheets and pillow cases.
- Keep green plants in the home to freshen and oxygenate the indoor air.
- To avoid a shower of radiation, limit television watching to a maximum half hour per day; minimize or avoid the use of a computer monitor.
- Change fluorescent lights to incandescent lights in the home and workplace.
- Avoid exposure to a chemicalized environment.
- Avoid artificial chemicals in cosmetics, soaps, toothpaste, etc. Use toiletries made from more natural ingredients from natural food stores.
- Maintain a happy, relaxed, and regular lifestyle.
- Chew very well, ideally fifty times or more for each mouthful.
- To refresh and enliven your physical and mental condition, sing a happy song every day.

These recommendations and those for external applications clearly indicate that the macrobiotic approach to cancer is not limited to dietary recommendations, although the diet is clearly the centerpiece.

Evaluating Macrobiotics as a Cancer Treatment

In addition to the accounts of individual recovery from cancer by Kohler and Sattilaro cited earlier, several other reports have been published in recent years. These include a book about a nurse's recovery from malignant melanoma,[145] a book about recovery from carcinosarcoma of the uterus with multiple metastases by a woman who subsequently went on to earn a master's degree in nutrition,[146] and compilations of case histories.[147] The Office of Technology Assessment noted, however, that "although these various accounts reflect the authors' beliefs that they were helped by following a macrobiotic diet, they are nevertheless inadequate to make an objective assessment of the efficacy of the diet in treating cancer."[148] Several attempts have been made to systematically assess the effectiveness of the macrobiotic approach to cancer. However, these studies are considered inconclusive or incomplete.

Summary

While there is substantial information about the role of diet in breast cancer, much of this information is not definitive. However, there is reasonably good evidence that fruits and vegetables offer preventive benefits, while increased body size and alcohol intake contribute to risk. Other suspected risk factors included inadequate folic acid and regular red meat intake. Foods that may provide protection against cancer include carotenoids, soy foods, and other plant foods such as whole grains.

The evidence at this point supports a dietary pattern that emphasizes whole plant foods and deemphasizes animal foods. This dietary pattern is the focus of guidelines provided by the American Cancer Society (1996)[149] and the American Institute for Cancer Research/World Cancer Research Fund (1997) for cancer prevention in general, not just for breast cancer prevention. It is probably a reasonable framework on which to base one's diet, whether for the prevention or the treatment of cancer.

Relatively few studies have looked at the value of comprehensive dietary change in the context of cancer treatment and the management of breast cancer. However, the few existing studies suggest that a similar dietary pattern—one that is relatively low in fat and animal food intake and high in plant foods—may be helpful. Indeed, the evidence is so strong that the National Cancer Institute has funded two separate studies to investigate whether such dietary patterns affect the survival rates of women with breast cancer. In addition, there are compelling case stories, like the one detailed here along with others featured in other publications, that illustrate how macrobiotics might be helpful for women with breast cancer (as well as other cancers). While macrobiotics and other comprehensive dietary approaches to cancer have not been evaluated adequately, these powerful case histories provide a reasonable rationale for diet in the context of management of breast cancer. This is especially true given the similarity of the Gerson therapy and the macrobiotic diet to more mainstream dietary recommendations for cancer prevention.

However, there remains substantial opposition among clinicians to the idea that dietary factors or substantial dietary change may be important for breast cancer patients. For example, in the case that introduced this chapter, the oncologist's dietary advice was to tell his patient not to lose weight and to consume a substantial amount of calories. Such advice often translates into a high-fat diet full of high-calorie foods like milk shakes. While the doctor's intention was to help the patient withstand the effects of chemotherapy, this dietary advice, like most aspects of diet in cancer management, has not undergone appropriate scientific investigation to determine whether it actually contributes to a better breast cancer prognosis. Indeed, one can argue that there is more information to support a diet emphasizing plant foods, as noted in Table 5-3 (and thus supporting these clinical trials) than one that favors a calorie-dense diet.

The idea that a diet emphasizing plant foods can affect breast cancer prognosis is also supported in part by many published reports. As noted previously, the mechanisms by which dietary factors may influence carcinogenesis may be important after diagnosis as well as before it. As importantly, the specific time of diagnosis is somewhat arbitrary, given the changes in diagnostic technology and screening patterns that have developed. More cases of breast cancer are being detected at earlier stages as mammographic screening practices become more widespread and are conducted at regular intervals from an earlier age. To suggest that dietary recommendations for cancer prevention may no longer be relevant after diagnosis ignores the semiarbitrary nature of the time of diagnosis.

When the lessons of the scientific literature and a reasonable interpretation of alternative dietary approaches to cancer are taken together, the following general recommendations can be suggested for the management of cancer, including breast cancer:

- *Choose most of your foods from the plant kingdom.* This is the first recommendation of the American Cancer Society's dietary guidelines for the prevention of cancer, and it is a strong foundation for a healthful diet.
- *Emphasize a variety of whole unprocessed grains, vegetables, and fruits.* There is growing evidence that the abundance of compounds that are found naturally in a variety of whole grains, vegetables, and fruits are important for cancer prevention and may also play a role in cancer treatment.
- *Eat foods according to tradition.* It is probably worthwhile to include regular consumption of sea vegetables and beans and bean products, including soy foods such as tofu, tempeh, and miso, such as those used traditionally in East Asian cuisines. It is much less clear whether isolated compounds derived from such foods with putative cancer prevention properties (e.g., genistein or bioflavonoids) are helpful.
- *Choose foods low on the food chain.* Animal foods, especially red meat and eggs, can be minimized or avoided altogether.
- *Eat real foods.* Choose organically grown and produced foods whenever possible to minimize exposure to pesticides, herbicides, and related chemicals.
- *Don't drink alcohol.* This recommendation is specific for breast cancer prevention, in which there is good evidence that alcoholic beverages increase the risk of breast cancer. If other chronic diseases, notably coronary heart disease, are also considered, modest (one drink a day or less) regular alcohol intake may be recommended.

- *Be physically active.* While this is not specifically a food-related recommendation and has not explicitly been reviewed in this chapter, there is growing evidence that regular physical activity may prevent breast cancer. This is also one of the guidelines for cancer prevention that is advocated by the American Cancer Society.

There are no guarantees that these recommendations will prevent the recurrence of breast cancer, increase survival, or prevent breast cancer in the first place, but they are generally consistent with guidelines for a healthful diet. They are likely to provide a sound foundation that may be modified or augmented with other treatments, including conventional therapies, with the guidance of appropriate health care professionals.

CHAPTER SIX

Food as Medicine: The Role of Soy and Phytoestrogens

Mary Tagliaferri, M.D., L.Ac.

MARY TAGLIAFERRI M.D., L.Ac., is one of the founders of the Complementary and Alternative Medicine Program at the University of California, San Francisco Carol Franc Buck Breast Care Center. She holds a master of science degree in traditional Chinese medicine, is a nationally certified herbalist and acupuncturist, and received an M.D. degree from the University of California, San Francisco. As one of the few practitioners dually trained in Eastern and Western medicine, she has spearheaded a number of laboratory and clinical studies to assess the efficacy of traditional herbal agents and soy to treat breast cancer, the side effects from cancer treatments, and menopausal symptoms. She has lectured to and taught physicians about alternative therapies used to treat breast cancer. She opened the first Traditional Chinese Medicine Clinic at UCSF and was the program manager for the UCSF Breast Care Center Complementary and Alternative Medicine Program for four years. At age thirty, Mary Tagliaferri was diagnosed with breast cancer.

> *Let your food be your medicine and your medicine be your food.*
> —HIPPOCRATES

At the age of thirty, four months after receiving my master's degree in traditional Chinese medicine, I received the news that I had invasive breast cancer.

What shocked me wasn't just the shattering news of the diagnosis. It was also my sudden loss of faith in an alternative system of medicine that, until then, I was sure I would turn to if I ever became seriously ill. Where had all my convictions gone? All the years of study and practice I'd poured into becoming a certified massage therapist, a licensed acupuncturist, and a devoted proponent of Chinese herbal medicine seemed inconsequential at the moment of this diagnosis. Listening to all the claims, directions, and scientific evidence offered by my Western medical doctors, I felt I could no longer rely on the alternative therapies I had once championed.

This feeling intensified when my surgeon walked in shortly after my diagnosis, hauling piles of mammograms, charts, and test results that he could barely fit under his arm, and began to recite an impressive list of clinical trials and other data detailing the statistics and scientific evidence for surgery, radiation, and chemotherapy. He assured me that with Western medical treatment, I had a 93% chance of being alive in five years. How could I argue with such certainty? The traditions in which I had been trained had no equivalent proofs, charts, and percentages. A part of me still held on to my long-standing belief in alternative therapies; but faced with all this medical "proof," I was wary about risking my life by relying on them alone.

However, as I underwent the difficult experiences of having someone cut into my breast and watching radiology technicians run out of the room while I was zapped by high-energy beams, I knew I needed more help than I was getting. I wanted to find my way back to alternative medicine and the other forms of therapy that had healed so many of the patients I met during my training and in my private practice. While I respected Western medical procedures for their precision and effectiveness, I realized that surgery and radiation would only treat the cancer. I would need other forms of medicine to feel better emotionally, to relieve the side effects of radiation, and to restore my overall sense of well-being. I decided, as many women do, to combine conventional Western treatments with selected complementary and alternative therapies—and with foods I knew would help to restore my health.

Making this decision was empowering. I regained confidence and hope. I decided that I would win over the cancer—not only by supplementing my Western treatment with a macrobiotic diet, Chinese herbs, and acupuncture, but also by continuing the activities I had pursued before my breast cancer diagnosis. So even while undergoing surgery, and throughout the subsequent six weeks of radiation, I began a very demanding, time-consuming macrobiotic diet, attended school full time, and treated patients in a busy acupuncture practice.

I was able to maintain most of this—except the diet. I probably ought to have realized that this was too much too soon. All the demands in my life made it too difficult to adhere to a strictly macrobiotic diet, which required hours of food preparation and cooking. Even when my best friend, Lila, agreed to eat organic sauerkraut three times a day with me, I still couldn't do it. So I investigated ways I could eat more sensibly with foods readily available in any grocery store. One of the most important of these foods was soy, which I learned provided multiple dietary benefits believed to prevent breast cancer and its recurrence. While the evidence for soy's benefits was persuasive, it was, of course, only one of the components in the full range of healthy foods (or herbal supplements, for that matter) that I learned could ward off breast cancer. However, I was so impressed by the innumerable studies detailing the benefits of soy for breast cancer that I made it a staple of my revised diet.

What began as a medical condition that had polarized my views of Western medicine and alternative therapies ended in my choosing a career in integrative medicine, which combines the best of both systems. A year and a half after being diagnosed with breast cancer, I began my first year of medical school at the University of California, San Francisco. During the first few years of course work, I reviewed hundreds of scientific articles on soy and the convincing evidence for its anticancer properties. These findings were so impressive that I spearheaded clinical research to determine the benefits of soy to prevent breast cancer in women at high risk for developing the disease. Our study comparing soy with tamoxifen (the only drug approved by the Food and Drug Administration for breast cancer prevention) has been funded by the Department of Defense and is currently under way at the University of California, San Francisco Breast Care Center under the directorship of Drs. Laura Esserman and Jeffrey Tice.

As for my health, we submitted the manuscript for *Breast Cancer: Beyond Convention* to Atria Books on the day of my five-year anniversary of being diagnosed with breast cancer. My most recent mammogram was negative, and I graduated from medical school this year.

Food as Medicine:
The Potential Anticancer Effects of Soy

Soy was not a foreign food to me, even before I'd begun to learn about its health-related properties. I first tasted tofu when it was still considered hippie food. In fact, when I was in college fifteen years ago, people chuckled at my telephone number, 272-TOFU, because they associated my roommates and me with the counterculture: we wore Birkenstock sandals, listened nonstop to the Grateful Dead, and ate at the premier vegetarian restaurant in Ithaca, the Moosewood. Growing up with an Italian grandmother whose *penne a la matricianna* rivaled the best in Rome, I was used to good food and was impressed by Moosewood's gourmet tofu dishes like ratatouille, lasagna, moussaka, and spanokopita.

After college, I learned that soy not only was a versatile food in terrific dishes but had a long history in Asia, evidently appreciated earliest in China, where for over three thousand years it has been revered for its nutritive properties. Traditional Chinese medicine teaches us that the ancient Chinese emperor Shen-Nong, whose name means "divine farmer," chose the soybean as one of the five sacred grains (along with rice, wheat, barley, and millet). Tofu, one of the most ancient soy products, appears to have been discovered by Buddhist monks in China and taken by Buddhist missionaries to Japan, where today it is consumed in greater quantity than in any other nation. The soybean as food in Western countries has a much more recent history, appearing in Europe only in the 1500s, and first used more as ship ballast in the early 1800s by trade ships to the United States than as food. Its health-enhancing value was not significantly appreciated in this country until the 1920s, when advocates of vegetarian diets like Dr. John Harvey Kellogg (founder of the well-known cereal company) began to produce high-protein soy-based meat substitutes and soy milk.

But soy's role as a potential anticarcinogenic food is what makes it most remarkable to me. Understanding how it may protect against breast cancer requires understanding the amazing and subtle ways it interacts with the body to produce this protection, particularly in terms of its interaction with the human hormone estrogen.

For over one hundred years, researchers have been aware of an association between the hormones in our bodies and breast cancer. In 1896, the renowned physician Dr. George Beaston demonstrated that removing the ovaries from premenopausal women with metastatic breast cancer caused tumors to decrease in size.[1] This concept was supported by the findings from a much larger study that took place between 1920 and 1940 (but published in 1968) in which a total of 6908 women who had undergone hysterectomies were compared with 1479 women who had gone through menopause "naturally" to investigate which group was more likely to develop breast cancer. The results were startling: women who had both their uteruses and ovaries removed before age forty had a 75% lower rate of breast cancer.[2] Women who had their uteruses removed but kept their ovaries showed no decrease in the incidence of breast cancer. These studies offered the first clinical data that implicated the role of hormones such as estrogen in breast cancer.

Today we know that women who begin their menstrual cycles earlier or who go through menopause later are at increased risk for breast cancer. Likewise, if a woman's first pregnancy happened before the age of thirty, she has a lower risk for breast cancer; women who never have children are at increased risk.[3] These risk factors are significant because the trend shows that less exposure to estrogen over a woman's lifetime correlates with a lower incidence of breast cancer. Because 70% of tumors in the breast have proved to be estrogen-dependent,[4] it becomes even more clear that controlling estrogen activity can dramatically reduce the risks and recurrence of breast cancer.

TABLE 6-1.   Risk Factors and Protective Factors for Breast Cancer[5]

RISK FACTORS (INCREASED EXPOSURE TO ESTROGEN)

Early menarche

Late menopause

Postmenopausal obesity

Hormone replacement therapy

Alcohol consumption   *(continued)*

TABLE 6-1. *(continued)*

PROTECTIVE FACTORS (DECREASED EXPOSURE TO ESTROGEN)

Early first full-term pregnancy

Lactation

Physical activity

The cumulative exposure to estrogen over the course of a woman's life has a significant impact on her risk of breast cancer. High levels of estrogen affect breast cancer by causing proliferation of the epithelial cells: the

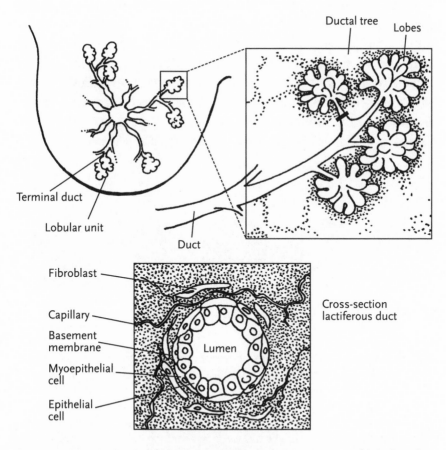

FIGURE 6.1. Structure of the breast. The breast consists of lobules that make milk, which drains through the ducts to the nipple. Each duct is lined by epithelial cells, the place where most breast cancers develop.

cells that line the six to eight ducts in each breast that carry milk to the nipple. If this growth becomes reckless, breast cancer tumors will form in the ducts. When the tumor extends outside the ductal wall, it becomes invasive breast cancer, or infiltrating ductal carcinoma.

The reason obesity is a factor in postmenopausal women is because the main source of estrogen after menopause is the conversion of androgens (other hormones including testosterone) to estrogen in fat tissue. This differs from premenopausal women, whose ovaries produce the majority of estrogen in their bodies. Therefore, increased fat in women who have gone through menopause leads to higher levels of estrogen and a greater risk for breast cancer. Alcohol consumption can increase the levels of estrogen in the body by interfering with the enzymes that metabolize estrogen in the liver. In fact, women who consume three or more alcoholic drinks per day have a 40% to 70% increased risk for breast cancer compared with nondrinkers.[6]

We have long known that the risk of breast cancer varies substantially throughout the world. Historically, there has been a sixfold lower breast cancer rate among native Japanese and Chinese women than in Caucasian women residing in the United States and Western Europe.[7]

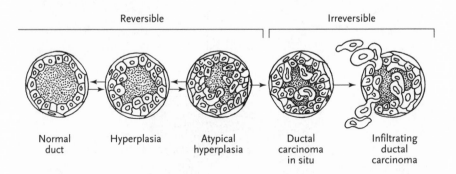

Reversible			Irreversible	
Normal duct	Hyperplasia	Atypical hyperplasia	Ductal carcinoma in situ	Infiltrating ductal carcinoma

FIGURE 6.2. Steps in the process of breast cancer. First there is an increase in the number of epithelial cells lining the milk ducts called hyperplasia. As the epithelial cells continue to replicate and divide, they begin to develop some of the architectural and cytologic features of a ductal carcinoma in situ. When the cells actually resemble breast cancer cells but are contained within the ductal wall, ductal carcinoma in situ forms. Once the cells break through the ductal wall to invade surrounding tissue, infiltrating ductal carcinoma develops.

However, the incidence of breast cancer in Japanese women who have migrated to the United States increases in one generation, and the second generation[8] will have a rate of breast cancer similar to that in American white women. This suggests that environmental factors such as diet, rather than genetic differences, are primarily responsible for the decrease in breast cancer incidence among women in China and Japan. Because Asian women consume twenty to fifty times more soy per capita than American women,[9-11] it has been speculated that soy products can ward off breast cancer or prevent a recurrence. Clinical studies support this hypothesis, and the data show that the more soy a woman eats, the less likely she will be to develop breast cancer.[12] Not only are differences between these breast cancer rates striking, but differences in mortality from the disease are also startling. As Table 6-2 shows, American women are almost three times more likely to die of breast cancer than Japanese women.

TABLE 6-2. Soy Consumption and Breast Cancer Deaths

COUNTRY	AVERAGE SOY PROTEIN CONSUMPTION (GRAMS/DAY)	BREAST CANCER DEATHS PER 100,000 WOMEN
Japan	30	7.7*
Korea	20	4
Hong Kong	10	8
China	9	5*
United States	<1	20*

*Statistics from National Cancer Institute's Surveillance, Epidemiology and End Results (SEER) Database, 1994–1997.

The chemical compounds in soy believed most to contribute to this phenomenon are the phytoestrogens—chemical compounds found in plants that have a structure similar to that of estrogen. There are three main chemical classes of phytoestrogens: isoflavones, lignans, and coumestans. Foods that contain these phytoestrogens are listed in Table 6-3.

TABLE 6-3.   Food Sources of Isoflavones, Lignans, and Coumestans[13-15]

ISOFLAVONES	LIGNANS	COUMESTANS
Tofu	Flaxseeds	Clover sprouts
Tempeh	Lentils	Alfalfa sprouts
Lentils	Dried seaweed	Soybean sprouts
Kidney beans	Oat bran	Mung bean sprouts
Lima beans	Wheat	Soymilk
Chickpeas	Barley	Tofu
Tofu yogurt	Hops	Split peas
Soy flour	Rye	Pinto beans
Soybeans (edamame)	Rice	Lima beans
Soybean sprouts	Kidney beans	Grapefruit
Soy noodles	Cherries	Orange juice
Miso soup	Apples	
	Pears	
	Carrots	
	Sunflower seeds	
	Fennel	

In this chapter, I will discuss only the isoflavones found in soy products. The two most potent isoflavones in soy are genistein and daidzein, and it is believed that these two compounds account for many of the anticarcinogenic effects of soy. Clinical studies and laboratory experiments in both animals and cell lines have shown that the phytoestrogens in soy have at least four mechanisms by which they can prevent breast cancer:

- Control of estrogen levels—estrogenic/antiestrogenic activity
- Prevention of free radicals—the antioxidant effect
- Cutting off the tumor's food supply—inhibition of angiogenesis
- Preventing tumor cells from dividing—inhibition of enzymes

Control of Estrogen Levels—Estrogenic/Antiestrogenic Activity

Estrogen has many functions in the body, one of which is to regulate cell growth in the breasts. Attaching to receptors on the inside of a cell, estrogen then moves into the cell's nucleus, where it acts like a drill sergeant telling the cell to replicate. Cells that are rapidly dividing under the influence of estrogen are susceptible to genetic errors. If the incorrect DNA sequence in a cell is not repaired, a mutant cell may develop. A buildup of these mutant cells can form a tumor in the breast ducts, where most tumors originate. This is one way estrogen fosters tumor growth and is the reason women with breast cancer often take antiestrogen drugs such as tamoxifen or raloxifene. A meta-analysis, wherein the results of fifty-one case-control and cohort studies were combined to include more than 52,000 women with breast cancer, found no increase in risk of breast cancer with short-term hormone replacement therapy lasting less than five years; however, the risk of breast cancer increased to 35% in women who used estrogen alone for more than five years.[16] A recent study of 46,355 postmenopausal women published in the *Journal of the American Medical Association* suggests that the combination of estrogen and progestin in hormone replacement therapy may increase the risk of breast cancer even more than estrogen therapy alone.[17]

Phytoestrogens, with a chemical structure similar to the estrogens we produce in our bodies, can have both estrogenic and antiestrogenic effects.[18,19] By exerting only 1/1000 to 1/100,000 the hormonal effect of estrogen, the phytoestrogens in soy can attach to the receptors that normally attract estrogen, keeping estrogen from exerting its effect on cell growth and inhibiting tumor formation. This may be important in premenopausal women, whose ovaries produce high levels of estrogen. Soy may also be important for postmenopausal women, who develop breast cancer because they still have high levels of estrogen around the tissue where the tumor has formed, even though they have low levels of estrogen in the blood. (Again, this is because androgens are converted to estrogen in the breast tissue, where there is a relatively high fat content.) Conversely, in these postmenopausal women, phytoestrogens may be able to *replace* the waning levels of estrogen and carry out some of estrogen's beneficial functions, such as preventing osteoporosis,

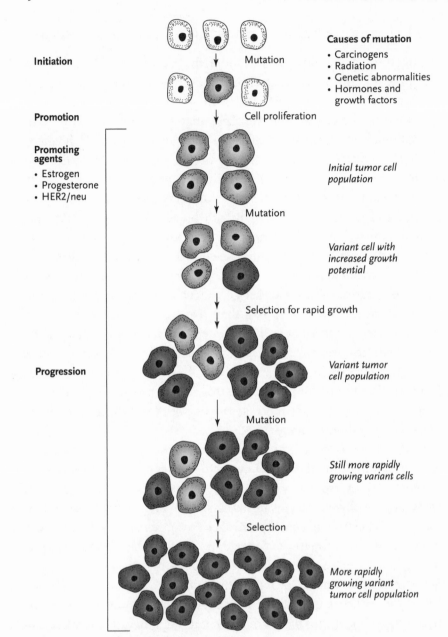

Initiation   Mutation

Causes of mutation
- Carcinogens
- Radiation
- Genetic abnormalities
- Hormones and growth factors

Promotion   Cell proliferation

Promoting agents
- Estrogen
- Progesterone
- HER2/neu

Initial tumor cell population

Mutation

Variant cell with increased growth potential

Selection for rapid growth

Progression   *Variant tumor cell population*

Mutation

Still more rapidly growing variant cells

Selection

More rapidly growing variant tumor cell population

FIGURE 6.3. Cancer initiation. The growth of a tumor in the breast occurs by a series of steps. First, a mutation occurs; then this mutated cell begins to divide. If the variant cell divides more quickly than normal cells, there will be selection for the more rapidly growing variant cell population, eventually leading to the development of a tumor.

heart disease, and possibly the undesirable effects of menopause such as hot flashes and depression. (However, I should point out that a recent study evaluating soy for hot flashes among 177 breast cancer survivors did not show that the soy isoflavones were any more effective than a placebo at reducing the number of daily hot flashes. It is also important to note that more than 77% of the women in the trial were concurrently taking tamoxifen, an antiestrogen drug that causes hot flashes. A final point is that the study examined only the effects of an isolated soy protein administered as a pill, not soy foods such as tofu.[20] Data from three other clinical trials have shown that soy can have a modest beneficial effect on hot flashes.)[21–23] Overall, it may be the dual nature of genistein to act as both agonist and antagonist at the estrogen receptor site that may account for soy's ability to decrease high levels of estrogen at harmful levels and to increase the levels when they are dangerously low.

The second potential benefit of soy on estrogen-related activity is its effect on the menstrual cycle. In this country, we refer to an "ideal menstrual cycle" as twenty-eight days, but as many women know, these cycles can be shorter or longer. Researchers at the Harvard School of Public Health studied the association between menstrual cycle length and the risk of breast cancer in an ongoing study that includes a total of 116,678 nurses. The results from this very large study showed that compared with menstrual cycles of 26 to 31 days, a cycle length of 32 to 39 days was associated with a decreased risk of breast cancer, and women with cycles longer than 39 days were 60% less likely to develop the disease.[24] These results were consistent with the hypothesis that the longer the menstrual cycle, the fewer cycles a women will experience each year, and the overall exposure to estrogens that are secreted naturally will be reduced, thus providing a protective benefit against breast cancer. At least four studies have shown that phytoestrogens can increase the menstrual cycle length by two to five days, which may have a protective benefit against breast cancer by reducing a woman's exposure to estrogen over her lifetime, significantly reducing the risk of breast cancer.[25–29] The amount of soy consumed by women in these studies varied. In one trial, women consumed three 12-ounce glasses of soymilk per day (or 200 mg of isoflavones per day). In a second study, the participants ate their usual diet and then received a powdered soy protein supplement. The maximum daily dosage of the isolated soy protein supplementation was calculated at 2.01 mg/kg of total isoflavones per day, or approximately 129 mg of total isoflavones per day. More details about isolated soy protein supplements versus soy foods and their respective amounts of isoflavones will be discussed later in the chapter.

Preventing Free Radicals—The Antioxidant Effects

Everyone has heard that taking supplements or eating foods rich in antioxidants helps lower the risk of cancer. This is because they protect against dangerous chemicals called free radicals, which are generated by exposure to ultraviolet radiation, sunlight, X rays, and certain chemicals in the environment as well as through normal metabolic reactions that occur in our bodies every day. Unstable molecules with one electron in their outer shells, free radicals seek completion by "stealing" a second electron from healthy molecules, producing a harmful domino effect that rampages through the body, potentially damaging DNA. Genistein, the major phytoestrogen in soy, has been shown in laboratory experiments to effectively "mop up" free radicals, thereby protecting DNA from harm and potentially reducing the risk of cancer.[30–35]

Cutting Off the Tumor's Food Supply— Inhibition of Angiogenesis

In cancer, tumor cells proliferate at a wild rate, using up an enormous amount of their "fuel"—oxygen and glucose. To obtain this fuel, tumor cells send out chemical triggers that result in the formation of new blood vessels sprouting from existing small capillaries like branches from a tree, a process called angiogenesis. If the tumor does not initiate this burst of new capillaries, it will be deprived of essential nutrients and cease to grow. Laboratory experiments have shown that genistein, in addition to its ability to act as an antioxidant, inhibits angiogenesis.[36,37] It cuts the cancer cell off from its "fuel," causing it to wither and die. Remarkably, in these laboratory experiments, soy doesn't keep healthy cells from their nutrition: genistein affects only the cells that are dividing abnormally or in wanton growth patterns.

Preventing Tumor Cells from Dividing—
Inhibition of an Enzyme Associated with Cancer

All the cells in our body are "programmed" to respond to a specific set of signals that command the cell to act in various ways. One signal may tell a cell to kill itself; another may instruct the cell to replicate. In the same way, hormones like estrogen can act as drill sergeants and tell a cell what to do. Enzymes behave similarly in the body. One enzyme that functions this way is tyrosine kinase, which attaches to the receptors on the outer surface of cells in a lock-and-key fit and sends a cascade of messages to the cell's nucleus, telling the cell how to behave (such as causing the cell to replicate and divide). In cancerous cells, this signaling pathway can spiral out of control. Since tyrosine kinase can trigger these signaling pathways that go haywire, inhibiting this enzyme is an effective way to prevent tumor growth. Specifically, in laboratory experiments, genistein, the main isoflavone in soy, blocks tyrosine kinase in tumor cells, inhibiting replication and thereby acting as a powerful anticancer agent.[38,39]

Clinical Trials with Soy

Dr. Bruce Trock and colleagues at Georgetown University completed a meta-analysis of all the epidemiologic studies examining the role of soy intake and breast cancer risk. This type of statistical analysis is used to combine the results from several different studies to increase the power (or ability) to determine an overall effect, which in this case is the relationship between eating soy and the risk of breast cancer. A total of nine studies were included in Dr. Trock's analysis. Five of the studies were completed in Asia, one of the studies involved women of Asian ancestry in the United States, and two of the studies were completed in non-Asian populations. The findings from the meta-analysis did show a decrease in breast cancer risk with a higher soy diet.[40] When the researchers further evaluated the data by looking at the effects of dietary soy intake and breast cancer risk among premenopausal and postmenopausal women, they found that the beneficial effects were limited to premenopausal women. Some laboratory data in animal models suggest that early exposure to genistein, the main isoflavone in soy, confers a protective benefit against the development of breast cancer.[41-42] It is still unclear whether dietary soy intake before puberty is essential for reducing the risk of breast cancer or whether early childhood exposure to a diet rich in soy foods bolsters a protective benefit. In addition to conducting randomized, placebo-controlled clinical trials to more precisely evaluate the effects of soy to reduce breast cancer (like the study under way at our comprehensive cancer center, the UCSF Breast Care Center), we will also have to examine *when* in a person's life soy must be introduced into the diet to maximize a protective benefit. We do know that recently published retrospective data indicate that exposure to soy infant formula early in life does not adversely alter either endocrinological or reproductive outcomes in young adulthood. These new data confirm that it is safe to begin consuming soy formulas early in life.[43]

How Best to Get Your Soy: Supplement or Food?

Is it better to get your soy through supplements or through food? Since the FDA does not regulate the contents of nutritional supplements, you cannot be guaranteed "quality control" when purchasing these products. In fact, what you read on a soy supplement label may not indeed be what you get. Various research laboratories have tested soy products on the market, and some of the soy supplements claiming to have phytoestrogens actually had no detectable levels of them (i.e., the anticancer isoflavones, genistein and daidzein) in the product. Recently, however, because isoflavones have been identified as at least one of the compounds in soy that protect against breast cancer and heart disease, many reliable nutritional supplement companies are now marketing products with high levels of isoflavones. But since ideal doses of isoflavones have not yet been established, and we still don't know enough about their effects on all organ systems, I would avoid dietary supplements of soy or isoflavones at this time. *Caveat emptor:* try to get your soy protein from food—preferably from traditional Asian soy products.

How Much Soy Should You Eat?

To date, we do not have sufficient scientific information to provide recommendations about the amount or frequency of soy intake that may be effective at reducing the incidence of breast cancer. On the other hand, the scientific literature regarding soy and its ability to reduce cholesterol (and ultimately the risk of heart disease) was so convincing that the FDA has announced that Americans should incorporate four servings of at least 6.25 grams of soy protein per day—equivalent to *25 grams* per day. This concurs with the amount of soy consumed daily for centuries by Japanese women, who have one sixth the amount of breast cancer as American women and are three times less likely to die of the disease. An intake of 25 grams of soy protein per day amounts to a daily intake of roughly 25 to 50 milligrams of isoflavones (genistein and daidzein). Since the recommended daily allowance for total protein intake per day is 44 grams for women, roughly 50% to 60% of your daily protein should come from soy. Luckily, a wide variety of foods are made with soy, and the versatility of soy products such as tofu makes it easy to include in many dishes. All the traditional Asian soy products such as tempeh, tofu, soy milk, and miso are rich sources of isoflavones. Secondary soy products such as soy franks, soy burgers, and soy ice cream have much lower amounts of isoflavones, since they usually contain considerable amounts of nonsoy ingredients. Table 6-4 shows the nutritional makeup of the most common soy foods.

To get your 25 grams of soy protein per day, you should eat on average at least four servings of soy food per day. Remember that most people tend to eat several servings in one sitting. For instance, a cup of soymilk constitutes two servings, not one. In other words, it's easier than you may think to consume the minimum requirement.

The Many Nutrients in Soybeans

The soybean is part of the legume family, like beans, peas, and lentils; yet, the soybean is unique because of its high protein content: 35% to 40%. The rest of the soybean is composed of roughly 15% to 20% fat,

TABLE 6-4. Nutritional Values of Popular Soy Foods

Food	Calories (Kcal)	Protein (Grams)	Isoflavones (Milligrams)	Carbohydrates (Grams)	Fat (Grams)	Saturated Fat (Grams)
½ cup soybeans	149	14.3	70	8.5	7.7	1.1
½ cup tempeh	165	15.7	60	12.5	6.0	0.8
¼ cup soynuts	202	15	60	14.5	10.9	1.6
½ cup tofu	94	10	38	2.3	5.9	0.9
¼ cup soy flour	81.7	12.8	25	8.4	0.3	0.02
½ cup soymilk	79	6.6	10	4.3	4.6	0.5
½ cup texturized soy protein (TSP)	59	11	28	7	0.2	Fat free

30% carbohydrates, 5% crude fiber from the hulls, and 5% minerals. As Table 6-5 illustrates, soy is a complete protein like beef or chicken, full of essential amino acids, necessary vitamins and minerals, and dietary fiber.

Soy Foods—a Sampling

Tofu

Tofu is possibly the most widely consumed soybean product in the world. It is usually found in the dairy food section or produce section of grocery stores, often packaged in a deep rectangular plastic container and sitting as a large white block soaked in water. The texture is like that of a soft cheese. Tofu's mild flavor accounts for its versatility: it tends to assume the flavor of any spice or food around it. That's why tofu is used as a main ingredient in such disparate foods as chocolate cheesecake, spicy Mexican fajitas, Italian pasta dishes, and Szechuan stir-fry. As a traditional Asian product, it is naturally processed from whole soybeans and therefore retains most of the important nutrients, including isoflavones. Softer tofu has a higher water content than extra-firm tofu and therefore less fat but also less soy protein. Tofu is prepared and eaten in a virtually infinite variety of ways: fried, baked, grilled, sautéed, marinated, raw—in salads, casseroles, snacks, main dishes, and desserts.

Green Soybeans (Edamame in Japanese Restaurants)

These green, pleasant-tasting soybeans can be found on the menu at almost any Japanese sushi restaurant, usually served steamed and lightly salted. They are more difficult to find in grocery stores but can be purchased fresh in the early fall or found in the frozen food section year round. They tend to be sweet, since they are picked at the peak of maturity when their sucrose levels are high. A simple way to prepare the bean is to boil or steam the pods for fifteen minutes, drain them, and break open the furry pod, which usually encases two to three

TABLE 6-5.   The Nutrients in Soy

Protein	The soybean is a complete protein like animal meat, such as chicken or beef. As such, the soybean contains all the necessary amino acids necessary to sustain life. Our bodies need twenty different amino acids to survive, and meat has traditionally been the source for these essential building blocks. Of the twenty amino acids necessary for the body to sufficiently build proteins, ten can be produced internally by our bodies, and ten are known as essential, meaning that these amino acids must be obtained through food sources. Soy is remarkable in that it contains all twenty of the necessary amino acids. Therefore, it is an excellent low-fat, high-fiber protein substitution for meat.
Isoflavones	Isoflavones are the phytoestrogen derivatives from soy that have gained the most popularity and have generated an enormous amount of scientific interest for their anticancer properties. Two isoflavones found in soy are genistein and daidzein.
Fiber	Fiber refers to the portions of foods that pass through our gut and remain virtually unchanged as they make that tortuous journey. The insoluble carbohydrates are the source of dietary fiber in the soybean. It is the fiber that helps to keep cholesterol levels low, maintain normal bowel movements, and potentially provide protection against colon cancer.
Fat	In comparison with other legumes, soybeans are slightly higher in fat. As we also know, certain types of fat are more damaging to our arteries, such as saturated fats. Of the fat in soybeans, 85% is the "good kind of fat," or unsaturated, and 15% is saturated. Roughly half of the fat in soybeans consists of a polyunsaturated fat, an essential nutrient our bodies cannot produce alone. Moreover, soybeans can have up to 8% omega-3 fatty acids, which are also believed to play a role in preventing cancer and heart disease.
Vitamins and Minerals	Soybeans are loaded with nutrients that we need to eat on a daily basis. Specifically, soybeans are an excellent source of iron, calcium, magnesium, zinc, thiamine, niacin, riboflavin, and vitamin B_6.

pea-sized beans. Green soybeans contain the same amount of protein as tofu (roughly 13%) and are naturally high in calcium.

Whole Dry Soybeans

Whole dry soybeans may be difficult to find in your supermarket, but natural food stores usually carry them as a prepackaged item or in the bulk food section. Dry soybeans should be rinsed before use and soaked overnight before cooking. It can take up to two hours for the soybeans to soften when they are boiled, so using a pressure cooker for one or two hours is the best method of preparation.

Soymilk

Today you can find soymilk in the refrigerator section of your local supermarket. Soy beverages, which are rapidly replacing cow's milk on the American kitchen table, are also packaged in aseptic cartons which have a nonrefrigerated shelf life of one year. Since there are no standards for producing soymilk, each product can have different amounts of fat, nutrients, soy protein, and isoflavones. So, check the label. A general rule of thumb is that the higher the protein level, the more isoflavones contained in the product. Another reason soymilk may become more popular is that it is free of both lactose and cholesterol. You can even find soymilk supplemented with calcium and other nutrients. Soy-based infant formulas are also becoming extremely popular. Approximately 25% of all infant formulas used today are soy based, and the American Association of Pediatricians claims that they are both safe and effective.

Tempeh

Tempeh is a fermented soy product with many of the same applications in cooking as tofu. Unlike tofu, though, tempeh has a distinct flavor frequently described as nutty, with a firm and slightly dense texture. Tempeh is rich in protein, fiber, and various vitamins and minerals. It is usually found in the produce section of grocery stores, often next to tofu.

Miso

Miso is the vegetarian bouillion cube of the East. Like tempeh, it is a fermented soy product made from aged whole soybeans, sometimes combined with rice, barley, or wheat to make a concentrated salty paste. It is traditionally used throughout Asia to flavor soup and salad dressings or enrich the taste of various dishes. In Japan, many people drink a bowl of miso soup for breakfast, prepared by adding 1 tablespoon of miso paste to 1 cup of hot water, simmered but not boiled. Although miso is rich in soy protein and isoflavones, it should be used in moderation because of its high salt content. It is difficult to find in conventional supermarkets, but most health food stores carry a variety of brands with varying amounts of soybean content.

Soy Sauces

Soy sauce is a well-known cooking ingredient that has reached the kitchens of many people in the West. It is a fermented soy product like tempeh and miso; when made exclusively from soybeans, it is called tamari. If a fermented wheat is added in the processing, the product is called shoyu. Today, soy sauces come in many different flavors, some sweet and others salty. Although soy sauce is high in protein and isoflavones, people who limit salt in their diets should note its high salt content.

Soy Flour

Soy flour is carried by natural food stores in the bulk food section. It is easily distinguished from wheat or white flour by its yellow color. It is produced from finely ground soybeans, is usually 50% protein, and is used in baked goods. Since soy flour is devoid of gluten, it cannot be the primary flour for baking recipes that require yeast for rising purposes, but you may substitute up to 15% of the flour called for in most recipes with soy flour.

Soy Protein Isolates

Soy protein isolates are the most highly refined soy products available and have the highest protein percentage of any soy product. They come from defatted soy flakes, and the protein content is usually 90%. For each gram of soy protein isolate, there are 3 to 4 milligrams of isoflavones. Since the sugars have been removed, the isolated soy proteins are carbohydrate free and very easy to digest. Originally these products were devoid of the valuable isoflavones, but with new processing techniques, the isoflavones are now retained, sometimes at very high concentrations. They can be ordered through the mail, on-line via the Internet, or purchased in health food stores. However, I do not recommend these products because we have no knowledge about their effects on the body.

Soy Nuts

If you like peanuts you will probably enjoy soy nuts. These snack products are dry-roasted or deep-fried after being soaked in water, and they are an excellent source of soy protein, fiber, and isoflavones.

Texturized Soy Protein

Texturized soy proteins (TSP) are made from defatted soy flour, come dehydrated, and when cooked in various dishes (like stews and casseroles) are used as substitutes for a variety of meats, poultry, and seafood. A great source of protein, fiber, and isoflavones, TSP can be purchased in the bulk food section of health food stores. In its dehydrated form, texturized soy protein is yellow and very light in weight. Hydrated TSP can be added to meat to reduce the fat content, caloric intake, and cholesterol and to add some omega-3 fatty acids as well as isoflavones to the meal.

Soybean Oil

Soybean oil, extracted from the whole soybean, is cholesterol free, low in saturated fat, and a source of omega-3 fatty acids. Light and with a very mild taste, soybean oil accounts for probably 75% of all the vegetable oil consumed in this country. Soy oils are not a good source of isoflavones or protein, and in processed foods they may be partially hydrogenated, increasing the saturated fat content and decreasing the omega-3 fatty acids. Soybean oil is a common ingredient in processed foods, baked goods, and salad dressings.

A Day in the Life

After reading about the intricate and dramatic ways that soy can influence and interact with your body, it's a particular perk to realize that it tastes good, too. Here are just some of the soy foods available for every meal and snack of the day, followed by recipes that will enable you to enjoy them right now.

Breakfast

Soymilk with toasted soyflake cereal; tofu added to smoothies; eggs and tofu in a delicious scramble; one of many variations of soy cheese on a bagel; miso soup; decadent fried soy breakfast patty, link, or strip.

Snacks

Steamed fresh whole soybeans; roasted soybeans; chocolate, vanilla, or strawberry soy drink; soy protein bar; dairyless soy yogurt; prepacked tofu that is baked or smoked; soy nuts.

Lunch or Dinner

Salad with soy sprouts topped with a soy salad dressing; miso soup; any of the hundreds of traditional Asian recipes (found in any Asian cookbook) such as tofu and vegetable stir-fry; more modern favorites such as tofu meatless meatballs, tempeh burritos, soy minestrone soup, stuffed pasta shells with tofu and soy cheese, chimichangas, moussaka, and shepherd's pie; meat substitutes such as meatless franks with catchy names like Smart Dogs, Tofu Pups, and Wonder-dogs; soy burgers in many brands, varieties, and flavors; tempeh sand-wiches, with tempting varieties such as barbecue, lemon, savory herb, garlic, sweet, and tangy; soy-based mayonnaise spreads; texturized soy protein (substitute for ground beef); prepackaged products rich in soy such as vegetarian chili, lasagna, penne pasta, ravioli, meatless meat-loaf, Thai tofu.

Desserts

Tofu ice cream, tofu chocolate mousse, tofu cheesecake, tofu pumpkin pie, and a slew of other baked goods prepared from soy flour.

Recipes

All recipes were created by Chef Holly Peterson Mondavi, owner of Sea Star Sea Salt.

Triple Soy Cereal
with Cranberries and Papaya
Serves 4–6

1 cup cranberries	¼ cup toasted slivered almonds (skin on)
2½ cups apple juice	
3 cups water	¼ cup soy nuts
¼ cup rolled oats	1 cup papaya (cubes)
¾ cup cracked wheat	½ cup blueberries
½ cup buckwheat kasha	optional: soymilk (to taste)
¾ cup soy flakes	optional: maple syrup or honey (to taste)

DIRECTIONS

In a little of the hot water, cook the cranberries until tender and juicy. Bring apple juice and water to a boil, then add rolled oats and cracked wheat. Cook 12–15 minutes. Add kasha and simmer 10 minutes. Add soy flakes, stir, and simmer until most of the liquid evaporates. Toss in toasted slivered almonds, soy nuts, fresh papaya, fresh blueberries, and the cooked cranberries. Serve with warm soymilk and a drizzle of maple syrup or honey.

Edamame

2 tablespoons Sea Star sea salt	1 pound raw soybeans or edamame

DIRECTIONS

It is simple to prepare these little jewels yourself and well worth the few minutes it takes. In a pot of water add 1 tablespoon of salt and bring to a boil. Add the rinsed edamame and cook 3–4 minutes or until tender and yet still bright green. Scoop out or strain, and plunge immediately into an ice bath to stop the cooking. When cool, remove and drain on a kitchen towel. Toss with crushed natural gray sea salt.

Fresh Soybean Salad with Grated Carrots, Beets, and Celery Root
Serves 4

2 cups edamame (beans only)	½ cup vegetable oil
2 cups grated raw carrots	3 sprigs fresh lemon thyme leaves
2 cups grated cooked beets	2 tablespoons fresh Italian parsley leaves
2 cups grated raw celery root	10 fresh basil leaves
¼ cup red wine vinegar	1 cup fresh broccoli sprouts for garnish
1 teaspoon Sea Star sea salt	8–12 fresh violets or nasturtiums for garnish
2 tablespoons Dijon mustard	
1 clove fresh garlic (pressed or freshly minced)	

DIRECTIONS

Place each of the four vegetables in a small bowl, keeping them separate. In a mixing bowl, whisk together red wine vinegar, natural gray sea salt, Dijon mustard, and crushed garlic. Once they are mixed, add the oil and whisk. Pour a little dressing in each vegetable dish, and toss. Add the lemon thyme leaves to the carrots. Roughly chop the Italian parsley, and toss with celery root. Slice the basil into fine ribbons, and toss with the beets. Arrange a little mound of each on a serving platter or individual plates, then garnish with fresh broccoli sprouts and edible flowers.

Tomato Basil Soup with Tofu
Serves 6

2 onions	vegetarians, use vegetable stock)
2 cloves garlic, chopped	
2 bunches basil	2 quarts ripe garden tomatoes, peeled, seeded
bouquet garni (parsley stems, bay leaf, thyme sprigs, leek)	10 oz silken tofu
	Sea Star sea salt to taste
splash of white wine to taste	black pepper
	2 cups arugula leaves
2 cups reduced homemade chicken stock (for pure	1 bunch Greek basil (for garnish)

DIRECTIONS

Sauté onions, chopped garlic, 1 bunch of basil, and bouquet garni in white wine and chicken (or vegetable) stock. Add peeled, seeded, chopped tomatoes, and simmer for 40 minutes. Puree, return to pan, and taste. Add chiffonade* of basil and silken tofu, whisk, and season to taste. Garnish with arugula and Greek basil.

---

*A chiffonade is fine ribbon slices. This technique is used predominantly for fine herbs.

Garden Carrot Soup with Mint
Serves 10

SOUP BASE

5 pounds young, tender carrots

4–5 cloves garlic, peeled

2 quarts bottled spring water

3–4 sprigs fresh lemon thyme

2 bunches fresh mint

1 cup Chardonnay

2 cups chicken stock or vegetable stock

Sea Star sea salt and freshly ground pepper to taste

1 cup silken tofu

GARNISHES

1 dozen baby turnip carrots

1 pound brussels sprouts

1 bunch small baby beets (with leaves)

2–3 tender celery ribs, peeled and julienned

1 pound French green beans

DIRECTIONS

Prepare soup base: Peel and roughly chop carrots. Peel garlic cloves. Combine carrots and garlic in a large pot, and add just enough water to cover. Bring to a boil, then reduce heat to a medium flame. Cook carrots until tender enough to puree. Puree carrots and garlic. Place puree back on stove. Place a bouquet garni of thyme sprigs and 1 bunch of mint (in cheesecloth) into the soup. Add the Chardonnay (to taste), chicken stock, sea salt, and fresh black pepper. Pluck the remaining bunch of mint, then cut the leaves into chiffonade. Simmer soup for 1 hour (or to desired flavor) before removing the bouquet garni. Add silken tofu and mix with whisk or hand soup blender. Add the mint chiffonade and stir gently to mix.

Prepare garnishes: Remove greens from carrots, peel, split in half, then blanch and refresh. (Cook in boiling salted water until just tender. Then plunge into ice water to stop the cooking.) Peel outer leaves from brussels sprouts, then remove the tender inner leaves. Blanch and refresh. Remove greens from beets, and wash well. Pick out small tender leaves, blanch, and refresh. Peel beet root and cut into long thin wedges, and blanch in just enough water to cover. Cool quickly, and cut in 3-inch julienne pieces. Snip stems from green beans, blanch and refresh. To service, heat all garnishes (except beets) in a steamer until fully hot.

To finish: Ladle hot carrot soup into warm bowls. Decoratively place all of the hot garnishes on top of the soup.

Corn and Edamame Salad with Cilantro Lime Dressing
Serves 6

VEGETABLES

2 pounds corn (cut off cob)	18 baby corn
½ cup water	½ pound edamame (shelled)
½ cup vegetable or chicken stock	3 bunches arugula
Sea Star sea salt	½ pint onion sprouts
1 lime	½ pint pea sprouts
½ purple onion	2 bunches cilantro
1 cup jicama (sliced)	1 bunch chervil

VINAIGRETTE

1 tablespoon balsamic vinegar	1 fresh young clove garlic, finely chopped or garlic pressed
1 tablespoon rice wine vinegar	1 tablespoon lemon zest
1 tablespoon Dijon mustard	½ cup vegetable stock
1 tablespoon shallots	freshly cracked pepper
	handful cilantro leaves

DIRECTIONS

Cut corn off cob and sauté in ½ cup water and ½ cup vegetable or chicken stock, until tender. Season with natural gray sea salt, juice of lime, chopped purple onion, and jicama. Toss. Remove the husk from baby corn, blanch in salted water, and slice in half lengthwise. Add edamame to corn mixture.

Prepare vinaigrette: In a mixing bowl, combine vinegars, mustard, shallots (chopped and rinsed), chopped garlic, lemon zest, then pour in vegetable stock a little at a time while whisking. Taste and correct seasoning with Sea Star natural gray sea salt and black pepper.

Prepare greens: Wash arugula and sprouts, snip ends if needed. Keep cool until you use them.

To finish: Dress corn mixture with vinaigrette and cilantro to taste, then arrange on top of arugula and garnish with sprouts, chervil, and additional cilantro to make this dish beautiful to the eye.

Beets with Creamy Horseradish Tofu Dressing

1 pound organic beets with a variety of colors:	1 tablespoon red wine vinegar
1 large or 2 small red beets	2 tablespoons virgin olive oil
1 large or 2 small chioga beets*	1 tablespoon soybean oil
1 large or 2 small golden beets	2 tablespoons silken tofu
1 large or 2 small orange beets	1 tablespoon prepared horseradish
pinch Sea Star sea salt	2 tablespoons Italian parsley leaves or fresh dill

DIRECTIONS

Wash beets, and remove leaves and roots. In a saucepan, cover beets with salted water and gently simmer until tender. While beets are hot, rub under cool water to peel. The skin will just slough off to reveal a perfectly smooth surface. (My mom's trick!) Slice each beet into quarters or eighths depending on their size. Cut them about the size of orange segments.

Dressing: Whisk together the vinegar, the oils, Sea Star natural gray sea salt, silken tofu, and horseradish. Adjust seasoning to taste.

To finish: Toss the beets with the dressing, and chill. Sprinkle with plucked Italian parsley leaves or fresh dill before serving.

---

*Chioga beets are marked by white and pink rings, very pretty. If unavailable, substitute more of the other beets.

Penne Pasta with Chickpeas, Edamame, Cauliflower, and Sweet Tomatoes
Serves 6

4–6 tablespoons extra virgin olive oil (or to taste)	Sea Star sea salt (to taste)
1 pound penne pasta	1 cup cubed firm tofu
1 cup cauliflower flowerets	1 cup vegetable stock (homemade if possible)
3 shallots (sliced)	1½ cups edamame
1 cup chickpeas	1½ cups small organic tomatoes

DIRECTIONS

Bring pot of salted water to a boil. Add a drizzle of olive oil, then pasta; cook until tender. In a sauté pan, heat 2 tablespoons olive oil, and sear cauliflower until golden brown on edges, then add shallots and chickpeas. Add more oil if necessary. Season with natural gray sea salt, and add tofu. Toss until mixed. Add some vegetable stock and continue to cook for several minutes, then add edamame and tomatoes. Add the rest of the vegetable broth and olive oil as needed. Feel free to add your favorite herbs, chili flakes, or seasoning. Toss with drained hot pasta.

Optional: Add grated parmesan cheese, chili flakes, or a little extra drizzle of olive oil to taste.

Thai Bean Thread
Serves 8

¼ pound soybean threads

¼ pound firm tofu

3 cups coconut milk

2 cups water

2 cups chicken stock

1 inch section thinly sliced young ginger

1–2 tablespoons fish sauce

¼ cup freshly squeezed lime juice

1 tablespoon green curry paste

4 ounces baby corn sliced in half

4 ounces asparagus sliced in 2-inch diagonal pieces

3 green onions sliced diagonally

Sea Star sea salt (to taste)

2 tablespoons cilantro

DIRECTIONS

Soak soybean threads in water for 15 minutes, and drain. Cut tofu in cubes. Bring coconut milk, water, and chicken stock to a boil, then reduce to a simmer. Add ginger, fish sauce, and lime juice, and whisk in green curry paste. Add baby corn, tofu, bean threads, and asparagus. Continue to simmer several more minutes. At finish, add green onion, natural gray sea salt, and cilantro, and arrange beautifully.

Sesame Asparagus and Edamame
Serves 4–6

1 pound asparagus

2 tablespoons peanut oil

dash of light sesame oil (to taste)

2 tablespoons green onion

1 teaspoon grated ginger (or finely minced)

1 tablespoon black sesame seeds

1 cup edamame (beans only)

1 teaspoon Sea Star sea salt (to taste)

2 teaspoons good organic soy sauce

freshly ground black pepper

1 bunch fresh chervil

DIRECTIONS

Blanch asparagus in a pot of salted boiling water until tender, and refresh in an ice bath. Drain when cool. In a sauté pan, heat peanut oil and sesame oil. Add green onion, minced ginger, and black sesame seeds. Swirl to mix, then add edamame and simmer several minutes. Slice asparagus lengthwise into long pretty half spears, and add to sauté pan. Toss with Sea Star natural gray sea salt, soy sauce, and freshly ground black pepper. Garnish with sprigs of chervil. Serve when hot and don't overcook.

Southwestern Soybeans
Serves 8

1 pound dried soybeans, soaked overnight	½ tablespoon whole cumin seed
1 white onion, finely chopped	1 bay leaf
1 red bell pepper, seeded, deveined, and chopped	3 quarts water
2 fresh jalapeño peppers, seeded and minced	2 teaspoons Sea Star sea salt (to taste)

DIRECTIONS

Soak soybeans overnight, and rinse. Combine with all other ingredients in a soup pot and bring to a boil, then reduce to a simmer in an uncovered pot until the soybeans are tender (approximately 1½ hours). Adjust the cooking liquid by adding water if necessary (the soybeans will need to be covered with liquid during cooking). You may also reduce the liquid at finish by turning up the flame so all of the flavor from the juice goes back into the soybeans.

From the base recipe, you can do many things. Use it as a side dish, as a main course, as the filling for burritos or enchiladas, or even pureed as a soup by adding more liquid or vegetable/chicken stock. Adjust the seasoning to taste at the finish.

Tofu in Wine Sauce
(Tofu au Vin)
Serves 4

1	tablespoon butter	1	sprig fresh rosemary
1	tablespoon olive oil	4	sprigs fresh thyme
1	cup pearl onions, peeled	1	leek, slivered
1½	cups mushrooms, quartered	3	carrots
		3	celery ribs
2	tablespoons soy flour	2	pounds firm tofu
1	cup white wine		nutmeg, grated (to taste)
1	quart vegetable stock		Sea Star sea salt (to taste)
2	leaves fresh sage	¼	cup parsley

Reader's note: A twist on a classic French dish, coq au vin. It has everything but the chicken and bacon . . . substituting tofu and several vegetables. When I recently served it side by side with the original dish, even the carnivores preferred the tofu version.

DIRECTIONS

To prepare the base: Melt butter in a casserole pot or French oven. Add olive oil. Peel pearl onions, trim to remove the roots, add them with the quartered mushrooms to the pot, sauté gently until just lightly colored. Add 2 tablespoons soy flour, then whisk gently while cooking until bubbly. Add white wine and whisk, then add vegetable stock and continue stirring with whisk until there is a nice smooth texture. Add sage, rosemary, thyme, and slivered leek. Continue to simmer to reduce for about 15 minutes.

To prepare vegetables: With a little kitchen tool called a channeler you can make your carrots look like little flowers. This of course is optional (I like to do it because we eat with our eyes, and it's the classic carrot preparation for coq au vin). With the channeler, cut long grooves the full length of the carrot, then give it a slight turn and make another groove. Make about five grooves, then slice carrots straight across to cut beautiful little flowers. Wash and peel celery with vegetable peeler. Then slice evenly.

To assemble: Slice each tofu piece into four lengthwise slices. Lay them in the simmering pot; add carrots, celery, freshly grated nutmeg, and

Sea Star natural gray sea salt to taste. Cover the tofu with the sauce, and gently mix the ingredients. Cover with lid, and continue to simmer for 10 minutes. Roughly chop parsley. Toss gently in at finish.

Truffled Soybean Soup
Serves 6

2 small shallots (choose nice firm ones)

2 ribs celery, finely chopped

¾ cup cooked soybeans

2½ cups chicken stock (home-made)

2½ cups vegetable stock (homemade)

1 cup silken tofu

2 sprigs thyme

1 whole black truffle (1½ oz)

Sea Star sea salt to taste

freshly ground white pepper to taste

DIRECTIONS

Finely chop shallots and rinse in cold water. Sauté shallots and celery in butter. Add half of the cooked soybeans, the chicken stock, vegetable stock, and silken tofu. Simmer several minutes, then add to a blender to puree. Return puree to pan and add thyme sprigs. Adjust desired thickness by adding more stock if necessary. Add the other half of cooked soybeans, and simmer. Clean the truffle carefully with a brush, then pound it to a coarse paste with a mortar and pestle. Whisk into the soup, and season to taste with natural gray sea salt and freshly ground white pepper.

Lemon Thyme Tofu Ravioli
Serves 6

PASTA (RAVIOLI DOUGH RECIPE)

½ pound all-purpose flour (can add 15% soy flour)

1 whole egg

1 ounce olive oil

½ tablespoon Sea Star sea salt

1½ ounces milk

semolina and unbleached organic flour (for dusting)

FILLING

- 1 pound tempeh
- 1 cup silken tofu
- 2 tablespoons parsley leaves
- 1 tablespoon lemon thyme
- ¼ cup basil, chopped
- 1 tablespoon lemon zest

- 1 onion (finely chopped)
- dry white wine (splash to taste)
- Sea Star sea salt
- freshly ground pepper

TOMATO CONCASSER

- 2 cups well reduced chicken stock (dark color and good flavor)
- 1½ cups orange tomatoes (organic, peeled, seeded, and chopped)
- 1½ cups yellow tomatoes (organic, peeled, seeded, and chopped)

- 1½ cups red tomatoes (organic, peeled, seeded, and chopped)
- basil stock to taste
- Sea Star sea salt to taste
- optional: extra virgin olive oil (to taste)

GARNISHES

- 1 bunch basil
- 1 bunch lemon thyme

- 1 bunch chives

DIRECTIONS

Prepare pasta: Sift flour (and soy flour, if used), and make a well in the center. Pour a mixture of egg, olive oil, natural gray sea salt, and milk into the well. Slowly incorporate the flour into the liquid ingredients with a fork, using a whisking motion. Form the pasta into one ball of dough and knead by hand for several minutes until dough is smooth but elastic. Wrap in plastic, and let it rest briefly. Pass the pasta through a pasta machine on each setting twice to get it as thin as possible.

Prepare filling: Combine tempeh, silken tofu, herbs, lemon zest, onion, white wine, natural gray sea salt, and black pepper. Mix just enough to incorporate ingredients.

Assembly and cooking: Cut squares from the sheets of pasta and place filling on one half. Brush edges with a little water or egg wash, then fold like a triangle or whatever shape you like. Place on sheet trays lined with kitchen towels dusted with semolina and unbleached organic flour. Do not cover. These are best when cooked within 20 minutes. When ready to cook, bring a large pot of salted water to a boil, and lower raviolis into water. Cook al dente for 2 to 4 minutes. Drain; do not rinse.

Melted tomato concasser: Heat chicken stock. While raviolis are cooking, quickly "melt" the chopped tomatoes by cooking them in the hot chicken stock. Season with the basil stock, natural gray sea salt, and herbs of your liking. You can always add a good extra virgin olive oil if you like.

To finish: Spoon a little tomato concasser onto each plate, then place raviolis on top and garnish with more concasser and herbs. Enjoy! For more color and style, you can cook each color of tomato separately and arrange on top of the ravioli. Season each with a different herb; for example, yellow with basil, orange with lemon thyme, and red with chives. This of course uses more pans, but sometimes it's worth it!

Delicate Lasagna with Tofu and Shiitake Mushrooms
Serves 6

PASTA

3 cups all-purpose flour
½ cup soy flour
3 whole eggs
4 tablespoons good-quality olive oil

1 tablespoon Sea Star sea salt, crushed
6 tablespoons whole milk

TOMATO SAUCE

½ onion, chopped
2 tablespoons olive oil
3 cups tomato concasser
¼ cup red wine
¼ cup chicken stock

1 clove fresh garlic, chopped
½ cup chopped basil
½ cup chopped parsley
Sea Star sea salt
black pepper to taste

Filling

1 cup steamed, chopped Swiss chard	¼ cup (splash) madeira
2 cups silken tofu or soft tofu	fresh thyme
	½ cup Italian parsley
freshly ground nutmeg (to taste)	1 clove garlic, chopped
fresh sage	3 cups Japanese eggplant (sliced, unpeeled)
Sea Star sea salt (to taste)	½ cup herbal or chicken stock
black pepper (to taste)	
3 cups shiitake mushrooms	1 bunch Italian parsley
1 cup reduced chicken stock (or vegetable)	oregano

Directions

Prepare pasta: Sift flours and make well in center. Pour mixture of eggs, olive oil, Sea Star natural gray sea salt, and milk into the well. Slowly incorporate the flour into the liquid ingredients with a fork, using a whisking motion. Form the pasta into one ball of dough and knead by hand for several minutes until dough is smooth but elastic. Wrap in plastic and let it rest briefly. Pass the pasta through a pasta machine on each setting twice to get it as thin and smooth as possible.

Prepare tomato sauce: Sauté onion in olive oil until tender. Add tomato concasser (prepared as in the recipe for Lemon Thyme Tofu Ravioli), red wine, chicken stock, chopped garlic, basil, parsley. Season with natural gray sea salt and black pepper, simmer for about 40 minutes.

Prepare filling: Steam and chop Swiss chard, mix together with tofu, and season with nutmeg, sage, Sea Star natural gray sea salt, and black pepper. Sauté cleaned mushrooms in reduced chicken stock, madeira; season with thyme and Italian parsley and chopped garlic. Simmer until flavors marry well. Set aside to cool. Slice eggplant and sprinkle with Sea Star natural gray sea salt. Let stand 5 minutes or so to remove some of the bitterness. Sear in a hot pan, sprinkle with a little herbal stock, and turn once to brown both sides. Layer lasagna with tomato sauce, pasta, mushroom mixture, pasta, Swiss chard mixture, pasta, eggplant, and pasta. Place some tomato sauce in between each layer as well.

To finish: Bake in oven at 350° for 45 minutes. Remove from oven and garnish with beautiful fresh herbs such as Italian parsley and oregano.

Seckel Pears in Red Wine with Silky Maple Tofu Sauce
Serves 6

FRUIT

18 Seckel pears (3 small per person)	½ cup sugar
	zest from 1 meyer lemon*
3 cups red table wine	

SAUCE

1 cup organic, plain silken tofu	maple syrup to taste

GARNISH

1 basket raspberries	flowers and mint

DIRECTIONS

Prepare fruit: Peel and core pears, being careful to keep their shape. Marinate in red wine for a day or so, making sure the pears are completely covered. Before cooking, remove pears from wine, add sugar, return wine to pot, and simmer until sugar is dissolved. Add pears, and simmer gently until just tender. Let cool in the wine to take on more color. Cut the zest from the lemon with a vegetable peeler, removing the yellow only—no white pith. Then cut the zest into fine ribbons, or use a zester.

Prepare sauce: Mix silken tofu and just enough real maple syrup to flavor it and mix until creamy. Add a splash of soymilk if necessary.

To finish: Place a ladle of sauce on plate, then arrange pears on top. Drizzle with maple tofu sauce, arrange some raspberries, and garnish with flowers and mint.

---

*Meyer lemon is actually a hybrid, a cross between a lemon and an orange. Its juice is less acidic and its zest has a more delicate floral flavor than regular lemons. It is just delicious; try it! If you can't find one, substitute regular fresh lemon.

CHAPTER SEVEN

The Will to Live
and Other Mysteries

Rachel Naomi Remen, M.D.

RACHEL NAOMI REMEN, M.D., is one of the earliest pioneers of mind-body medicine and the bestselling author of *My Grandfather's Blessings* and *Kitchen Table Wisdom*. She is clinical professor of family and community medicine at the University of California, San Francisco School of Medicine and a co-founder and medical director of the Commonweal Cancer Help Program in Bolinas, California.

The will to live is not a preference. It is a mysterious impulse toward life, which is hidden in the heart of all living things. Buried deep in the unconscious, it shapes our instinctive behaviors, influencing our conscious choices and even our physiology. The will to live is unconditional. The wish to live, on the other hand, is highly particular. It has its reasons and even its terms. It is conscious and personal rather than cellular and universal. It is bounded by the attachments of our individual lives. But the will to live is larger than ourselves. We may find ways to collaborate with it, unblock it, and even strengthen it, but it is a force of nature, an intimate experience of the life force itself.

I was fourteen years old when I first noticed the will to live. It was a Saturday morning in New York City, and I was window-shopping on Fifth Avenue with two of my friends—which was what young girls did on Saturday mornings in the 1950s. As we walked up the street a flash of green caught my eye. There, growing right through the cement of the New York City sidewalk, were two tender green blades of grass. We all stopped and stared in amazement. We were only fourteen, but we were New Yorkers and we were all pretty sophisticated about power.

Just from living all my life in New York, I knew a lot about the power of money. I knew quite a bit about the power of knowledge, too; my medical family had taught me that. But I had never seen this other kind of power before. At the time, it struck me as a kind of a miracle.

About a year later, when I was fifteen, I was diagnosed with Crohn's disease, the chronic condition that I have lived with for most of my life. At the time of my diagnosis, many experts in white coats gathered around me and my family and told us the facts: The cause of this disease was unknown, and there was no cure for it. As the disease progressed I would have surgery after surgery, and I would die by the time I was forty.

At fifteen, this was not my idea of the future. It was a time of great darkness and despair. The nine physicians and three nurses in my family never questioned what these experts told us. And so, neither did I. It would be years before I would make a connection between myself and the two little blades of grass I had seen the year before.

Thinking back on this, I realize that if only one of the many doctors around me had told me it was possible that there might be something in me that could break through this obstacle—something medicine could not measure or even understand—it would have made a great difference to me. But no one did. Now that I am a physician myself, I realize they did not tell me because in all probability, they did not know. This is not something you learn from reading a medical textbook. Knowing this requires you to know life itself. Strange as it may seem, it is actually possible to study *about* life for many years without knowing life at all.

Over all these years the facts have not changed. There is still no known cause of Crohn's disease, and no known cure. I have had eight major abdominal surgeries and no longer have most of my intestine. But I have not been dead these past twenty-four years. So I suppose the moral of the story is this: what was in those two little blades of grass is in us all.

The will to live cannot be measured. That puts it beyond the reach of science. But we cannot allow science to define life for us. Science defines life in its own ways, but life is larger than science. Many things happen that science cannot explain. These things are not replicable or quantifiable: they are touching, moving, inspiring, strengthening, and powerful. They are also profoundly mysterious. In truth, we all experience many things that we cannot explain or measure. In many circumstances, experiencing may be far more important than understanding or measuring. It is important to consider the possibility that science may have defined life in terms that are too small, that life may best be defined not by science but by Mystery.

The will to live is part of life's Mystery. The first time I came across the word *Mystery*, I did not understand it. As both a physician and an addicted reader of mystery stories, I had the idea that something is a mystery only when the answer to it has not yet been found. But Mystery is not something that you solve. When mystery has a capital M it becomes something different—something that by its very nature cannot be solved or understood or even known. Mystery can only be lived.

Whenever there is a difference between the facts and the story, we are in the presence of Mystery. It has been said that the world is not made up of facts; the world is made of stories. Each of our stories is as unique as our fingerprints. Each of us is a story that has never happened before, a story that has not yet been written. Perhaps because our lives touch so many other lives, our stories may never be completely written.

In the presence of Mystery, life becomes more filled with possibility, more inspiring, somehow larger. In allowing a larger and more mysterious definition of life than science offers us, we may discover one of Mystery's greatest gifts, which is hope. Perhaps it might be good to acknowledge the Mystery in things a little more, to be able to know that the diagnosis is Crohn's disease or cancer, and to remember that what this will mean remains to be seen. To recognize that every diagnosis is a process of discovery.

We have all encountered far more Mystery than we have experienced. Life is full of Mystery. Perhaps we often miss this because our culture does not help us to cultivate a comfort with Mystery and the Unknown. We tend to see the Unknown as an insult to our competence, a personal failing. "I don't know" has become a statement of inadaquacy or even shame. Few people over the age of seven can say it with a sense of adventure. As a young physician I was trained to view every instance of the unknown as an emergency, like a hemorrhage: something out of control that required immediate action. My job as a physician was to make things known as quickly, as efficiently, and—of course—as cost effectively as possible. But some things cannot be known. Mystery does not require action; Mystery requires our attention. It requires us to listen. If we listen long enough, Mystery may offer us the wisdom we need to live.

My friend and colleague Marion Weber has taught me to sit before the Unknown as an artist sits before a blank canvas. As an artist she is patient with the Unknown. She waits. She knows a blank canvas is a place where something may happen that has never happened before. It is a place of revelation. We may never understand what is revealed in such places. No matter. We can witness it anyway.

Knowing life often requires us to surrender the drive to understand, to realize that all our hard-won knowledge may only be provisional and that life may be far different from what we believe it to be. This can be humbling and even stressful, but it is also deeply rewarding. Befriending the Unknown can give us a sense of wonder and aliveness. Perhaps we all need to know less and wonder more.

Sometimes the more we know the harder it is to see something we cannot understand. This happens often in medicine. A medical culture clearly mirrors the values of the larger culture it serves. In fact, the values of the dominant culture are often intensified in its medical culture. Our whole culture is based on the pursuit of control and mastery—and so is our medicine. We have become so deeply concerned with mastery that we may not even recognize Mystery when it happens right in front of us.

A friend who is the director of research at a nonprofit institute became interested in the spontaneous remission of cancer. As his interest became more widely known, people would call or write him to tell him their stories of unexplained recovery from serious illness. Many of these stories fell into a gray zone: people had completed a single treatment of radiation or chemotherapy before quitting, or they had used extensive but unproven alternative treatments alone. Perhaps those measures were enough to effect a cure.

But there was one man whose story was definitely outside the box. As a youth in college he had been diagnosed with osteogenic sarcoma, an aggressive bone cancer. His doctors had offered him the standard treatment, which involved the surgical removal of his leg at the hip.

Despite pressure from them and from his family, he had refused this surgery and had gone back to his home town to die. The only intervention was that the pastor of his church had asked people to pray for him every evening if they were so inclined, and people had prayed for almost two years. Over time, the rock-hard mass in his thigh had grown smaller. Ultimately it disappeared. It was now twenty years later.

My friend was captivated by this story. Through his work he had developed a researcher's healthy skepticism, but the man seemed so genuine and matter-of-fact that he could not get the story out of his mind. Finally he called to ask me a favor. Would I mind trying to track down the doctor who had made the original diagnosis and see if he would confirm this story or had kept the biopsy report?

The man had been diagnosed at a major cancer center, and the physician who had made this diagnosis was still practicing there. I called him, hoping to get more information. Despite the passage of so many years, he recognized the man's name immediately. When I expressed my surprise he said, "Of course I remember him! Who could forget a thing like that? What a tragedy!" Then he asked me if I was calling for the family. When I told him that the man himself had asked me to call, he was deeply moved. "Thank God," he exclaimed. "Where did he have his surgery?" I told him that he had not had surgery. There was a surprised silence. Then, cautiously, he asked me what had happened. I told him the story much as it had been told to me. He greeted this information with a long silence. Then, without another word, he simply hung up the phone. I called him several times, but he never returned my calls.

It can be difficult and even frightening when our basic assumptions about life are called into question. But knowing life may require a willingness to not understand, a willingness to listen. Life is often not limited by the facts; life is filled with Mystery. If we are not willing to at least wonder, we may have to hang up the phone on life.

The will to live is common, although in most instances it is not as dramatic as this. Yet, many people who are living examples of it may not recognize it or trust its power. Over the years, countless people have told me that they have recovered from cancer because of radiation, chemotherapy, or surgery. But perhaps this is not completely accurate. Such approaches may have the same effect on us as pruning has on a rose bush. They create the conditions that give the will to live the best chance to express itself, but they are not *why* we recover. When challenged with a life-threatening illness, we may need to mobilize the full power of science and to draw on the wisdom of the world's healing traditions as well. But we cannot forget the power of the will to live in us, the Mystery at the heart of our lives and all other lives.

Perhaps we often do not recognize the power of the will to live because of the way we have learned to deal with our wounds. In a culture that sees woundedness as a weakness, many of us feel ashamed to be wounded and even hide our wounds. It is only natural that we try to put our wounds behind us and get on with the rest of our lives, but we do this only at a price. The power of the will to live is buried in the depths of any wound that we have survived, and we may need to revisit our wounds in order to know our strength. The secret to this may lie in how we look at our wounds. We need to look, not as victims but with a certain curiosity, as a witness to the hidden power in us to move past obstacles.

Most commonly, the will to live shows itself in subtle ways, taking forms that we do not expect or recognize. At the beginning of a disease, the will to live often looks like anger or even an unexplained, self-destructive behavior, but it is the will to live just the same.

David was diagnosed with diabetes just after his seventeenth birthday. His response was rage. He refused to take care of himself, to hold to a diet, or to take his insulin daily. Not surprisingly, in the first year after his diagnosis he was brought to the emergency room over and over again in diabetic coma. His behavior was so extreme that his parents became afraid for his life and insisted that he enter therapy. He did not want to do this, but he obeyed them.

For the first six months he made little progress. But then he had a dream, so real that he did not realize he had been asleep until he awoke. Something deep and unsuspected in him had pointed his way to freedom. In his dream David found himself in an empty room sitting before a little statue of the Buddha. While he was not a spiritual young man, he had seen many pictures of the Buddha and recognized the statue immediately. What surprised him was the sort of kinship he felt with it, perhaps because this Buddha was a young man, not much older than himself. The statue had an odd effect on him. It seemed to radiate a sort of peacefulness, and in its presence David felt more and more at peace himself. He had been sitting for a while, enjoying this unfamiliar feeling, when suddenly, from somewhere behind him, a dagger was thrown. It plunged deep into the Buddha's heart.

David was stunned. Powerful feelings of anguish and despair rose up in him, and from the depths of these emotions a single question emerged: WHY IS LIFE LIKE THIS? And then, despite his distress, he began to notice that the statue seemed to be slowly getting larger, so slowly that at first he was not really sure it was happening. But it was. And somehow David knew that this growing was the Buddha's response to the knife. As the statue grew larger and larger the knife remained exactly the same size. Gradually it became a tiny dot on the breast of the enormous peaceful Buddha. Watching this, David felt something release him and found that he could breathe deeply for the first time in a long time. He awoke with tears in his eyes.

At first David did not understand this dream, but as he told me about it he recognized the feelings of despair and anguish. They were the same feelings he had had in his doctor's office when he was told of his diagnosis. Even the question WHY IS LIFE LIKE THIS? was familiar. But David's response had been very different from the Buddha's.

David saw this dream much as the opening of a door. When he had been told that his disease was incurable, his response had been anger and despair, as if the life in him had been stopped and there was no way to move forward. But the dream showed him that he had the power to grow in such a way that his physical problem could become a smaller and smaller part of the sum total of his life—that perhaps he might yet have a good life even if it would not be an easy life.

I have seen many women whose bodies have been changed by cancer come to this same conclusion. We may become trapped and invalidated less by our disease and its treatment than by our beliefs about it. Disease is at various times brutal, lonely, constricting, and terrifying. But the life in us may be stronger than all that and may ultimately free us even from whatever we must endure. Sometimes someone dreams a dream for us all. I think of David's dream as one of those dreams.

One of the most subtle and powerful manifestations of the will to live is a certain shift in values, a change in what we think is important that may free us from life-long limitations and help us live more deeply, passionately, and fully. Wounded, we may become more whole. A life-threatening illness may shuffle our values like a deck of cards. Sometimes a card that has been on the bottom of the deck for most of our lives turns out to be the top card, the thing that really matters. Having watched people sort their cards and play their hands in the presence of death for many years, I would say that rarely is the top card perfection, or possessions, or pride, or even power. Most often the top card is love.

Sometimes love reconnects us to the will to live, and those who love us can evoke and restore our wholeness far more powerfully than even the most skillful of surgeons. On first meeting Clare, I would not have thought that this would have been her story. In her beige linen suit and white silk blouse, she appeared flawless, competent, and totally in control. In contrast to her elegance, my waiting room looked shabby. When I said her name, she rose and shook my hand. Without another word she followed me into my office and folded herself into a chair, crossing her long, beautifully shaped legs at the ankles. I settled myself opposite and smiled at her. Without any warning whatsoever, she burst into tears. The contrast between her tears and her self-possession was so extreme that I was caught completely by surprise. For a moment I was stunned. Then I reached forward and took her hand between my own as she sobbed. We sat like that for a long time, until she had cried enough. Turning a tear-stained face toward me, she commented, "How embarrassing. I have not cried in years."

"These are special times," I said. She nodded. "Would you tell me about it?" I asked her.

She had come to see me because eight weeks earlier she had undergone surgery to remove her right breast. After much discussion, she and her doctor had made this decision together. She felt certain that it was the right choice, and she had healed nicely. "And how has this been for you?" I asked her. "I don't know," she told me.

Clare was in her late twenties, unmarried, and successful as a businesswoman. Until her surgery she had worked out daily and had been very proud of her body. Men had always found her very attractive, and having a man in her life was important to her. She'd had many lovers, mostly colleagues she had met in the business world. "But that is over now," she told me. "I could never allow anyone to see me disfigured like this." After the surgery she had ended her relationship with the two men she had been seeing. Both had accepted it gracefully and moved on. No one at work and none of her friends even suspected that she had cancer, she told me. She had gone through the surgery and its aftermath entirely alone. So obsessed had she been with secrecy that she had told everyone she was going on a vacation to Europe and had even made arrangements to have cards sent to them from abroad. Even her parents did not know. But she was here with me because the pressure of keeping this secret had become too much, and she needed a place to talk and to be herself. "I can't come very often," she told me. "People would begin to suspect." "Come whenever you need to," I told her.

For the next few years I saw Clare every three or four months. On the surface, her life was much as it had been, except that she lived as a celibate, putting all her energy into her work. During one of her infrequent visits I called this to her attention and asked her if she planned to be alone for the rest of her life. "Only for five years, Rachel," she told me. Seeing my look of surprise, she explained that her oncologist was very conservative. She had picked him because she too was conservative. Early on they had discussed a breast reconstruction. He had encouraged her to put off having this surgery until the fifth anniversary of her diagnosis. "And this is so that any recurrence can be easily seen?" I asked. She nodded. "Yes," she said. "After five years the chances are I will be home free."

A little more than a year before this important anniversary, we had one of our sessions. During the hour, she told me that she had gone to an opening at an art gallery and had struck up a conversation with a painter named Peter, who had asked her to join him for a cup of coffee. "He is a very attractive man, but obviously totally unsuitable as a lover," she told me. "So I said yes." "Because he is unsuitable?" I said, puzzled. "I thought we could become friends," she replied. Surprisingly, she had a very good time. "Will you see him again?" I asked her. "Yes, I think so," she told me. "He is such good company." Three months later, when she returned for another session, Peter's name came up frequently in our conversation. They had gone to the zoo. She had visited his studio and had been very impressed with his work. By now, she had met several of his friends who were artists and sculptors and found that she liked them very much. It had surprised her to discover that she fit in so well with these people and was even more comfortable with them than with people she knew from her own work. "Perhaps it's because you are creative yourself, Clare," I told her. "Business can be as much an art form as paint or stone." She thought this over for several moments. She had never seen herself in this way before.

About two months later she called to schedule an urgent visit. She came into the office looking somber. "It's the end," she told me. I thought that perhaps she had suffered a recurrence, and my heart jumped into my throat. But this was not what she meant at all. "Peter left a message on my voice mail, inviting me away for the weekend. I will have to tell him now," she said. "It is over." Relieved, I said, "Perhaps once he knows he might not feel that way about things." "I doubt it," she replied. "He is exactly the wrong sort of man. Beauty is his whole life. He will be completely repulsed." "When will you tell him?" I asked, my heart sinking. "Tonight at dinner." "Call if you need to," I told her. I found myself thinking of her all evening, but she did not call. As the weeks went by I continued to wonder what had happened, but I resisted calling her to see how things had gone. As was her way, she came in again three months later. In response to my questioning look she laughed. "I was wrong," she said. "He still wants to be friends."

It turned out that Peter wanted to be more than friends, but Clare had refused. She was convinced that her body was too ugly, too maimed. "My fifth anniversary is less than six months away, and I will have my reconstruction," she told me. "Perhaps then." She went on to tell me her plans. She had scheduled the date of her reconstructive surgery more than a year earlier and had interviewed several surgeons and some of their patients before deciding on the surgeon she would use. She had arranged vacation time at work. As her insurance did not cover this sort of surgery, she had begun saving the money for it right after her mastectomy, and over the past five years she had put enough away. The surgery would be very expensive and difficult, but she hoped it would return her to wholeness. She looked down at her hands clasped in her lap for a few minutes. Then she looked up. "I hope it works, Rachel," she said. I was not sure, but I thought there were tears in her eyes.

I did not see her again until a few days before her fifth anniversary. She came in looking excited and happy. I was delighted to celebrate this milestone with her and asked her about the upcoming surgery. She smiled and told me that she had canceled it. I looked at her in surprise. "How come?" I asked her. She returned my look for a long moment. Then slowly she unbuttoned her blouse and shrugged it off her shoulders. She was not wearing a bra, and her left breast was exquisite. But its beauty was overshadowed by the radical change in her body. Her mastectomy scar was now covered over with a mass of tiny exquisite tattooed flowers. They looked real. In the most delicate of pastel shades they climbed to the top of her right shoulder. As she turned away from me I could see that they fell across her shoulder and down her back, as if scattered by gravity or the wind. She stood, pulling her slacks down over her hips. Her body was beautiful. One little tattooed flower had come to rest in the small of her back, and another lay against her right buttock. Under it was the tiny initial "P." My mouth dropped open in shock while at the same time I experienced a pang of envy. She was indescribably erotic. Men encountered women like her only in their dreams.

Shrugging back into her blouse and buttoning her slacks, she sat down again, laughing aloud at my look of astonishment. "Isn't it beautiful?" she said. "Peter painted it, and we went to Belgium to have it done. Then we used the money I had saved for the surgery for a honeymoon. I am so happy, Rachel," she said, blushing slightly. "My husband has convinced me beyond the shadow of a doubt that anything of real beauty is one of a kind."

The will to live responds to the people around us—the very people who may feel that they are powerless to help us because they have no knowledge of our disease or no expertise. But evoking the will to live is not a matter of expertise. We all have the power to affect those around us. We can strengthen the will to live even in total strangers with a word or a smile, often without even realizing it. We evoke the will to live in others not by what we know but simply by being who we are.

Recently I had the opportunity to meet a colleague, a master storyteller whose work is with women who have been victims of domestic abuse and whose stories about these women help others still trapped in such circumstances find the strength to free themselves. I asked her how she had become interested in this field, and she told me that she had once been one of those women. Her first husband had been a very violent and abusive man. He was a professional, a pillar of the community, and had treated her well in public. No one had dreamed that she did not have the perfect marriage or that her life was a living hell. In a rather classic way he had told her that she caused his abusive behavior by the stupid things she said and did. She had tried harder and harder, but her efforts were never good enough. Over the years she had become so diminished that she came to believe him and felt that she deserved to be treated in this way.

All this ended abruptly one day on a street corner during a visit to New York City. She and her husband were standing on the corner waiting for the light to change when she looked across the street and noticed a beautiful building with Art Deco architecture. She turned to him and called his attention to it. "Honey, look at that beautiful building!" He, thinking that they were alone, responded in the tone of utter contempt that he reserved for their private conversations. "Do you mean the yellow one?" he sneered. "The one that anyone who wasn't blind would know was just the same as every building on the street?" Humiliated, she fell silent. But a woman standing next to him, a total stranger who was also waiting for the light to change, turned to him and said, "Why, what do you mean? That's a perfectly beautiful building! She's absolutely right, you know . . . and you, sir, are a horse's ass!"

And then the light changed, and this total stranger crossed the street and went on about her business. My colleague smiled and told me that her life had changed in that moment as well. Suddenly she realized what had been happening over the past seven years of marriage; she knew beyond any doubt that she had not deserved any of this abuse. Even more important, she knew that she was going to leave him. It would take some time and some planning, but she could feel something new inside, an unfamiliar strength that told her she would be able to leave.

Somehow I doubt that this outspoken New Yorker ever had any idea of the effect of her chance remark or that she might have quite literally saved another woman's life. The web of relationship is part of life's Mystery, and because of it we all have strengthened the will to live in others far more often than we realize, simply by being who we are. Strengthening the will to live is not the work of experts, it is the work of human beings.

When we define life too small, we may define ourselves too small as well. The will to live may have a trajectory far longer than any of us may have dreamed. If life is Mystery, every life is a Mystery, and perhaps every one of us is a Mystery as well. Medicine is a front row seat on life's Mystery. In the practice of medicine, Mystery can present itself to you when you are least expecting it.

Ahiro, a very elegant Japanese man, came into my practice at the end of a long struggle with prostate cancer. He came with a very clear agenda for our sessions together. Knowing he did not have long to live, he wanted to invite those who had made his life meaningful and worthwhile to meet with us, one at a time, so he could thank them. And so began a series of very moving sessions. About halfway through our work together, as we were sitting and talking about the session we had just completed with one of his sons, Ahiro suddenly changed the subject. "Rachel," he said, "I am an educated man . . . and so I believe that death is the end. And you, as an educated woman, you must believe the same. Don't you?"

Taken completely by surprise, I told him that I had once believed much as he did, but now I simply did not know. Perhaps death was the ultimate Mystery at the heart of life. He raised his eyebrows and looked at me for a long moment. Then he abandoned the subject, but not before I saw something shift in his eyes and realized that there might be an even deeper agenda for our meetings than the one he had proposed in his first session.

In every session after this, usually when I was least expecting it, he would raise this question again, and I would respond in the same way. This led to a series of far-ranging discussions about death. He had read extensively, and so had I. We explored much of the world's wisdom on such matters and shared our own experiences. Some of these conversations were very moving; others were hilariously funny. I began to look forward to them. Close to the last of our sessions, he once again raised this issue. With some frustration he repeated that he was a rational man and must believe that death is the end. Then he smiled. "But just in case it isn't, Rachel, I will return as a great white crane and show myself to you to let you know that I have lost this argument." We both began to laugh, and I told him that dropping in as a white bird seemed rather obvious and somehow out of character for him. Still laughing, he agreed. "I am much more of a minimalist," he told me. Then suddenly he became quite serious. "If I can, I will do something in my own way," he said, meeting my eyes squarely, "something that you will recognize."

Sadly, within a month or two this remarkable man went on to die. A few months afterward, I found myself in the TransAmerica Building in downtown San Francisco, waiting for an elevator. As the building is tall, the wait can be long, and often one has a few minutes to reflect. As I waited my mind turned to Ahiro, and I felt once again a sadness about his death. Standing there, I realized how much I missed our conversations and remembered the many things I had discovered about this remarkable man. Then the elevator arrived; it was empty. With my heart and mind filled with memories of this relationship, I stepped in. The doors closed, and suddenly the elevator started upward so abruptly that I lost my balance. I looked down hurriedly to get my feet under me, and there, lying on the floor of the elevator, was a perfect large white feather.

In a matter of speaking, one might say that Ahiro had raised the level of the dialogue. But in all honesty, if he were to ask me today whether death is the end, I would not change my answer. The feathers that fall into all of our lives don't prove anything. They are simply reminders to pay attention, to stay awake, because the Mystery at the heart of life may speak to you at any time.

So what does the will to live really ask of us? I suspect it is something my grandfather showed me years ago. My grandfather was an orthodox rabbi, a dedicated student of Kabbalah, and a very special person in my childhood. Often when he came to visit he would bring me a present. These were never the sorts of things that other people brought, but my grandfather was not an ordinary sort of person.

Once he brought me a little paper cup. I looked inside it, expecting something magic, but saw only that it was filled with dirt. I was disappointed. But Grandpa seemed not to notice. He took me into the kitchen and showed me how to put a little water into the cup. "If you water this every day, something may happen, Neshume-le," he told me.

I was four years old at the time and lived on the sixth floor of an apartment building in the heart of New York City. I could not imagine what might happen, but my grandfather was very special to me and so I promised. At first, filled with curiosity, I watered the little cup every day with enthusiasm. But as the days passed and nothing changed, it got harder and harder to remember to water the cup. When he visited me the following week, I asked him if it was time to stop yet. Shaking his head no, he reminded me, "Every day, Neshume-le." The second week was even harder, and I became resentful of my promise to water the cup. When my grandfather came again, I tried to give it back to him but he refused to take it, saying simply, "Every day, Neshume-le." The third week was very hard indeed but one morning, there were two little green leaves in the cup that had not been there the night before.

I was completely astonished. I could not wait to tell my grandfather, certain that he would be as surprised as I was. But of course he was not. Carefully he explained to me that life is everywhere, hidden in the most ordinary and unlikely places. I was delighted. "And all it needs is water, Grandpa?" I asked him. Gently he touched me on the top of my head. "No, Neshume-le," he told me. "All it needs is your faithfulness."

I thought of this often in the years when I was a pediatrician and watched mothers tending their children, moment by moment, day by day. I think of it now when I see someone going through a difficult chemotherapy, radiation, or surgery, moment by moment, day by day. Or when someone walks this difficult path with a person whose life matters to them, step by step by step. All life needs is our faithfulness. We already have the power to nurture the will to live in ourselves and in others.

Sometimes the ways in which we have been taught to live conceal our real power, and we may know only a small part of who we are. My mother was a woman who owned her full power. Born at the turn of the century, she was a highly trained nurse, a professional woman who was well versed in the science of her day. But she was not limited by her scientific expertise. Like life itself, she was full of surprises—something that my father on certain occasions found trying.

Almost everyone in the family was drafted at one time or another to be my father's opponent at cards. My father was a scientific player, and he practiced constantly. Often after the first five or so cards were played he would be able to tell you with a high percentage of accuracy what you held in your hand and what cards you probably needed to win. He based his conclusions on the cards that had been discarded and what he held in his hand. He was rarely wrong. He would hold back the cards you needed in his own hand until he picked the cards he needed to declare victory. He played with his buddies, filling the kitchen with cigar smoke and winning almost every hand.

My mother played by pure intuition. She ignored every rule of the game, blithely breaking up lays and discarding matching cards, throwing back the very cards she had picked up only moments ago. He was never able to beat her.

I remember his outraged howls when she would discard one of the three Jacks he knew she must be holding and pick another card. "Gladys, you can't do that," he would bellow. My mother would look at him with the most innocent and wicked of smiles. "But I have, Ray," she would tell him. "I have." Eventually he refused to play with her. "She does not play fair," he would tell me.

My parents' kitchen table card games are among my favorite family memories. They were often hilariously funny. But they were important in other ways as well. These were some of my earliest lessons in the fact that the game may lie beyond the rules, that we can know many things we can never explain, and that following our own deepest wisdom may be the best way of all to live.

CHAPTER EIGHT

Natural Products in the Management of Breast Cancer

Heather Boon, BSc.Phm., Ph.D.

HEATHER S. BOON, BSc.PHM., PH.D., is an assistant professor in the Faculty of Pharmacy, University of Toronto. In addition, Dr. Boon is cross-appointed to the Department of Family and Community Medicine and the Department of Health Policy, Management and Evaluation, Faculty of Medicine, University of Toronto. Dr. Boon co-authored the textbook *The Botanical Pharmacy* and has founded the Toronto Complementary and Alternative Medicine Research Network. Her primary research interests are patients' use of complementary or alternative medicine, the safety and efficacy of natural health products, and complementary or alternative medicine regulation and policy issues.

It is astounding how many women turn to complementary and alternative medicine after receiving a diagnosis of breast cancer. Recent surveys of women diagnosed with breast cancer reveal that as many as two out of every three women use some kind of alternative or complementary product or therapy.[1-6] In our recent study involving a group of Canadian women diagnosed with breast cancer, we found that the most commonly used complementary/alternative medicine (CAM) therapies included vitamins and minerals (49.6%), herbal remedies (24.6%), green tea (17.3%), special foods or diets (15.3%), and Essiac (14.8%). Since vitamins and minerals and special foods or diets are covered elsewhere in this book, this chapter will focus on herbal remedies, including Essiac, green tea, the Hoxsey treament, Iscador (mistletoe), reishi mushrooms, shiitake mushrooms, and another popular nonherbal natural health product called shark cartilage. I shall begin with a discussion of why women in our study chose to use these products and then review the scientific evidence available to support the usefulness of each product, including any potential known side effects from these therapies. The chapter will conclude with general advice about using natural health products in combination with conventional Western medicine.

Why Women Diagnosed with Breast Cancer Choose to Use CAM

We asked women who had been diagnosed with breast cancer to describe their perceptions, ideas, and feelings about CAM in an attempt to understand why women choose to use it.[7] We talked with thirty-six women, aged forty-one to seventy-three years, in a series of six focus groups. On average, the women had been diagnosed with breast cancer five years beforehand, although the range spanned from eight months to fifteen years. Most of the women, twenty-five of the thirty-six, identified themselves as "users" of CAM, and eleven had not tried any type of CAM when they attended our group discussion.[8]

Many different reasons for using CAM surfaced during our focus groups, but it was possible to identify four of the most common: (1) survival, (2) reacting to bad experiences with conventional medicine, (3) being proactive in an attempt to prevent further illness or a recurrence of breast cancer, and (4) a belief that there was nothing to lose by trying CAM.[9] Despite the widespread interest in CAM, almost everyone in our group chose to have surgery, and many had follow-up treatment with radiation and chemotherapy. Complementary and alternative therapies were seen by almost everyone as an additional treatment rather than a true substitute for conventional medical therapy.[10,11]

Many women felt that using CAM increased their overall chance of surviving breast cancer. One woman commented:

The reason why I got into it after the cancer was because of
the statistic that more people were dying of cancer now than
ever. I think that there's been a lot more success out there,
whether the doctors want to admit it or not, [with] people
using complementary or alternative [approaches].

Some women described turning to CAM after a disappointing experience with conventional therapies or to help alleviate the adverse effects
of Western medical treatments:

> My sister's always been trying to get me to take the Essiac. And
> I knew that shark cartilage was dealing with the blood, but I
> didn't start taking anything at all until the damage from the
> chemo[therapy], which in my case was severe fatigue. . . . So
> then people started saying, "You should take this," and "You
> should take that," and so I did.

Other women described their reason for trying CAM as a desire to be
more proactive. They talked about using CAM to "boost" the immune
system, "stabilize" their current condition, prevent recurrence of disease,
aid the conventional medical treatments, allow action during waiting
periods, and "treat" the cancer directly. The perception that CAM had the
ability to boost or enhance the action of the immune system gave many
women a sense of control over both their lives and the cancer:

> I think that the two basic differences in approach are (1) attack the
> disease, the problem itself, or (2) support the body to attack it. . . .
> I compare the medical approach at the moment to the napalm
> bombing of Vietnam. I think that this is the kind of mind-set—
> we have a problem and we're going to eradicate it. . . . What are
> you aiming at: Do you want to kill the cancer cells, or do you want
> to strengthen my body?

Overall there was a widespread perception among the women that we
talked with that there was nothing to lose by trying CAM because it
could not be harmful:

> One of the gals in the support group had mentioned barley green.
> I thought, "Hey, I don't think you can lose by trying it. Let's give it
> a shot." It's minerals, I would think, and vitamins. And it
> certainly can't hurt.

Why Not Use CAM?

A few of the women we talked with decided not to try any of the readily available complementary and alternative therapies. Their reasons usually fell into one of two categories: lack of information and fear that the therapy might actually cause some harm:

> I belong to a breast cancer support group, and I heard many, many of our members talking about the alternative medicine that they had taken. . . . They just said, "What have I got to lose?" So they were on shark cartilage and Essiac tea and vitamins to no end. And I just made a comment once, "Could all this combination be too much for your body?"

Some women wanted to try CAM, but since these therapies are generally not paid for by either government or private insurance plans, the costs involved made it impossible:

> I'd be ready to take it as long as it doesn't cost too much money. I haven't been to a naturopath and I'd love to go, but I heard the price and I thought, well, do I really want to spend that much? I know once you walk in there they will tell you, "Take this, take that," and it's a lot of money, you know.

Other barriers to CAM use included lack of access (for example, it was not possible to purchase the product in their town or city) and the time-consuming nature of many CAM therapies:

> It's also time. I don't want cancer to be my life. . . . So things that I can sort of integrate into my life are more likely to find a place in my life than something that requires that I live as a cancer patient.

Does It Work?

One question asked by all the women in our study was, "Does it work?" They wanted to know which CAM therapies "cured" cancer and which ones had positive effects on their quality of life. They also wanted to know what would relieve the adverse effects they were experiencing from their conventional therapies, and they wanted to be reassured that these products were safe. Some of the more common CAM products used by the women in our study are reviewed below with these questions in mind.

Essiac

Essiac is an herbal tea named after an Ontario nurse, Rene Caisse, who was reportedly given the formula by an Ojibwa healer in 1922. Essiac is her last name spelled backwards. The Essiac brand (manufactured by the Reserpin Corporation of Canada) contains four herbs: burdock root, rhubarb, sheep sorrel, and the inner bark of the slippery elm. Another brand, Flor-Essence (Flora Manufacturing and Distributing Ltd.), contains the four herbs listed above as well as four additional herbs (watercress, blessed thistle, red clover, and kelp), which are reported to enhance both its taste and its activity.[12–15]

Essiac is thought to work as a cleansing and strengthening tonic that supports the body in resisting the cancer. According to Flora Manufacturing, the herbs clear mucous membranes, relieve inflammation, break down tissue masses that are foreign to the body, strengthen the stomach, and cleanse the lymphatic glands. None of the herbs in either Essiac or Flor-Essence has been shown to have direct anticancer effects. Burdock root shows an antimutagenic effect (the ability to prevent chemically produced chromosomal aberrations) to some chemicals, and rhubarb has immune modulatory effects.

Essiac is popular among North American cancer patients, who use it both in attempts to cure their cancer and to increase their quality of life. However, the evidence of the efficacy of this herbal product is currently limited to patient testimonials.[16–18] Although patient testimonials are important in identifying the therapies we should study in more detail, they are not sufficient to prove that a product is effective. This is because it is not possible to assess how each of the patients would have responded to the disease if they had not taken Essaic tea in the first place.

Several attempts have been made to systematically assess the effects of Essiac in the management of cancer. However, all have been abandoned, most commonly because of an inability to collect sufficient data. Overall, the incomplete results of these studies appear to indicate that Essiac has little or no effect on the natural progression of cancer, although some patients have experienced improvements in their overall quality of life.[19,20] One unpublished study of 162 patients conducted by a marketing company in Israel reported that 50% of those taking Essiac had reduced adverse effects associated with chemotherapy, 20% showed tumor regression, 5% healed completely, and no one complained of adverse effects of Essiac.[21] As scientists we are critical of this study, since it has never been published and therefore the medical community cannot accurately judge whether the results stem from a properly designed clinical trial. This review process is particularly important, since the study was conducted by the manufacturer, who will reap direct financial gain from the sale of Essiac. In addition, the study report does not provide any information to confirm that the individuals in the trial who were taking Essiac actually had cancer. These problems lead the medical community to be very skeptical about the purported benefits of Essiac. However, a group of Canadian and American researchers is currently planning a well-designed clinical trial to investigate the effect of Flor-Essence on the quality of life of cancer patients.[22]

The only adverse effects experienced by humans who drank Essiac tea were reported as mild nausea and diarrhea.[23,24] Some people have suggested that any adverse effects that have been associated with any of the individual herbal ingredients (such as allergic reactions, kidney damage, and liver injury) are possible;[25] however, none of these has ever been documented. To be safe, it is recommended that all pregnant or nursing women avoid Essiac, as well as anyone with a bowel obstruction[26] because of the tannins present in some of the herbs and their laxative effects. Red clover, one of the herbs in Essiac, is classified as a phytoestrogen, and some authors suggest that it should be used with caution by women with estrogen-positive breast cancer.[27] Although no interactions with any other drugs have been reported to date, Essiac appears to have the potential to interact with laxatives, cardiac glycosides (for example, digoxin), diabetic medications,[28] and conventional estrogen antagonists such as tamoxifen.

Commercially available Essiac products that are sold in dried powdered form are usually prepared as a tea that is taken twice a day. To minimize the potential for gastric irritation, the tea should be consumed on an empty stomach (one hour before eating or two hours after eating). The Flor-Essence liquid preparation is also ingested twice daily. The typical daily dose of Flor-Essence is 60 milligrams.

There is currently *no* evidence that Essiac can be used as an alternative to conventional cancer treatment. The proponents of Essiac claim that its use in addition to conventional therapy will result in increased quality of life; however, further research is necessary to confirm this claim.

Green Tea

There is growing interest among the scientific and lay communities in the association between green tea (unfermented tea) consumption and the prevention of cancer. Specific components of green tea, called polyphenols, are thought to be the most important in its suggested anticancer actions.[29,30] These particular chemical structures are destroyed during the fermentation process that is used to make black tea. Animal studies lend support to claims that green tea may help prevent cancer, including breast cancer.[31–33] In addition, several epidemiological studies have reported a correlation between lower cancer rates (primarily cancers of the digestive system) and increased consumption of green tea, but other studies have failed to confirm these findings.[34–37] One clinical trial is currently under way at the M. D. Anderson Cancer Center in collaboration with Memorial Sloan-Kettering Cancer Center to investigate the safety and possible efficacy of consuming the equivalent of a minimum of ten cups of green tea per day to reduce the risk of cancer.

Only a few studies have investigated the effects of green tea with respect to breast cancer. One study of 472 patients with Stage I, II, or III breast cancer reported that increased consumption of green tea *before* breast cancer diagnosis was associated with an improved prognosis of Stage I and II breast cancer.[38] These promising results need to be confirmed in a randomized, controlled trial, because the effects noted by the researchers in this study may have been due to factors other than simply the consumption of green tea. Likewise, the number of years that one consumes green tea, or the age at which an individual begins to drink green tea, may play a role in the protective benefits.

The medicinal use of green tea has not been reported to be associated with any adverse effects. However, green tea does contain caffeine (the amount varies depending on the type of tea and the way in which it is prepared), and caffeine can cause insomnia, nervousness, and irregularities in heart rate, especially in sensitive individuals. It has been suggested that pregnant or nursing women and anyone with cardiac disease should drink no more than two cups of green tea daily.[39] Overall, moderate consumption of green tea appears to be safe.

Green tea taken for medicinal purposes is usually prepared by steeping 1 or 2 teaspoons of dried herb in 1 cup of boiling water for approximately 3 to 15 minutes. The amount of green tea consumed can vary widely from one to ten or more cups per day.

In summary, there is some evidence to support a diet that includes drinking green tea to prevent cancer, but significantly less evidence exists that supports green tea's role as an anticancer treatment.

Hoxsey Treament

Harry Hoxsey, often described as intelligent, boisterous, and charismatic, lived from 1901 to 1974. His passionate advocacy of his family's anticancer treatment triggered one of the greatest controversies in the American medical community of the twentieth century. For nearly forty years, much to the chagrin of the American Medical Association, Harry Hoxsey treated cancer patients with an herbal formula passed on to him by his great-grandfather.

The legend is that Hoxsey's great-grandfather was a horse breeder in the 1840s, and one of his stallions developed a tumor. Instead of dying, the horse began to graze on a select group of plants in the pasture, and the cancer went into remission. Harry Hoxsey's great-grandfather wrote down the herbs and treated other horses afflicted with cancer, using both an external salve and an internal herbal mixture. The family secret was passed down from generation to generation, and while Harry Hoxsey was working as a coal miner he treated his first cancer patient.

Word spread of Hoxsey's treatments, and he eventually opened his first medical clinic in Taylorville, Illinois, in the 1920s. Hostile encounters with the American Medical Association forced him to move to Dallas. At the peak of his career, Hoxsey was managing clinics in seventeen states, but ultimately he was forced to close them because of his legal battles with the Food and Drug Administration. When he closed the last clinic in Dallas, he gave the formula to one of his nurses, Mildred Nelson, whose mother had been "cured" of cancer at the Hoxsey clinic. Nelson then set up a clinic in Tijuana, Mexico, where she and a full medical staff treat cancer patients today. About 1200 new patients and 3500 follow-up patients (not all are cancer patients) come to Mildred Nelson's clinic each year. That clinic has been operating since 1963. Therapy at the clinic costs $3500, which includes a lifetime supply of tonic, visits, medications, and doctor's fees.

The Hoxsey treatment is available as two different remedies: (1) a red paste to be applied externally, consisting of antimony trisulfide, zinc chloride, bloodroot, and a yellow powder containing arsenic sulfide, sulfur, and talc; and (2) a tea made from a combination of herbs (red clover, licorice, burdock root, bayberry, poke root, stillingia, prickly ash bark, cascara, and buckthorn) and potassium iodide. The exact formula remains shrouded in secrecy, and many different adaptations of the original formula are available. The anticancer properties of the Hoxsey formula are passionately maintained by its proponents, but to date, there is no objective evidence to support these testimonials. A few animal studies and laboratory data suggest that some of the herbs in the formula, or components of those herbs, may have immunostimulant and/or anticancer properties.[40] Despite these findings, currently there is no evidence that these effects are seen in humans, especially at the doses recommended to patients taking the Hoxsey formula. Only two attempts to evaluate the effects of the Hoxsey formula in humans were found for this review. One was a description of nine cancer patients who had been "successfully" treated with the Hoxsey formula. However, seven of the nine patients were also receiving conventional medical cancer treatments either before or during their Hoxsey therapy.[41] A second small study of thirty-nine cancer patients taking the Hoxsey formula noted that after an average of forty-eight months of therapy, six individuals (two patients with lung cancer, two with melanoma, one with recurrent bladder cancer, and one with labial cancer) claimed to be disease free. However, only sixteen of the original thirty-nine patients were available for interview (there is no record of the outcomes in the other twenty-three) and ten of those who were followed up died after an average of 15 months. Documentation of any other therapies the patients may have been taking was not reported. The authors acknowledge that their study has many limitations, but suggest that further studies are warranted.[42,43]

There is no good documentation regarding the adverse effects associated with either the external salve or the internal Hoxsey formula. However, some of the herbs included in the formula (pokeroot, for example) are considered to be potentially toxic.[44]

Given the lack of information about the Hoxsey formula and the potential safety concerns, women diagnosed with breast cancer are cautioned against using this treatment until further information is available.

Iscador (Mistletoe)

Mistletoe (*Viscum album* L.) is a semiparasitic plant that lives with several tree species, including oak, pine, fir, elm, and apple. Although mistletoe is found in America and Korea, to date only the European species is used in the treatment of cancer. In traditional Chinese medicine, mistletoe (*Viscum album* L. var. coloratum) is used for low back stiffness, lumbar pain, and vaginal bleeding during pregnancy. In Native American medicine it was used for calming. It is claimed that mistletoe preparations can be used to stimulate the immune system, kill cancer cells, and improve the quality of life of breast cancer patients. Extracts of mistletoe are marketed under several trade names, most of which are available primarily in Europe. Iscador is a commercially available product made by fermenting an extract of European mistletoe (*Viscum album* L.) and the probiotic *Lactobacillus plantarum*. Slight variations of the Iscador formula have been produced and marketed to individuals with specific types of cancer. For example, Iscador M (made from mistletoe grown on apple trees) is thought to be for women only. In addition, very dilute concentrations of various metals may be added to enhance Iscador's action on specific parts of the body (for example, silver is sometimes added for the treatment of breast diseases and diseases of the urinary tract).[45]

The use of mistletoe products in the management of cancer was originated by an early twentieth-century scientist, Rudolf Steiner. Steiner blended scientific and spiritual concepts to create the theory of anthroposophy, which he then applied to the treatment of disease, especially cancer. He was highly influenced by homeopathic medicine, which was very popular in his time and whose guiding principle is that "like treats like." Steiner extended the homeopathic theory to include medicines that seem to allegorically emulate disease processes. Since mistletoe shows "strong antagonism towards regular organization," he thought it would be able to stimulate the "higher organizational forces" that, according to the theory, cancer patients need.[46] In more simple terms, mistletoe seems, like cancer in the human body, to defy the normal rules of growth and distribution. It is a semiparasitic plant, which does not have roots and therefore depends on another living tree for some of its nutrients. Yet, unlike full parasites, it is green and therefore converts gases from the air for its energy source. In addition, mistletoe produces berries all year round, unlike most plants that respond to seasons. Although the use of Iscador is relatively rare in North America, it has been a popular cancer treatment in Europe, especially Germany and Switzerland, for over fifty years.

The effectiveness of Iscador in the management of cancer is currently unclear. Animal and laboratory studies suggest that some of the chemicals in mistletoe may have both immunostimulant and anticancer properties.[47-49] In addition, several case studies and clinical trials designed to evaluate the effects of Iscador in cancer patients have been published.[50-52] Although some studies have reported improvements in patients' quality of life, length of survival, and immune function, a recent detailed review of all the trials conducted before 1994 concluded that serious flaws in the trial designs made their results inconclusive.[53] A more recent nonrandomized case-control study of 396 matched pairs of cancer patients reported that those treated with Iscador lived approximately 40% longer (mean 4.23 years) than those who did not receive Iscador (mean 3.05 years). The patients diagnosed with breast cancer in this study who took Iscador lived statistically significantly longer than those who did not.[54] These findings were confirmed by two small randomized, prospective, matched-pair studies by the same research team.[55] One key limitation of these studies was that the patients were not blinded to the treatments they received. Since they knew that they were taking Iscador, their beliefs about the product may have influenced their survival. Overall, these data suggest that Iscador may increase the survival time of individuals diagnosed with cancer and warrants further investigation.

Iscador is given by injection subcutaneously (just under the skin) near the tumor or into the tumor itself, depending on the location of the mass. Injections may be given daily, usually the first thing in the morning, or three times per week. Treatment with Iscador may continue for many years and often begins before surgical intervention.

The known adverse side effects associated with Iscador include fever, headache, nausea, skin irritation, and inflammation at the injection site. These effects are often considered to be signs that the therapy is working. There is a potential for serious allergic reactions to Iscador; in fact, several cases of anaphylactic reaction, a very serious side effect, after the use of mistletoe products have been reported.[56] In addition, mistletoe itself is a potentially poisonous plant.

There is currently *no* evidence that Iscador can be used as an alternative to conventional cancer treatment. There is some evidence that when Iscador is used in addition to conventional treatment it may contribute to an increase in length of survival. Given the potential for adverse effects associated with this product, its use cannot be routinely recommended at this time.

Reishi Mushrooms

Reishi mushrooms *(Ganoderma lucidum* [Leyss. Ex Fr.] P. Karst.) have a long history of use in traditional Chinese medicine for a variety of conditions, including low immunity and cancer.[57] Although some immunostimulatory and anticancer activity has been documented in animal and laboratory studies, these effects have not been demonstrated in humans. There are no clinical trials evaluating the role of reishi mushrooms in the treatment of cancer.

The usual dose of reishi for cancer patients is 90 to 120 grams of mushrooms soaked in 500 milliliters of rice wine. The usual daily dosage is 60 milliliters of extract twice a day. Reishi is also available as 300-milligram capsules (containing a 50:1 extract). The dosage varies from 1 to 9 capsules daily. Finally, 1 to 2 milliliters of the commercially available aqueous-alcoholic extracts (1:2) are recommended to be taken up to three times daily.

The adverse effects associated with ingesting reishi for three to six months include skin rash; dryness of the mouth, throat, and nasal passages; upset stomach; and bloody diarrhea.[58–60] In addition, reishi mushrooms should be used with caution by individuals taking angiotensin-converting enzyme inhibitor drugs, drugs that affect the blood's ability to clot (for example, aspirin and warfarin), or drugs used in the management of diabetes.[61] Women who are pregnant or nursing should also use reishi mushrooms with caution because of the lack of information about their potential effects on the unborn or newly born child. Further research is necessary before reishi mushrooms can be recommended in the management of cancer.

Shiitake Mushrooms

Shiitake mushrooms *(Lentinus edodes* [Berkeley] Singer) have a long history of use in traditional Chinese and Japanese medicine to stimulate the immune system. Lentinan, a compound found in shiitake mushrooms, is approved in Japan for the treatment of gastric cancer; it is thought to increase the efficacy of conventional cancer treatments.[62] Several clinical trials suggest that lentinan may act as an immunostimulant and may be beneficial in the management of a variety of cancers, including cervical cancer, uterine cancer, prostate cancer, and stomach cancer.[63–65] This is supported by the findings of animal studies that have documented antitumor and immune-stimulating activity. However, the poor quality of the studies led researchers to recommend further studies to determine whether or not lentinan is in fact effective.

In many of the studies to date, lentinan was injected intravenously at a dosage of 2 milligrams per week, administered as either one or two doses. Dried powdered shiitake may be given in a dosage of 400 milligrams three times a day. However, fresh shiitake mushrooms are thought to have little medicinal value because they contain very little lentinan.[66]

A variety of adverse effects have been reported by patients taking lentinan. They include flu-like symptoms, heartburn, chest pressure, muscle pain, joint pain, nausea, vomiting, constipation, coughing, sinus pain, mouth ulcers, lightheadedness, and difficulty breathing. Allergic reactions have also been documented. Lentinan may decrease the body's ability to metabolize some drugs (those using the cytochrome P450 pathway) and may decrease the blood's ability to clot. Given these potential interactions with drugs, lentinan should be avoided by anyone taking drugs that affect blood clotting, like aspirin and warfarin. In addition, women who are pregnant or nursing should avoid taking lentinan until further information about its safety is available.[67] Further research is necessary before lentinan can be recommended for use by breast cancer patients.

Shark Cartilage

In the early 1950s, Dr. John F. Prudden, a surgeon at Columbia Presbyterian Medical Center, began using bovine cartilage to accelerate wound healing in surgical patients. In 1972, Dr. Prudden used cartilage powder to treat a woman with ulcerated breast cancer. Her cancer appeared to completely regress, and she was in remission for twelve years before dying of causes unrelated to her breast cancer. In addition, several laboratory studies suggested that cartilage had the ability to cut off the blood supply of tumors and thus inhibit their growth. These reports led to the popularization of shark cartilage as an anticancer treatment in the 1970s. Patient testimonials and the widely publicized claim that "sharks don't get cancer" fueled the popularity of this agent.[68]

Commercially available shark cartilage products are made from the cartilage of three shark species found in the Pacific Ocean: spiny dogfish shark, hammerhead shark, and blue fish shark. The dried powdered cartilage contains a variety of components, including protein, glycosaminoglycans (mainly chondroitin sulfate), and calcium. There are no standards for shark cartilage products sold in North America; thus, the composition may vary dramatically among manufacturers and from batch to batch from the same manufacturer.[69]

Despite the commercial hype surrounding shark cartilage, its use as an anticancer treatment is not supported by objective evidence. Several early studies reported that shark cartilage powder increased the length of survival of terminally ill cancer patients. However, the studies were poorly designed, and additional studies could not confirm those early results.[70,71] A recent clinical trial reported that shark cartilage powder had no activity in patients with a variety of advanced cancers.[72] Two small studies of the effectiveness of shark cartilage for the management of breast cancer have had disappointing results. In one study of twenty breast cancer patients, only ten of whom completed the study, there were no significant changes in quality of life, pain scores, or performance status after the women had taken shark cartilage for at least two months.[73] A second study designed to analyze the effects of shark cartilage in a group of fourteen women with Stage IV breast cancer also had unconvincing results. Only four of the fourteen women completed the twenty weeks of treatment. Two women had no response to the shark cartilage, one woman's disease appeared stable, and the fourth participant had evidence of a reduced neck metastasis and disappearance of a lung metastasis.[74] Currently, a clinical trial sponsored by the National Cancer Institute is under way to investigate the effect of shark cartilage in patients with metastatic lung cancer whose disease has failed to respond to conventional treatments.

The typical dosage of shark cartilage varies greatly, depending on the manufacturer and the patient's condition. Research studies have used doses of approximately 1 gram per kilogram of the patient's body weight (1 kilogram = 2.2 pounds) per day. For example, a 150-pound woman would take approximately 70 grams of shark cartilage per day. Dosage directions provided on product labels should be followed. No serious adverse reactions associated with ingesting shark cartilage have been reported. However, some patients have experienced nausea, vomiting, dizziness, a bad taste in the mouth, weakness, fatigue, and constipation.

It is currently recommended that shark cartilage be avoided by children, patients who have recently experienced a heart attack or undergone surgery, and women who are pregnant, trying to become pregnant, or nursing. Shark cartilage contains calcium and may cause hypercalcemia (calcium levels that are too high) if taken together with calcium supplements.[75] Currently, the scientific evidence suggests that shark cartilage will not help patients with cancer.

Using Natural Health Products with Conventional Cancer Treatments

There is little or no research to determine what happens when patients take natural health products together with conventional cancer treatments. Although it is possible that the combination may be beneficial and synergistic, it could also have negative effects. Thus, many practitioners recommend that patients avoid natural health products while undergoing radiation or chemotherapy. However, if you do decide to take a natural health product at the same time as your conventional therapies, it is very important that all your caregivers know about your decision. Your choices may have profound effects on your medical outcome, and any positive results will spark curiosity from the medical community and hopefully lead to further investigation of these unconventional modalities. Also, in the event that you suffer an adverse reaction, especially a new or uncommon side effect to the treatment, your health care team will be fully aware of the potential causes and in the best position to adequately help you recover.

Conclusion

Unfortunately, there are no magic bullets. Because the evidence is so scarce that any of the natural health products reviewed here will prevent or cure cancer, it would be premature to routinely recommend them to patients. However, some of these products look promising—for example, green tea for the prevention of some types of cancer and Iscador as an adjunct to conventional cancer treatment—and many are currently being investigated in research centers across North America.

Suggested Additional Resources

A GUIDE TO UNCONVENTIONAL CANCER THERAPIES
Ontario Breast Cancer Information Exchange Project
Toronto, Ontario, 1994
416-480-5899

CANADIAN BREAST CANCER RESEARCH INITIATIVE
Suite 200
Alcorn Ave.
Toronto, Ontario
Canada M4V 3B1
www.breast.cancer.ca/english/e_frame.htm

Information packages on Iscador, Essiac, green tea, hydrazine sulfate, vitamins A, C, E, and 714-X (1996, Canadian Breast Cancer Research Initiative).

CENTRE FOR ALTERNATIVE MEDICINE RESEARCH IN CANCER
www.sph.uth.tmc.edu/utcam/therapy.htm

CHAPTER NINE

Micronutrients: Vitamin and Mineral Supplementation

Keith I. Block, M.D.

KEITH I. BLOCK, M.D., is a cancer specialist and the medical-scientific director of the Block Center for Integrative Cancer Care, a research and treatment center integrating the best of conventional medical care with scientifically sound alternative therapies. For over twenty years, Dr. Block has been developing innovative, comprehensive treatment programs that provide custom-tailored, individualized care. Block and his staff of specialized caregivers treat patients with a diverse array of therapies, including chemotherapy in continuous and fractionated doses, chronochemotherapy (circadian timing of treatment in order to reduce toxicity while improving efficacy), personalized mind-spirit strategies, acupuncture, aromatherapy, prescriptive therapeutic exercise, nutritional counseling with disease-specific modifications, herbal and botanical supplementation, and micronutrients such as multivitamins, antioxidants, and other dietary support. Dr. Block is the editor-in-chief of *Integrative Cancer Therapies*, a peer-reviewed medical journal published by Sage Science Publications, and a clinical assistant professor in the University of Illinois College of Medicine and in the department of medicinal chemistry and pharmacognosy in the Program for Collaborative Research in the Pharmacological Sciences at the University of Illinois at Chicago. Dr. Block serves as a facilitator for the POMES Project at the National Institutes of Health in Washington, D.C., and is a member of the American Society of Clinical Oncology.

Sydney was in her mid-forties when she had a mastectomy to remove a 4.5-centimeter breast tumor that had metastasized to ten of her thirteen axillary lymph nodes. With a diagnosis of Stage III breast cancer, her prognosis was poor.

Although her doctors strongly recommended chemotherapy, Sydney instead chose to explore treatment solely with nutritional alternatives. When she came to my clinic six months later, we created a full nutritional program, and I explained some strategies for protecting all the healthy cells in her body. I also recommended fractionated dosed chemotherapy.

Sydney ultimately decided to combine chemotherapy with integrative approaches that included an individually tailored diet, a supplement program, stress care strategies, "mind fitness" training, and therapeutic exercise (yoga and qigong). She went through careful clinical, nutritional, and lifestyle assessments while figuring out what was right for her and for her particular situation. With all this in place, Sydney succeeded in bringing about a complete remission.

Five years later, Sydney is still cancer free.

Marcia's story also has a remarkable ending—from an even worse beginning. Just shy of age 40, Marcia was diagnosed with inflammatory breast cancer, a less common and more aggressive type of breast cancer. Her tumor was 5 centimeters in size, and the cancer had invaded her lymph nodes. The skin of her breast became extremely red and hot to the touch. The pathology report confirmed that Marcia had an aggressive type of cancer, which led to an unfavorable and most worrisome prognosis. Marcia was told that she had a mere eighteen months to live.

Marcia underwent eight cycles of a five-drug chemotherapy regimen, a bone marrow transplant, and radiation. She also followed an integrative care plan, which included therapeutic nutrition, a customized supplement regimen, and mind-body and lifestyle interventions. Certainly more research is needed to prove the value of these treatments. Nonetheless, Marcia's success story speaks for itself. Seven years later, she is alive and well with no signs of cancer.

These cases exemplify the possibilities with truly integrative treatments for breast cancer. It is the path we take and a course we help breast cancer patients navigate at the Block Center for Integrative Cancer Care in Evanston, Illinois. We've developed our approach over the course of twenty-plus years. By relying on precise clinical, nutritional, and lab assessments, we tailor treatments to the biological, social, and emotional needs of each individual patient. Our modified approach to conventional Western medical care includes a wide range of innovative, experimental, and complementary strategies. At our center the emphasis is always on the responsible and scientifically reasoned use of alternative treatments. Additionally, our central focus is on helping women follow nutritious diets along with specific combinations of vitamins, minerals, botanicals, and phytochemical supplements. These are intended to be integrated with, rather than substitutes for, conventional therapy. Our overall aim is to enhance the efficacy of conventional treatments, improve survival, diminish or eliminate the toxic side effects of the anticancer therapies, improve a patient's capacity to heal, and empower patients and families to more effectively confront the challenge of illness.

In this chapter, I have been asked to discuss one aspect of our center's care, micronutients. Over the past twenty years, there has been a dramatic surge in the interest in and use of micronutrient supplementation by patients with breast cancer. Micronutrients are the vitamins and minerals found in foods that our bodies require in relatively small amounts. They are among the most popular complementary therapies for cancer patients.[1] Today, as many as 60% of all cancer patients in the United States begin to use vitamin supplements at some point during their treatment.[2-5] There has also been a rise in the popularity of nutritional supplements in the United States. Between 1987 and 1992, retail sales of vitamins increased by 19%, to a $3.7 billion business.[6] In 1997, Americans were estimated to spend $27 billion dollars every year on alternative medicine, of which $5 billion was spent on megavitamins and dietary supplements.[7] By the early 1990s, one in every four Americans was taking vitamins daily,[8,9] and about half took them more sporadically.[10] Today, close to half of rural America is using supplements; yet, more than two thirds of the people surveyed were lacking vitamins and minerals in their diet.[11] It is also interesting that half of the female physicians in this country take at least one multivitamin supplement regularly.[12] Unfortunately, only 15% of our teenagers use supplements on a daily basis, and those who take supplements tend to have a more nutritious diet than their counterparts who tend to have a high-fat diet and more problems with obesity.[13] Supplement users tend to be white, female, affluent, college-educated, and of normal weight. They also tend to eat fewer high-fat, low-fiber foods, and they often avoid alcohol and tobacco as well.[14-16] Most people who use supplements do so without telling their doctors about it.

In this Information Age, you can easily access websites about breast cancer and the available supplemental treatment options. Much of the information on the Internet, however, may have no scientific basis, and may be inappropriate to your particular clinical situation and unique biomedical needs. Of course you can also obtain medical and scientific information through Medline and other academic databases, but the technical details can easily overwhelm even a knowledgeable lay person. My patients frequently discover contradictory and misleading information on the Internet. While supporting their search for useful therapies, I have found serious limits in the information they have collected, particularly when it comes to drug interactions between supplements and chemotherapy. This can include enhancing effective treatment while mitigating side effects. It also can include concerns of either stimulating tumor growth or interfering with conventional treatment.

Many health care providers—even proponents of supplement use—may not have the time for ongoing evaluation of the literature and thus may be insufficiently informed about the optimal and safe use of micronutrients and their complex mechanistic roles in cancer control and recovery. In part, that knowledge gap is understandable, given that new "nutriceuticals" are constantly being introduced, and physicians generally get little or no education on nutrition and nutritional pharmacology in medical school. On top of that, more research is necessary to fill the information gaps presently existing with micronutrients in the context of cancer and how best to use them.

For all these reasons, it is important to work with a health care professional to make the best use of supplements—to make sure the compounds are as risk free as possible while being maximally effective. The information presented in this chapter can steer you in the right direction, but in a book I obviously cannot tailor my recommendations to your particular set of circumstances. No two patients, and no two breast cancers, are exactly alike, and prescriptions should vary accordingly. That is not something you can do entirely on your own. This chapter will help you understand how you, working with your health care team, can take advantage of the powerful effects of micronutrient supplements while keeping an eye on any possible downsides. I'll review the micronutrients that have helped my patients combat breast cancer and give you guidelines for using them in conjunction with other treatments while recognizing they are only one aspect of a fully integrative treatment plan.

What Are Micronutrients?

As mentioned above, micronutrients are the vitamins and minerals found in foods. The need for micronutrients may fluctuate as conditions inside the body change. In contrast to micronutrients, macronutrients represent the host of foods that contain proteins, fats, and carbohydrates that are consumed in large amounts for the production of energy and support your physiology and functioning. You are probably already familiar with micronutrients such as vitamins A, B-complex, C, D, E, and K, and minerals like calcium, magnesium, selenium, and zinc. The body can make some vitamins, including vitamins D and B_{12}, though supplements may still be required if your diet provides inadequate amounts. Some vitamins, such as vitamin C, are needed in larger quantities in times of psychological or physical stress, such as major surgery, receiving a serious diagnosis, or undergoing invasive treatments.

Scientists identified the first micronutrients in the early 1900s when they discovered the role of vitamins B_1, B_3, and C in the prevention of diseases such as beriberi, pellagra, and scurvy. Understanding grew from there. More recently, a nonclassical, or secondary, category of micronutrients has emerged. These include molecules called biologics, which the body requires and can, in many cases, manufacture in small amounts to fulfill its biochemical needs. Examples include the amino acid glutamine, coenzyme Q10 (CoQ10), and melatonin. The body may also need more of these when under stress, and supplements can help bring the body back into balance with increased metabolic demands.

Many micronutrients are antioxidants, meaning they counteract the harmful effects of oxidants and free radicals, which can promote the growth and progression of cancer, among other things. Oxidants and free radicals may also harm tissues, damage cell membranes, destroy organelles, cause mutations to the DNA, or inhibit the body's ability to eliminate cancer cells through programmed cell death (apoptosis).

Supplements provide micronutrients in doses that are physiologic (smaller amounts similar to what your body makes) or pharmacologic (larger amounts, more equivalent to drugs). They all come in many different forms, some of which are more potent and/or tolerable than others. Just what form to use (buffered or not, natural or synthetic, capsule, tablet, or liquid, and so on) should be part of the plan you make for yourself with a practitioner who has expertise in this field.

Oxidants, Antioxidants, and Cancer

Oxygen is essential to life, enabling the body to produce large amounts of energy from a limited amount of food. Yet, sometimes the oxygen we consume turns into reactive molecules that are unstable and can interact with many signaling mechanisms. These molecules are sometimes called oxidants, reactive oxygen species, or free radicals. Some of this interaction is negative and can interfere with normal processes like DNA repair, growth factors, gene transcription, or the activation of oncogenes (genes capable of stimulating cancer cells to replicate). Large amounts of oxidants can result in tissue, DNA, and cellular damage that can lead to cancer and its progression. It is important to recognize that oxidants are crucial to some normal metabolism and immune functions. For example, they act as an alarm to attract phagocytes, the cells of our immune system, to eliminate invading bacteria.

To control the damaging effects of oxidants, the body has an elaborate system to neutralize and render them nonreactive. This system uses antioxidants that provide a chemical defense team systemically, mopping up oxidants and free radicals. The balance between oxidants and antioxidants is therefore crucial for the maintenance of normal health. On the other hand, any excess buildup of oxidants can cause modifications to DNA, such as strand breaks, that may cause cell mutations and initiate malignancy.

How Much Do You Need?

Much information on supplement doses is based on the Recommended Dietary Allowances (RDAs) the Food and Drug Administration established in 1941 (see Table 9-1). But most Americans take supplements in doses well in excess of those levels. And rightly so, since they are widely considered outmoded. Recently, the National Academy of Sciences' Institute of Medicine released a series of reports updating and expanding the general recommendations. The new dietary guidelines are called Dietary Reference Intakes and are far more comprehensive—and complicated—than the old RDAs. They add an upper tolerable intake figure, for example, defining the highest level of daily nutritional intake that is unlikely to cause negative side effects. These guidelines are more useful, but they still don't take into account critical information on larger, therapeutic doses of micronutrients. For breast cancer patients, the more general guidelines below can provide a place to begin, but many clinical factors are needed to determine optimal ranges when designing an integrative cancer care plan.

TABLE 9-1. U.S. Food and Drug Administration, Recommended Daily Dietary Allowances (revised 1989)

Protein	44 grams
Vitamin A*	800 micrograms
Vitamin D*	5 micrograms
Vitamin E *	8 milligrams
Vitamin K*	65 micrograms
Vitamin C†	60 milligrams
Thiamine†	1.1 milligrams
Riboflavin†	1.3 milligrams
Niacin†	15 milligrams
Vitamin B_6†	1.6 milligrams
Folate†	180 micrograms
Vitamin B_{12}†	2 micrograms
Calcium	800 milligrams
Phosphorus	800 milligrams
Magnesium	280 milligrams
Iron	15 milligrams
Zinc	12 milligrams
Iodine	150 micrograms
Selenium	55 micrograms
Total recommended calories	2200 calories with regular physical activity

*Fat-soluble vitamin.
†Water-soluble vitamin.

An Integrative Approach

The program at our clinic, on which this chapter is based, starts with the premise that an optimal biochemical environment, combined with target-specific therapies, will maximize the potential for overcoming cancer if all of the systems in the human body—immune, endocrine (hormonal), nervous, digestive, circulatory—work together to help create the biochemical environment for recovery from cancer. On the other hand, when one system is out of balance or dysfunctional, it can affect other systems in ways that promote the growth and spread of cancer, contributing to a biochemical atmosphere that can influence the ultimate course of the disease. Restoring balance is a major pathway to optimal health and maximum disease resistance. Our clinical program focuses on establishing the conditions that best support conventional treatment and sustain long-term remission.

Modern scientific medicine generally attacks disease with aggressive treatments. By contrast, our program strives to lay a solid foundation of gentle, natural, nurturing self-care practices that reinforce the treatment and recovery process. These practices are meant for use even before standard therapies begin, and they are also vital during and even after treatment. Its general principles apply to everyone, but our plan is then tailored to each person's specific symptoms, conditions, and biological, physical, social, mental, emotional, and spiritual needs. The program can work for anyone, but one size definitely does not fit all.

Diet

If you are not eating a nutritious diet, supplements will not be sufficient to counteract poor eating habits. More important, they enhance the foundation already created by good eating habits. I recommend a diet designed to remove toxins from the body while rebuilding your body's stores of nutrients and antioxidants. That means a largely vegetarian diet (with limited animal foods, preferably fish) centered on whole grains, land and sea vegetables, legumes, and fruits. Forget about the fad-of-the-month "diet" books aimed only at losing weight, sometimes at the cost of good health. You don't need any elaborate or confusing system. There's no magic bullet or secret formula. All it takes is a commitment to a balanced selection of nutritious foods. These are the macronutrients:

- Fats should constitute 10% to 20% of total calories and be mostly omega-3 (polyunsaturated) and omega-9 (monounsaturated) fatty acids like those from cold-water fish, nuts and seeds, canola oil, and high-quality virgin olive oil. The fat range is determined based on clinical condition, weight and appetite, disease, and laboratory considerations. Keep in mind that while malnutrition is always worrisome, weight gain with breast cancer, and particularly while undergoing chemotherapy, is associated with a poorer prognosis.
- Protein should make up 15% to 20% of the total calories each day and should come mostly from soy and other legumes, as well as fish. (As you are making the transition to this new way of eating, small amounts of skinless chicken can also be included.)
- Carbohydrates, then, are 60% to 75% of the diet, all from unrefined sources, including whole grains, vegetables, and fruits. Choose foods high in bioactive compounds like carotenoids and flavonoids. In other words, eat your vegetables! I encourage twelve-plus servings of fruits and mostly vegetables daily. This can take work to do, and I have developed a phytochemically rich, organically grown, vegetable-based product to assist my patients in meeting this need.

Steer clear of refined carbohydrates, especially white sugar and white flour. The same goes for stimulants (like caffeine), tobacco, artificial sweeteners, red meat, and dairy products. Alcohol, if you drink it at all, should be used only occasionally and taken only in small quantities. Both alcohol and smoking have been shown to fuel the development and progression of tumors.

For best results, this general diet should be individualized just for you and your specific biochemical needs. The type of disease you have, your body composition and condition, the phytochemical assessments of your body, your allergies or food sensitivities, and your ethnic, cultural, and personal preferences should all be taken into account when designing an optimal regimen for your personal requirements to challenge your illness. The types and amounts of proteins, fats, and carbohydrates that make up your diet all need to be considered in the design of your individualized micronutrient regimen. To this end, unrefined whole-food, vegetable-based sources are best.

Lifestyle

In addition to diet, regular exercise and good stress management are key components of a healthy lifestyle, and all three are necessary to take the most advantage of supplements and more disease- and target-specific treatments, including conventional approaches. Studies have indicated that exercise and stress reduction, along with an assertive, proactive "fighting spirit" and actively involved attitude, might positively influence the prognosis for women with breast cancer. Active involvement in a life-affirming system of care, together with attention to adjustments in severe stress-producing personal and environmental factors, can all contribute to the optimal conditions for cancer recovery.

The Truth about Cancer-Fighting Vitamins

As I've mentioned, your supplement regimen should be specialized for you and you alone. That will require working closely with a health care provider who is both knowledgeable and adept at designing a plan for you. Such a design should ideally take into account your type of cancer, any conventional medications being considered, laboratory assessments going beyond routine analysis, and your personal condition and needs. Later in the chapter I'll get more specific about how that kind of tailoring happens. Here I'll start by covering the most commonly used vitamin supplements to give you an idea of what they do—and what they can't do.

Vitamin A enhances and supports chemotherapy and radiation treatments.[17,18] It induces programmed cell death (apoptosis) of cancer cells and cell differentiation. (Differentiation, or full maturity, is a good thing: the less differentiated a cell, the higher the risk that it will become a cancer cell; the less differentiated a cancer cell, the poorer the prognosis.)[19–22] Vitamin A boosts the immune system, stimulating natural killer cell activity, and inhibits the creation of new blood supplies to tumors, a process called angiogenesis. It is important to work closely with your health care provider about an appropriate daily dose of vitamin A, because at very high levels, some particular forms of vitamin A may stimulate growth in some kinds of tumors and can cause toxic effects.

Carotenoids (carotene, lutein, lycopene) are molecules that can be converted to vitamin A. They boost the effects of some kinds of chemotherapy such as the alkylating agents (cytoxan is an example of one), particularly in combination with vitamin E. Carotenoids are effective antioxidants. I should also note that in two large studies synthetic beta-carotene seemed to actually promote lung cancer in smokers and/or asbestos workers, while one study of nonsmokers found no adverse effect.[23] It is not implausible that people with high oxidative burdens (i.e., excessive free radical activity due to smoking and a high-fat diet) would respond adversely to a single beta-carotene supplement. Beta-carotene becomes a pro-oxidant in the presence of such oxidative stress. Conversely, the pro-oxidant impact will more likely be abolished by avoidance of tobacco smoke, a low-fat diet, and supplemental use of other antioxidants, such as vitamin E, glutathione, and mixtures of carotenoids.

TABLE 9-2.   Preferred Food Sources of Vitamin A and Carotenoids

Milk and dairy products
Egg yolk
Fish oils
Dark green leafy vegetables (spinach, chard, kale)—not easily digestible
Carrots—not easily digestible
Mango
Papaya
Pumpkin
Sweet potato

B-complex vitamins enhance the function of both the immune system and the central nervous system. These vitamins are B_1—thiamine, B_2—riboflavin, B_3—niacin, B_5—pantothenic acid, B_6—pyridoxine, B_{12}, and folate. They act as coenzymes involved in cellular metabolism and are essential in maintaining normal cell function and ample energy production. B-complex vitamins can also reduce the negative side effects of chemotherapy. Niacin can enhance the efficacy of radiation treatments by temporarily increasing blood flow to tumors.

It is important to realize that breast tumors can be stimulated by certain B vitamins, even those found in low doses in foods.[24] However, prolonged use of high doses of niacin can stimulate the supply of blood and nutrients to growing tumors. Moreover, taking more than 500 mg of niacin daily over a long time can damage the liver. Niacin can also cause uncomfortable "flushing," though the ester form of the vitamin avoids this problem in most people. On the favorable side, the ester form provides inositol, an important cellular messenger that can boost the positive effects of properly used niacin.

TABLE 9-3. Preferred Food Sources of B Vitamins

Thiamin (vitamin B₁): wheat germ, whole wheat, yeast, nuts, pork, duck, oatmeal (in descending order)

Riboflavin (vitamin B₂): dairy, eggs, yeast extracts (almost all food contains some vitamin B₂)

Niacin (vitamin B₃): meat, poultry, fish, brewer's yeast, yeast, peanuts, bran, whole wheat (in descending order)

Pyridoxine (vitamin B₆): meats, whole grains, vegetables, nuts; available in unprocessed foods

Biotin: nuts, whole grains, dairy, vegetables, brewer's yeast

Pantothenic acid (vitamin B₅): whole-grain cereals, eggs

Folate: green leafy vegetables, beans, beetroots, bran, peanuts, avocados, bananas, eggs, fish

Vitamin B₁₂: food fermented by bacteria, meat, shellfish, fish, eggs, dairy

Vitamin C, like vitamin A, enhances and supports chemotherapy and radiation,[25-27] induces cell differentiation and apoptosis, and boosts the body's immune response by activating natural killer cells. Although some concerns were raised by the recent finding that cancer cells take up large amounts of vitamin C, this may in fact explain the widely reported *selective* killing effect of the vitamin on cancer cells, while normal cells are spared and apparently protected. Vitamin C can act as an anti-inflammatory and analgesic agent, providing pain relief. In a clinical trial, the combination of vitamin C (500 mg) and vitamin E

(400 mg) supplementation administered during tamoxifen treatment for women with breast cancer reduced the levels of cholesterol and lowered the risk of tamoxifen induced hypertryglyceremia.[28] Although these positive effects are noted for women with breast cancer, data suggest that leukemia cells may be stimulated by vitamin C.

High doses of vitamin C (> 3000 mg) can cause diarrhea and abdominal bloating, but decreasing your dose resolves such problems immediately. You can avoid the problem by using divided doses, and gradually increasing your total daily dose over the course of a week.

People who have had kidney stones or have kidney disease or are on dialysis should use caution with high doses of vitamin C. Don't take vitamin C supplements if you have hemochromatosis or other iron overload diseases. Discontinue supplementation if you are being screened for blood in your stool or sugar in your urine, as high doses can lead to erroneous results.

If you are using high doses of vitamin C, you should have your iron level checked, as high levels of both can cause oxidative damage in the body.

TABLE 9-4.   Preferred Food Sources of Vitamin C*

Blackcurrant
Kiwi
Cauliflower
Broccoli
Honeydew melon
Oranges
Strawberries
Grapefruit
Spinach
Pineapple
Sea vegetables
Tomatoes
Cabbage
Potatoes
Peaches

*In descending order.

Vitamin D inhibits the development of blood vessels to the tumor (which any tumor needs to survive), and induces cell differentiation and apoptosis in many types of breast cancer cells. It may also increase the number of vitamin A receptors on cells, allowing that vitamin to do its best work. Although there isn't enough clinical information to fully understand the phenomenon, very high doses of vitamin D can cause the loss of calcium from the bones. Therefore, vitamin D should not be taken without calcium.

TABLE 9-5. Preferred Food Sources of Vitamin D

Fish liver oils (cod, halibut)
Fish (sardines, tuna, salmon, and other fatty fish)
Milk is fortified with vitamin D in the United States.

Vitamin E can boost the effects of chemotherapy and protect cell membranes and mitochondria against the effects of free radicals that can damage cell integrity. It also helps improve the functioning of the immune system and the central nervous system. Vitamin E can protect against any negative side effects from high doses of vitamin A and preserves the supply of that vitamin, thereby boosting its beneficial potential.

On a cautionary note, vitamin E reduces platelet aggregation and platelet adhesion to collagen, thereby reducing the effectiveness of the blood clotting system. When it is combined with blood thinners like aspirin and coumadin, vitamin E in dosages of more than 300 IU a day (1 mg = 1.5 IU) can cause dangerously low platelet counts that can result in internal bleeding. Anyone with low platelet counts identified during chemotherapy should use less than 600 IU of vitamin E per day. If you have diabetes, rheumatic heart disease, or an overactive thyroid, keep levels below 600 IU daily. If you have high blood pressure, start with no more than 200 IU and increase gradually only while obtaining regular blood pressure monitoring.

TABLE 9-6. Preferred Food Sources of Vitamin E

Wheat germ oil (richest source)
Whole cereal grains

(continued)

TABLE 9-6.   *(continued)*

Leafy vegetables
Many other vegetables
Raw almonds
Peanuts
Other nuts and seeds

Anticancer Minerals

Naturally, whatever minerals you use should also be prescribed specifically for you. But to get you started in the right direction, I have listed some of the most commonly used choices.

Selenium is an antioxidant and an essential ingredient for the immune system. At higher doses it helps suppress tumor formation and metastasis. Many kinds of chemotherapy result in selenium deficiency, requiring repletion of this micronutrient. Selenium works best in conjunction with vitamin E. Since high doses of selenium may make some tumors more resistant to chemotherapy, I recommend 200 micrograms a day as the official safe upper limit. Higher amounts may be considered only with a full working knowledge of when this is safe and supported by data and experience. Dosage ranges as high as 600 to 800 micrograms per day have been used.

TABLE 9-7.   Preferred Food Sources of Selenium

Fish (the most stable source of selenium)
Grains and vegetables (vary greatly depending on the richness of selenium in the soil where they are grown)

Zinc is another good antioxidant and supports normal cell metabolism, immune system function, and central nervous system operation. It is often depleted in people with cancer. Additionally, the zinc/copper ratio is often low in cancer patients, which can contribute to inflammation and the formation of new blood vessels, including those that feed a tumor. High doses of zinc (above 100 mg/day) can actually suppress immunity. While I recommend 30 to 50 mg/day, exceptions do exist. Too much zinc can also counteract the effects of selenium.

TABLE 9-8. Preferred Food Sources of Zinc

Zinc from animal products is more readily absorbed by the body, but it may also be found in seafood (oysters) and organically grown whole-grain cereals, whole-grain breads, green vegetables, legumes, and nuts.

Magnesium is essential to cell metabolism (it is a component of adenosine triphosphate, a substance that provides energy to the cell) and is important for proper immune system functioning. Of concern is that some tumors may be stimulated by magnesium.

TABLE 9-9. Preferred Food Sources of Magnesium

Green vegetables
Cereals
Legumes

Iron is one of the few minerals that women with breast cancer should use with considerable caution, though iron is sometimes necessary in low dosages (10 to 20 mg/day) for someone recovering from chemotherapy-induced anemia. Iron can contribute to oxidative damage in the body—it can act like an "antiantioxidant," particularly if you already have too much iron and then take high doses of vitamin C. (Copper has a similar effect and should not be added as a supplement.) Cancer patients undergoing chemotherapy often have high levels of iron, which can cause excessive oxidative stress.

Furthermore, many types of bacteria require iron for growth, and the body "hides" large amounts of iron in the liver and other storage sites when an infection is present. Iron supplements can be a risk for anyone with an infection, and they may encourage an outbreak of a latent infection. With infection being a common cause of concern and associated with treatment-related marrow suppression and low white blood cell counts, iron supplementation may increase unnecessary risk of morbidity and mortality. It may also promote cell proliferation, which can be a risk for cancer growth when disease is present.

Other Beneficial Micronutrients

Melatonin, CoQ10, and other nonclassic micronutrients may also improve the clinical course of breast cancer, though their use, too, should be based on your specific constitution and disease involvement, determined with the help of an experienced expert.

Glutamine is the most abundant amino acid in human blood and muscle, and is made by healthy bodies. However, when a breast cancer patient undergoes major surgery or intensive radiation treatments, glutamine usually becomes severely depleted, so I recommend carefully timed supplemental use.[29–31] Glutamine is helpful in regenerating intestinal tissues and strengthening immune function in cases of advanced cancer.

Coenzyme Q10 (CoQ10) is an antioxidant that works closely with vitamin E and enhances several important biochemical functions in the human body. When all goes well, your body makes what you need, and it helps protect against free radical damage. But when a particular organ (most often the heart) or the body as a whole is overwhelmed by oxidation and free radicals, the body can't meet its own needs, and I will encourage supplemental dosing.[32,33]

Women with breast cancer tend to be deficient in CoQ10[34] because their bodies are not making sufficient quantities. Furthermore, CoQ10 protects the heart against the toxic side effects of some chemotherapy, particularly doxorubicin/adriamycin. Thus, women with low levels of CoQ10 are at greater risk of developing heart problems following treatment with adriamycin.[35,36] Supplementation can help to counteract these possible treatment after-effects.

Melatonin is another powerful antioxidant that helps modulate the immune system. The body produces its own supply, and supplements are derived from grains and beans.[37] As a hormone, melatonin has been shown to be effective against breast and other types of cancers.[38–40] Many women with breast cancer have low levels of melatonin, and research shows that low melatonin levels are associated with other indicators of poor prognosis, such as being estrogren receptor negative or having cells that are dividing very quickly ("high nuclear grade").[41] Melatonin levels in the body normally shift over the course of a day, usually peaking at night. Low nighttime levels have been implicated in breast cancer, as well as in menopausal symptoms such as insomnia and general signs of aging. For these reasons, women with low levels can benefit from melatonin replacement therapy.[42]

In addition to the direct beneficial effects, melatonin is also useful in combating the negative side effects of conventional treatment. It can inhibit peripheral nerve damage resulting from chemotherapy and can also help reverse the thrombocytopenia (low levels of platelets in the blood) commonly induced by chemotherapy.[43] Additionally, melatonin can enhance the effects of various chemotherapy regimens, although the chemotherapy drug 5-FU can inhibit the anticancer effects of melatonin.[44]

N-acetylcysteine (NAC) helps deactivate carcinogens and defuse toxicity. It protects healthy cells against the negative effects of chemotherapy and radiation (by increasing the normal cells' internal production of glutathione, a potent antioxidant) and helps prevent metastasis.

Arginine, another amino acid, has been shown in laboratory studies to enhance immune function and inhibit tumor growth. Many of its effects on the immune system have been reproduced in humans, but few studies have shown a direct effect on human tumors.

One study examining the effects of arginine in women with breast cancer has generated concern about recommending its use. In the study, the women were randomly assigned to receive either a standard diet or an extremely high dose of arginine (30 grams/day in four divided doses for three days before surgery).[45] At the time of surgery, tumor protein synthesis (a measure of growth stimulation) was significantly higher in the patients receiving arginine supplements. Although these results suggest that arginine should be avoided after a diagnosis of breast cancer, the amount used in the treatment group was quite large, and therefore the findings may not apply to the more typical dose of a few grams per day taken as a supplement under medical supervision.

Flavonoids are a group of antioxidant compounds that include quercetin, soy genistein, rutin, hesperidin, kaempferol, and myricetin, which are most abundant in brightly colored fruits and vegetables. In addition to ridding the body of harmful free radicals, many flavonoids are also toxic to cancer cells. They exhibit anti-inflammatory, antiestrogen, and antimetastatic effects. Soy genistein (isoflavone) helps modulate the immune system and can work synergistically with tamoxifen in blocking the growth of estrogen receptor–negative breast cancer cells.[46] Cell culture studies show that genistein and quercetin together can kill a wide range of cancer cell lines.[47]

The flavonoid tangeretin, found in citrus fruits, interferes with tamoxifen's inhibition of mammary tumors in animals (the equivalent of human breast cancer).[48] The soy flavonoid (isoflavone) genistein diminished the effectiveness of tamoxifen in a study of cell cultures.[49] Until more research is done, it may be best to avoid using pharmacologic doses of tangeretin and other flavonoid compounds if you are taking tamoxifen. The FDA recommends 25 grams of soy protein per day for its ability to lower cholesterol levels and protect the heart. Each gram of soy protein has an estimated 1 to 2 milligrams of isoflavones, so you should limit yourself to 40 to 70 milligrams of isoflavones a day to make sure you don't exceed what you might get in a normal diet. (For further discussion about soy, see chapter 6). Lastly, patients with breast cancer face many challenges. Having worked with patients suffering from this disease for more than two decades has provided the experience necessitating our development of a specific set of micronutrient, phytochemical, and botanical formulations. While space does not allow me to cover this vast array of valuable therapies, it is important to note that for the patient looking for evidence-driven low-invasive treatments, such answers do exist.

How to Make the Program Your Own

The key to making good nutrition and supplements work for you is to match your plan to your specific biochemistry. At Block Center for Integrative Cancer Care, we do this with clinical observation, careful histories, and comprehensive laboratory and tumor tissue analysis to evaluate all the systems that contribute to the internal environment of the body and the disease. The molecular markers assessed for targeting control and down-regulate further growth of breast cancer cells. We also assess each patient's medical history, diet, physical habits, and lifestyle habits as well as her emotional and mental well-being. We then select the specific micronutrient and botanical combinations that enhance and support the specific needs of each patient to more effectively combat her illness.

Our goals include supporting, stabilizing, adjusting, and optimizing the body's internal environment while targeting the disease with conventional, experimental, and nutritional compounds. We consider four important general factors when creating an individualized supplementation program:

- A breast tumor can significantly change a person's nutritional status. That is, the disease itself can alter the body's biochemistry, affecting several systems, including the immune system, and making it hard for the body to combat the cancer. Breast cancer patients are vulnerable to a range of micronutrient imbalances, and the deficiencies are highly dependent on the stage of disease (along with specific treatments). It is common to see low levels of vitamin A, C, and E in women with breast cancer as well as low levels of selenium, CoQ10, melatonin, and DHEA. Supplementation, when used with the foods listed in Tables 9-2 to 9-9, can bring the body back into balance to restore its immune system and cancer-fighting abilities.

- Surgery, chemotherapy, and radiation can further stress the body, leading to nutritional imbalances and deficiencies, which in turn can interfere with the full effectiveness of these treatments. When properly put together, our micronutrient supplementation regimen, in combination with dietary plans, can enhance the effectiveness of conventional treatments and reduce their potential for toxic side effects.

- Treatment with most chemotherapy drugs (such as Doxorubicin/ Adriamycin) carries an increased risk of DNA damage in normal cells—a mutagenic effect. That can lead to an increased risk of cancers or more aggressive recurrences. Research shows that specific supplementation strategies can reduce the risk of these long-range problems.

- After the removal and/or eradication of a tumor, therapeutic supplementation and nutrition can be used to activate the body's anticancer defenses, inhibiting the growth and spread of tumors, helping to prevent recurrences and metastases, and sustaining remission.

Because of the many favorable synergies and worrisome interactions, it is best to work under the guidance of a practitioner with expertise in both conventional care and in nutrition and supplements who can evaluate with some precision your personal biochemistry and tumor markers and assist in orchestrating a precise and optimal regimen, including the most advantageous selection of supplements. To accomplish this, one needs to analyze four broad areas: the cancer itself, other medical conditions, more advanced biochemical conventional treatments being used, and the results of testing.

Disease and Condition

I often see two women on the same day with the same diagnosis of breast cancer, at the same stage; yet, the two patients will have very different conditions and constitutions that demand different supplementation regimens. For example, Susan may be weak, with decreased muscle mass as a result of her breast cancer and having undergone aggressive interventions—so weak she comes into the clinic in a wheelchair. We'll develop a very different plan for her than for Jess, who is well nourished and full of vitality despite her disease and treatment. In fact, Jess goes jogging every day. By contrast, Susan's digestive system and metabolism are so weak that she needs to supplement her diet with nourishing foods that are easy to digest and in quantities that will not overwhelm her system. This demands dense caloric intake while still maintaining a cancer-resistant dietary approach. Susan's treatment emphasis may initially need to focus on regaining strength, vitality, and adequate nutrition intake before readdressing her primary focus, the treatment of her malignancy. Whereas Susan must be very conscientious in addressing her food and supplement intake, Jess is able to handle a large volume of intake and thus a calorically dilute dietary plan allowing for more flexibility to achieve similar aims. Additionally, Jess's supplement plan may have an emphasis on different priorities such as overcoming her illness, enhancing her treatment impact, and establishing a sustained remission instead of contending with the dangers of malnutrition.

To discover the best regimen in any given case, you need to make adjustments depending on the analysis of your tumor and the stage of the disease. In our assessment we review several factors, including a woman's menopausal status at the time of diagnosis, estrogen receptor and HER2/neu status, the DNA histogram (another measure of tumor proliferation), lymph node involvement, and any metastatic spread to sites beyond the breast and lymphatics. Additionally, tumor tissue profiling provides further direction in determining which molecular sites to target.

All other co-existing medical problems must also be taken into account in the decision making process. Diabetes, for example, must be addressed along with breast cancer, since women with diabetes are at a higher risk of recurrence.

As just one example, let me tell you about Stephanie. She came to us with treatment-related thrombocytopenia. She had been dealing with mitral valve prolapse, a heart condition for which she had taken the blood thinner warfarin (coumadin) every day for years before being diagnosed with breast cancer. She had heard about the benefits of vitamin E for the heart, and when she read that it was also thought to fight cancer, she wondered whether she should begin to take it as a supplement. But high dosages of vitamin E (over 400 IU a day) in combination with blood thinners would have increased her risk of excessive bleeding or hemorrhaging. (Taking garlic, ginkgo, and/or ginseng would have also amplified the risk.) So for Stephanie I recommended just 200 IU a day of vitamin E, with careful ongoing evaluation, to let her reap as much of the benefit as she could without causing any potential harm. For Stephanie, even with the relatively low dosage, regular follow-up visits were particularly important to make sure her regimen was both safe and effective.

Biochemical Testing

A basic clinical exam should be the starting point for creating your micronutrient supplement plan. Just the appearance of your tongue, the search for any cracks around your mouth and lips, and the color of your fingernails can provide experts with ample information to determine your nutritional status and overall deficiencies. Beyond observation, the standard complete blood count (CBC) and other chemical panels may provide further insight and at times crucial information. By looking at various aspects of your blood count and your chemistry, we can evaluate how your liver and kidneys function, whether your bone marrow is producing sufficient blood cells, and how well equipped your body is to fight off disease. In addition, more in-depth tests (as detailed in Table 9-10) can ascertain several important facts, including your specific nutrient needs and antioxidant status. By analyzing specific cell types, like subsets of lymphocytes or level of natural killer cells, we can determine how well your immune system is functioning.

At the Block Center we use an array of advanced lab tests (see Table 9-10) that give us a detailed picture of the biochemical conditions in a patient's body, which in turn gives us an idea of the aggressiveness and impact of her cancer on her internal environment and what is needed to change it. The three most important results we consider are micronutrient status, degree of oxidative stress or free radical damage, and the supply of certain antioxidants available for the body to use in its own defense. We rely on the findings from these tests to design an individualized micronutrient plan. Table 9-10 summarizes the most common tests we perform. You may prefer to discuss this type of testing with your nutrition expert.

TABLE 9-10.   Testing Your Body's Cancer-Fighting Potential

STATUS	TESTS
Tumor characteristics	Tumor markers (CEA, CA-15-3, CA 27,29, etc.) indicate the presence of cancer; tumor resistance factors (GST, MnSOD) indicate the resources the body has to fight the initiation and/or spread of cancer; overexpression of RAS, telomerase, Her2-neu, and others
Antioxidant/pro-oxidant ("redox") balance	Oxidative stress panel measures total oxidative protection (TOP) and the extent of oxidative damage: oxidized low-density lipoproteins, DNA oxidation, and lipid peroxidation (isoprostanes, urinary lipid peroxides)

(continued)

TABLE 9-10. *(continued)*

STATUS	TESTS
Micronutrient balance	Classic micronutrients: vitamin C (ascorbic acid), vitamin A and carotenoids, vitamin E (tocopherols), retinol, zinc/copper, calcium, magnesium
Immune competence	Natural killer (NK) activity, NK numbers, CD-4/CD-8 ratio, lymphocyte numbers
Toxin clearance capacity (TCC) and chemical burden	Measured by caffeine clearance (using acetaminophen and salicylic acid) and chemical burden (caused by exposure to toxins in the home and workplace)
Micrometastatic burden (MMB)	Measures number of circulating cancer cells in the blood with sensitivity up to 1 in 10,000,000 cells

Treatment-Induced Nutritional Deficits

With all this information in hand, I can then develop a strategic plan for each patient, adapting her nutrient program to the treatment protocols she is undergoing or will undergo. As I've mentioned, conventional treatments such as surgery, chemotherapy, and radiation can have major effects on the body's micronutrients. Each drug has a different mode of action and its own set of side effects and impacts the body's biochemistry differently. Therefore, each drug protocol requires different nutritional support. Likewise, radiation and surgery have very specific consequences on the body's nutrient reserves, and create different needs.

Many common breast cancer chemotherapy drugs have specific nutritional consequences. For example, adriamycin tends to deplete zinc, selenium, vitamin A, and vitamin E.[50,51] Cisplatin adversely affects the body's supply of vitamin D and magnesium.[52,53] Treatment with fluorouracil (5-FU) often leads to insufficient amounts of vitamins C and B_1. Whether these problems are part of the disease process or are due to the treatment—or both—in each instance, good nutrition and a wise supplement strategy can help restore the necessary nutrients to the body and enhance the overall efficacy of treatment.[54,55]

From the opposite direction, numerous combinations of micronutrients can enhance the effects of chemotherapy. For example, vitamins A, C, and E can improve the tumor-killing activity of adriamycin, the drug most commonly used to treat advanced breast cancer. After research in cell cultures pointed the way,[56-60] studies of mice treated with the drug showed that the combined action of the three vitamins boosted its therapeutic effects against tumors and also protected normal tissues.[61-66] Selenium proved similarly effective.[67,68] (Though no data yet exist to support the claim, some believe that selenium may also increase a tumor's resistance to chemotherapy over time, and more work needs to be done to establish whether or not the concern is warranted.) N-acetylcysteine also dramatically enhances the antitumor and antimetastatic effects of adriamycin.[69,70]

Another study looked at just vitamin A in conjunction with chemotherapy, using doses of 350,000 to 500,000 IU a day directly to the vein—far more than anyone would advise in the U.S., outside of a trial, due to toxicity concerns. In a trial of one hundred women with metastatic breast cancer, patients who received chemotherapy plus megadoses of vitamin A had a 38% response rate, compared with just 15% in those taking chemotherapy alone.[71] An impressive 93% of patients receiving the vitamin A had a projected survival rate of four years—more than three times as many as those who had chemotherapy alone. When only the postmenopausal women were compared, the advantage went up to four times as much.

Vitamin A is also helpful in conjunction with tamoxifen. Tamoxifen is the leading treatment for metastatic breast cancer, but tamoxifen resistance often leads to tumor recurrence.[72] A series of clinical trials in Italy showed that vitamin A supplements improved the outcome for breast cancer patients taking tamoxifen, particularly when combined with interferon, a protein produced by the immune system to make cells resistant to viruses.[73-77] The triple combination extended the length of response to the treatment beyond what tamoxifen alone produced.

You have no doubt noticed that the studies I'm describing focus on vitamin A as the sole nutrient. Discussing nutrients individually might be more manageable for researchers but does not reveal what will be most effective. In my experience, vitamin A is much more beneficial, is easier to use, and has fewer negative side effects when used in combination with other micronutrients, particularly mixed tocopherol vitamin E. By combining vitamin A with vitamin E, as well as vitamins B_2, B_{12}, and C, you can get most or all of the benefits with more moderate doses of vitamin A.

Some oncologists have their patients specifically *discontinue* the use of micronutrients, particularly antioxidants, during chemotherapy, out of concern that the antioxidants will protect cancer cells against chemotherapy just as they can protect healthy cells. Chemotherapy drugs work mainly by generating free radicals, which then damage cancer cells, so it is not unreasonable to fear that antioxidants might interfere with treatment. Radiation also relies on the deployment of free radicals, so the same concern has been voiced.

However, when used at high doses in combination with chemotherapy drugs, antioxidant supplements appear to act as pro-oxidants, which are toxic to cancer cells while retaining their antioxidant activity in normal cells.[78,79] Furthermore, many antioxidants have been shown to increase apoptosis, or programmed cell death, in cancer cells,[80,81] as do most chemotherapies.[82] The bottom line is that the preponderance of the existing evidence has shown that dietary antioxidants do not reduce the anticancer effects of either chemotherapy or radiation therapy. The best evidence to date simply does not support discontinuation of antioxidant therapy. There are, however, a few select areas of potential interaction between specific antioxidants and chemotherapy agents that warrant consultation with cancer specialists who have an in-depth knowledge of nutritional oncology.[83]

High-Dose Micronutrients

At very high pharmacological (with effects similar to those of a drug) or supraphysiologic (larger than what would occur naturally) doses, some micronutrients have been shown to be able to directly inhibit the growth of tumors, including breast tumors. At this level, it is absolutely necessary to work with practitioners who have expertise in nutritional therapy and understand the subtleties of host-tumor interactions. When drugs are mixed into the body's usual environment, there is both real potential for additive or synergistic effects and for conflict or interference between the drug and with micronutrients, which can reduce the efficacy of the drug.

Vitamin C was the first micronutrient used to fight cancer. To date, six clinical studies have reported better survival in patients with advanced cancers treated with high-dose vitamin C (5 to 30 grams/day).[84–89] Combining vitamin C with other vitamins (retinoic acid, beta-carotene, and vitamin E) enhances its ability to inhibit tumor growth, according to one study of cell cultures.[90] (Intriguingly, in the same study, low doses of vitamin C alone actually stimulated cancer cell growth, while high doses killed cancer cells.) Although many studies look at single micronutrients for the sake of the study design, in clinical use, combinations of micronutrients tend to be more therapeutic than any single one alone.[91,92]

The cell-killing, or cytotoxic, effects of vitamin C and other antioxidants are highly selective for cancer cells and spare—or even protect—normal cells.[93] For example, adding vitamins C and B_{12} to the diet of mice led to the regression of a kind of cancer known as Ehrlich carcinoma while enhancing the activities of immune cells.[94] Similarly, cell cultures enriched with vitamin C resulted in DNA damage and growth inhibition of cancer cells (human neuroblastomas), while normal neurons were spared.[95]

How Safe Are Micronutrients?

In general, micronutrient supplements have a large margin of safety compared with pharmaceutical drugs. The widespread use of supplements and the scarcity of reports of negative effects indicate that most preparations are safe for the majority of people. However, the fact remains that most medical professionals, including pharmacists, are not adequately prepared to address potential drug interactions with supplements. And as you've read in this chapter, some concern is justified: there *are* complicated interactions that must be addressed, especially with complex disorders like breast cancer. In most cases, there is a lack of clinical trial data on adverse effects, so it is usually difficult to quantify just how frequently, or infrequently, negative reactions occur.

Safe dosages have been established for many micronutrients. Only a few can easily reach toxic levels. In general, water-soluble vitamins such as C and B-complex are safe in high doses, as they are easily excreted. Still, even water-soluble vitamins in high doses can lead to problems in susceptible people.

More caution is warranted with trace minerals and fat-soluble vitamins such as A and D, as they become concentrated in tissues over time. Furthermore, trace elements like zinc, manganese, and chromium provide their many benefits only within a relatively narrow range of doses. Vitamins A and D become toxic at relatively low levels. Still, the numbers are far above what most people reasonably take: if you were to take 65,000 IU of vitamin D over several years, you'd get a toxic effect. Over time, the development of new forms of supplements of these vitamins, in fact both natural and synthetic, should help resolve potential problems. Some of these formulas are presently in the works.

While most supplements on the market today do provide micronutrients that breast cancer patients need, many also contain substances in doses that could be ineffective or, worse yet, unsafe. On top of that, many products contain potentially harmful contaminants such as microorganisms, heavy metals, and pesticides. Still others don't contain enough active ingredient to be meaningful, or fail to label all ingredients. Some don't dissolve appropriately.

Unfortunately, outside of a few facilities such as ours, supplements specifically designed to meet the special needs of cancer patients are quite rare. For patients and practitioners alike, regulations and standards are long overdue. Until that time comes, the burden unfortunately falls on you and your health care provider to sort out the best available products for you.

While we're waiting for universal standards and appropriate regulation, what is at risk is fully effective clinical care for all patients. In addition, research can be compromised. At our clinic, we address these issues by controlling every aspect of design, formulation, and manufacturing of the supplements our patients use. We've developed a core of micronutrient formulations to address the needs of women with breast cancer and to ensure that our patients get supplements made from only pure, high-quality ingredients—in the appropriate quantities—intended to protect healthy cells, improve the body's ability to battle the disease, and enhance treatment effects while diminishing negative side effects.

Trish

For the most part, I recommend micronutrients to breast cancer patients for their direct and immediate benefits, as we've been discussing. There's one other angle: prolonging your survival until a breakthrough therapy that might be right for you becomes available. That's just what happened to Trish, whom we kept stable long enough to be able to reach what was a new option to reverse her metastatic breast cancer.

Trish was in her mid-40s when she found a lump in her breast, which turned out to be cancerous. She had a mastectomy that revealed a 4.5-centimeter tumor, followed by five months of chemotherapy. She then took tamoxifen but stopped because of the side effects. It all seemed to work: no trace of cancer could be found.

But just over two years later, she began to show signs of what turned out to be extensive liver metastases. Her prognosis wasn't good. That's when she came to the clinic. Trish was not an active person, and she had a pretty typical American diet, which is high in fat and calories—the kind of diet we believe could be harmful in her fight against cancer. Furthermore, a history of breast cancer was in her family.

The program we designed for Trish included a second round of chemotherapy administered on a chronomodulated fractionated dosing schedule. Due primarily to the circadian timing and seventy-two-hour infusion method, along with IV micronutrients, Trish was able to tolerate the regimen with negligible toxicity. These innovations are documented to reduce adverse effects while improving treatment benefits. Additionally, we provided a comprehensive dietary regimen, which led to favorable changes in her eating habits to a low-fat, plant-based diet, and an individual stress care plan including biofeedback, our life strategies program, and cognitive restructuring, which help the mind and body have healthier physiological responses. Physical practices like yoga and qigong, designed to strengthen her body as a whole and especially her immune system, were also included in her program. Along with this regimen, we recommended specific oral micronutrients. As an example, Trish took CoQ-10 and magnesium citrate, a specific form of magnesium, among several others described in this chapter, in order to further diminish chemotherapy toxicity.

With these cutting-edge integrative methods, especially an advanced nutrition program, Trish was able to live a vital life substantially beyond what survival statistics would predict. That bought her enough time for Herceptin to become available to her. As it happened, Trish responded to Herceptin better than most patients do. I attribute her good response to her full program's building up optimal health in all her body's systems.

In a period of just over a year, Trish's metastases decreased significantly in size and number, and they continued to shrink until scans showed that her body was essentially free of disease. She will need medical monitoring for some time to make sure she remains disease-free. Trish's new diet has become a regular way of life for her now, and she still sticks carefully to her supplement regimen. The most remarkable change in Trish since we first met is her positive vision of the future, which she looks forward to with energy and enthusiasm.

Don't Go It Alone

Each woman's precise biochemical status is unique. Each breast tumor is different. Each course of conventional treatment is distinct. For every benefit of micronutrients, there is a potential downside if used inappropriately. Thus, this chapter cannot serve as a proper prescription for every woman. You will need to work with an experienced health care professional to design a program that is right for you, taking into account the interactions between and among your dietary choices, your condition, your biochemistry, and particularly your nutrients, herbs, and medications or chemotherapies. *"General use"* of supplements (i.e., not designed with cancer in mind and not tailored specifically for you) will *not* automatically enhance the treatment process. Misuse of micronutrients wastes time and money at best; at worst, it can be harmful to your health, interfere with treatment, and adversely impact your clinical outcome.

The safest and most effective way to use micronutrients is to combine them strategically and aim at multiple targets as determined by laboratory testing. Only a program carefully tailored for your needs can have the maximum biotherapeutic effect. Using multiple anticancer treatments, each with cancer-fighting properties but different mechanisms of action, is your best bet. To optimize your results, this means not only a full range of micronutrients but also a full range of conventional and complementary therapies. Just ask Trish.

CHAPTER TEN

Naturopathic Medicine

Leanna J. Standish, N.D., Ph.D., L.Ac.; assisted by Cheryl Grosshans, N.D.; Jennifer A. Lush, N.D.; and Michelle Robeson, N.D.

LEANNA J. STANDISH, N.D., PH.D., L.AC., is the principal investigator of the Bastyr University AIDS Research Center and Bastyr University Senior Scientist. She is a licensed naturopathic physician with a twenty-five-year career as a research scientist in experimental neuroscience who has spearheaded research on the efficacy of naturopathic medicine to treat breast cancer.

CHERYL GROSSHANS, N.D.; JENNIFER LUSH, N.D.; AND MICHELLE ROBESON, N.D., are recent graduates of Bastyr University.

I am a woman at high risk for breast cancer. No matter how much scientific understanding I gained, I had always been afraid of cancer, especially breast cancer—particularly because current scientific understanding is actually quite limited. No matter how much we've discovered about why and how it occurs, and what to do when it does, much remains to be learned.

When I am afraid of something, my standard practice is to dive straight into it. So I concentrated much of my research and my practice on breast cancer. I wanted to know as much as I could about this disease, not just from professional training, textbooks, and cutting-edge science, but also from sitting with and talking to women in my exam room. I wanted to learn from them what it is really like to be diagnosed, to break the news to loved ones, to make the decisions about conventional therapy, to learn to ask others for help, to sort through the ever-expanding options from complementary and alternative medicine (CAM), to have your world turned upside down, to find ways back to "normal" life.

Such a completeness of vision, I think, is crucial in being able to assess a woman's particular situation and so guide her in making the right choices. In this chapter, I bring to bear what I've learned about the most promising science-based natural medicine approaches for treating breast cancer, preventing its recurrence, and coping with the side effects of conventional therapy. I don't intend to cover everything in use for cancer treatment—just the treatments with the best evidence backing up effectiveness and safety.

As a naturopathic physician I am usually a member of my patients' health care team. I communicate with their surgeons, medical oncologists, and radiation oncologists. Many women choose to use both standard and CAM therapies, but they do so without cooperation among all their care providers. But you can't get optimal treatment without having everyone on the same page, sharing information and working collaboratively. Fortunately, I think almost all practitioners involved in breast care now strive for integrated care, or at least understand their patients' willingness to try the combination and the importance of the open exchange of information.

For my part, I see myself as a sort of coach for my patients, someone to help them develop a comprehensive game plan. I am outside of, but knowledgeable about, the conventional oncology realm, so women value my perspective on the options they are offered. I also make it my business to investigate available CAM treatments so I can help my patients sort out useful, science-based therapies from treatments that may be based more on self-delusion, wishful thinking, or marketing hype than on fact. Much of CAM has been practiced for a long time on the strength of trial and error, personal experience, and tradition. Many of those approaches may in fact be helpful, but now we're building a solid base of scientific studies and systematic clinical observation to validate the best approaches. Those evaluated therapies are the ones I'll present here. More work remains to be done, but the program in this chapter is supported by varying degrees of evidence of its effectiveness and safety in helping women heal from breast cancer and tolerate conventional treatments, minimizing and treating the side effects and maximizing the benefits.

Ronnie

Artist. Wife. Physical therapist. Mother. School board member. To her many and varied roles in life, Ronnie had just added breast cancer patient when I met her a few years ago. In her late 40s, she'd been recently diagnosed with Stage II breast cancer. She was facing a mastectomy in a few days, and chemotherapy the next month, followed by radiation.

Like every woman entering this brave new world, Ronnie's life was suddenly turned inside out and upside down. She fought back the best she knew how, though a lot of the time it felt as if all she could do was just get through the day. There's nothing special about her case—no miracle cure or unexplained recovery or unique symptoms. In fact, though every woman has her own story to tell, in brief outline Ronnie's case unfolds much like any other. That's why I'm going to keep coming back to her throughout this chapter, to make sure there's a human face to all the science I'm discussing. Of course, she didn't use or need every method in my toolbox, but she did benefit from many different natural medicines. The specifics of your situation won't match exactly, naturally, but I hope you'll see a little of yourself in her. Just as I do.

Goals and Principles

Naturopathic medicine is primary health care that emphasizes the prevention and treatment of disease and the promotion of optimal health with methods that support the body's own healing ability. Naturopathic physicians focus on treatment of the whole person, use natural medicines, encourage personal responsibility for one's health, and provide education about healthful lifestyles. Naturopathy blends centuries-old knowledge of natural, nontoxic therapies with current advances in the understanding of health and the human body. That includes herbs, nutrition, hydrotherapy, homeopathy, physical medicine, yoga and other forms of movement, and psychological counseling for total health.

Comprehensive Exams

Naturopathic medicine takes a more comprehensive, whole-person approach to breast cancer, and the differences from conventional medicine start with the diagnostic tools your naturopathic physician uses to determine your overall health. I use a blood "pesticide panel" to assess my patients' exposure to pesticides, for example. Few insurance companies will cover the costs of the test.

Listed below are the basic tests I see as crucial to the complete evaluation of a woman with breast cancer. In women currently receiving chemotherapy, I often wait until six months after the course is completed to do some of these tests, especially those of the immune system.

- Complete blood count with sedimentation rate and platelet count
- Blood chemistry panel
- T/B/natural killer cell immune panel (T-lymphocyte, B-lymphocyte, and natural killer cell immune panel)
- Natural killer cell activity test
- Thyroid panel
- Dehydroepiandrosterone (DHEA) serum test
- Bone density scan and/or n-teleopeptide urine test (for women who are peri- or post-menopausal)
- Complete digestive stool analysis and occasionally immunoglobulin G food allergy panel for women with a history of food intolerance or gastrointestinal complaints, with or without chemotherapy (see resources for these tests at the end of this chapter)

I was glad to begin working with Ronnie before her mainstream treatment began, so I could do these tests before surgery, chemotherapy, and radiation took their toll on the various measurements. Because she was experiencing severe fatigue, I also ordered a test for Epstein-Barr virus. It turned out to be negative.

Many diagnostic methods are common between naturopathic and conventional medicine. We use standard lab tests and clinical signs, including blood work, computed tomography, magnetic resonance imaging, and so on. It is the philosophy behind the information we choose to gather and what we then do with it that set naturopathy apart from the mainstream. Naturopathy searches for the cause of symptoms, not just ways to suppress them. It is a mind-body medicine aimed primarily at prevention and wellness, and committed to using the gentlest approach possible. The healing power of nature is central; the doctor is a teacher, not a boss. We do share with standard medicine the commitment expressed in the Hippocratic oath: "First, do no harm."

The Eight Principles of Naturopathic Medicine

- Use the healing power of nature
- Identify and treat the cause
- First, do no harm
- See the doctor as teacher
- Treat the whole person—mind, body, and spirit
- Focus on prevention
- Promote wellness
- Use the least force to obtain each therapeutic goal

All eight principles apply in treating breast cancer naturopathically, but there are also more specific treatment guidelines for breast cancer. We have identified ten goals for the treatment of breast cancer that follow the basic philosophy of treating the whole person as an individual, taking into account physical, mental, emotional, genetic, environmental, social, and spiritual factors. Later in this chapter we will walk you through each of these goals, providing you with the best known strategies for reaching each one, with specific treatments and state-of-the-art scientific knowledge about each.

Ten Goals of Naturopathic Breast Cancer Treatment

1. Prevent metastases
2. Block cancer cell cycle, induce apoptosis (cancer cell death), and reduce tumor cell division
3. Prevent mutation
4. Inhibit blood vessel growth in tumors
5. Enhance immune function
6. Decrease effect of estrogen on tumor

7. Remove initiators and promoters of malignancy
8. Provide nutritional support aimed at cancer prevention
9. Help patient access "the healer within"
10. Minimize side effects of conventional oncologic treatments

Art and Science

Naturopathic medical treatment for breast cancer is not standardized, and each practitioner may have his or her unique approach. In conventional breast cancer therapy there is far greater standardization. Conventional approaches are finite, whereas in natural medicine there are literally hundreds of different therapies that might be worth trying. The art of natural medicine is knowing which therapies are right for which patients, and in which combinations.

Still, naturopathic medicine is not just an art but also a science. Though much research remains to be done, many of the treatments used by naturopathic physicians have been evaluated in clinical trials, animal studies, and/or laboratory tissue culture experiments just as conventional therapies approved by the Food and Drug Administration (FDA) have been.

Ideally, we'd have huge, long-term, placebo-controlled clinical trials pinpointing the efficacy of all the treatments in the naturopathic toolbox. We have that for much (though by no means all) of conventional medicine, with drugs that go through a rigid step-by-step process from test tube studies through research in animals to multiple phases of human studies before gaining FDA approval and becoming generally available.

Most FDA-approved cancer drugs take seven to twenty years to develop and typically cost the pharmaceutical companies that ultimately patent them $75 million to $400 million to bring to the market. Because many natural products cannot be patented, there is little financial incentive to spend the millions of dollars required to get FDA approval as a cancer (or any other) therapy.

Many natural medicines, available by prescription and/or over the counter, have a long history of folk use and therefore a long history of being safe for humans. Many are what the FDA considers "generally regarded as safe." So when scientists do turn their attention to natural medicines, they often skip right over the test tube and animal testing in favor of clinical studies.

Positive results, even from small studies, tend to increase public confidence in a particular natural medicine, and are often used in marketing them. Nutriceutical companies often cite whatever laboratory and animal research exists in favor of their products as well. Sometimes the evidence is slim indeed.

But there is an impressive body of knowledge out there. Although even naturopathic physicians recommend natural medicines about which we have only incomplete scientific evidence, we often have more to go on than you might think. My colleagues and I have systematically searched the scientific literature to evaluate which CAM therapies have the strongest evidence backing up their use. This chapter presents the cream of the crop. All the recommendations here have either laboratory, animal, and/or clinical data showing efficacy: slowed disease progression, tumor shrinkage, and/or increased length or quality of life. Furthermore, they are known to have very low toxicity, based on those studies and long traditional use.

The big important question still remains to be answered definitively: Does CAM for breast cancer improve the final outcome? Almost all women who use CAM to cope with breast cancer do so in combination with conventional therapy. That makes sense to me. The available evidence certainly doesn't back CAM alone for breast cancer. I advocate for the studies that will give us the hard facts about the benefits of combining the best of conventional standard therapy with the best of CAM therapy. In the meantime, I'm more than convinced by my patients' experiences that someday those studies are going to show that we are on the right path.

Naturopathic Treatments for Breast Cancer

In the rest of this chapter, I'm going to take you through each of the ten naturopathic goals for breast cancer, with the best naturopathic treatments of choice for each, and a look at the science backing them up. If you have breast cancer, you should not try to be your own natural medicine doctor. Naturopathic physicians are licensed as primary health care providers in eleven states—Alaska, Arizona, Connecticut, Hawaii, Maine, Montana, New Hampshire, Oregon, Utah, Vermont, and Washington—and many practice in states that do not yet have a licensing procedure. Be aware that some people who call themselves naturopathic doctors have not received training from an accredited four-year institution. Rather, they paid for a correspondence course, and whereas they may have good information about natural medicine, they are not doctors. Find a qualified and licensed professional experienced in treating breast cancer, who works with conventional oncologists and surgeons. See Resources at the end of this chapter for guidance.

Goal 1: Prevent Metastases

MODIFIED CITRUS PECTIN

Once you've been diagnosed with breast cancer, the name of the game is preventing the spread or recurrence of the disease. That's a main goal of standard surgery, radiation, and chemotherapy, though they are not always completely effective. After standard treatment, or with it, modified citrus pectin (MCP) might help prevent recurrence. It was just about the first thing I gave Ronnie, so she could start on it immediately, to help prevent micrometastases, possibly released by surgery from adhering to other tissues and developing tumors.

MCP is just what it sounds like—a starch derived from the pectin in citrus fruit. It works by binding to a cancer cell protein, thereby preventing it from helping the cell to invade nearby tissues and spreading the disease.[1-3] Interfering with that process, then, can help prevent metastases.[4]

The protein that MCP binds to is produced at lower rates in late-stage breast cancer, so it is probably most effective when used in the early stages. I particularly recommend it to my patients with carcinoma in situ and to those who are about to have, or have just had, surgery.

Clinical studies have not yet been done to show the effectiveness of MCP in preventing metastases in humans. But animal studies give credence to its use. In one study, metastatic disease in the lungs of mice given MCP decreased 90%, compared with mice given unactivated citrus pectin as a placebo.[5] In another study, rats injected with prostate cancer cells, then given MCP in their drinking water, showed fewer metastases to the lung, compared with untreated rats.[6]

MCP PRESCRIPTION

Dosage: 1 teaspoon MCP powder mixed well in juice, taken twice a day.

Contraindications: There are no reports of toxicity or adverse drug interactions with MCP.

Goal 2: Block Cancer Cell Cycle, Induce Apoptosis (Cancer Cell Death), and Reduce Tumor Cell Division

It is possible to slow tumor growth in two ways. First, you can block the growth cycle and division of individual cancer cells. Second, you can

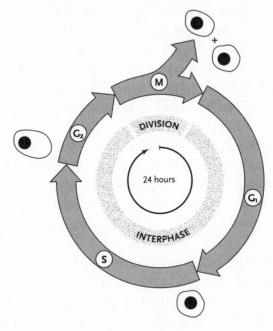

FIGURE 10.1. Cell cycle and division. During the S phase, the cell will replicate its DNA. In the M phase, the cell will divide its DNA into two identical parts and separate to become two new daughter cells.

accelerate the programmed cell death process called apoptosis, a process that all normal dividing cells possess and activate when they have lived out their useful purpose. Naturopathic medicine offers three prime treatments that can do one or the other—or both.

COENZYME Q10

Coenzyme Q10 (CoQ10), also known as ubiquinone, is an enzyme assistant crucial to the mitochondria, the energy-producing units of the cell. The human body makes its own CoQ10, but stress and illness can create deficiencies.[7,8] When you have breast cancer, you want to make sure you get plenty of CoQ10 to keep your healthy cells active. That's why I prescribed it for Ronnie.

CoQ10 supports healthy cellular function all over the body, benefiting the body in three specific ways. First, it supports the immune system. In fact, CoQ10 supplements have been proven to particularly affect the most metabolically active cells—including the immune system cells.[9,10] Second, CoQ10 is a potent antioxidant and thus protects the body from mutation-causing free radical damage. Third, cancer cells are real energy hogs and may monopolize the available CoQ10, leaving all the other cells in the body without what they need to function normally.

Most of the studies of CoQ10 have focused on its benefits for heart health. Heart cells are also among the most metabolically active in the body, so the heart is one of the places where CoQ10 is especially important. Published breast cancer studies have reported impressive results, but with less than impressive methodology. Still, the findings are promising and—at least until we get better data—compelling. In one instance, doctors reported that 390 milligrams of CoQ10 daily produced complete remission in five women with breast cancer.[11] In another study, thirty-two women with breast cancer that had spread to their lymph nodes took 90 milligrams of CoQ10 daily, along with 2840 milligrams of vitamin C, 2500 IU of vitamin E, 32.5 IU of beta-carotene, and 1.2 grams of gamma linoleic acid. After eighteen months, when statistics predict there would have been four deaths among them, all were still alive. Six had partial remissions (incomplete and temporary remission of cancer). None had metastatic recurrences.[12]

Two other studies, better designed and thus even more noteworthy, found that CoQ10 protected the heart from adriamycin, a chemotherapy drug known to be potentially damaging to the heart.[13,14] I recommend CoQ10 to many of my patients with breast cancer, and always to those taking adriamycin.

The vast majority of people have no side effects from CoQ10. As with all drugs or supplements, it is important to be mindful of possible interactions. CoQ10 can be depleted by 3-hydroxy-3-methylglutaryl-coenzyme A (HMG-CoA), reductase inhibitors (lovastatin, provastatin), beta-blockers (propranolol, metaprolol), phenothiazines, and tricyclic antidepressants.[15] Make sure you discuss possible interactions of all your medicines, both natural and conventional, with your doctor.

CoQ10 Prescription

Dosage: 200 milligrams twice a day, with meals. I often recommend taking cod liver oil at the same time, because CoQ10, which is fat soluble, is better absorbed along with fat. The best absorbed form of CoQ10 is an oil-based preparation, although powdered forms are effective, optimally so when taken with some kind of fat.[16,17] CoQ10 studies have mostly used the widely available powdered form.

Contraindications: None.

Garlic

I'm particularly excited by research at Bastyr University showing that in the laboratory, garlic can trigger apoptosis (programmed cell death) in breast cancer cells in a fraction of the time required for chemotherapy drugs to do the same job—in about two hours, compared with two to three days. Furthermore, the effect seems to be specific to hormone-sensitive breast cancer cells; prostate and colon cancer cells under the same conditions showed very little apoptosis (Sivam, unpublished results).

But that's just one of garlic's charms. According to a range of studies, garlic has a host of positive effects on the body when it comes to fighting breast cancer. It slows blood clotting, by an antiplatelet aggregation effect that may also interfere with the initiation of metastasis.[18] It enhances the immune system in ways that may have a significant impact on breast cancer.[19] Garlic is also an anti-inflammatory agent and inhibits the proliferation (division) of cancer cells.[20-33] It also has antioxidant properties, and high levels of antioxidants have been associated with a lowered risk of cancer.[34,35] Garlic protects the liver and stimulates the enzymes involved in eliminating carcinogenic substances from the body.[36,37] Increased intake of garlic (and fiber and onions) decreased the risk of recurrence of breast cancer significantly in one study of French women treated for early-stage breast cancer.[38] Furthermore, two epidemiological studies suggest a protective effect specifically against breast cancer.[39,40]

Garlic contains several chemical components that are potentially antitumor and anticarcinogenic.[41,42] Most studies zero in on garlic's organosulfur compounds allicin and allicin-derived thiosulfinates.[43] Despite numerous studies, we're still waiting to definitely define the biological and chemical mechanisms of garlic's therapeutic role.

The source and preparation of garlic are important in its effectiveness in preventing and treating breast cancer. Both European and American brands of garlic supplements vary greatly (twentyfold or more) in their composition.[44] One study, for example, found crushed garlic and microwaved crushed garlic to have anticarcinogenic activity—but not uncrushed garlic either microwaved or heated in an oven.[45] In another study, fresh garlic in the diet of mice bred to be at high risk of breast cancer tumors produced a greatly decreased incidence of tumors, while for allinase-inhibited mice, resulting in lower production of the active constituent, allicin, garlic did not yield the same positive results.[46]

I recommend either fresh crushed whole garlic or a water-extracted garlic powder standardized for high levels of allicin content. One product I use has 350 milligrams of dried whole garlic extract per enteric-coated tablet, which is equivalent to 1000 milligrams of fresh garlic (fresh garlic is 65% water). Perhaps the best way to take garlic as a medicine is to also use it as a food. I recommend that my patients use olive oil mixed with lots of fresh crushed garlic cloves rather than butter as a condiment.

Garlic is obviously a very common food and is generally regarded as safe by the FDA. In extremely high doses—over 25 milliliters of garlic extract—vomiting, and burning of the esophagus and stomach, may occur. Some people are sensitive to garlic and may experience allergic reactions, such as contact dermatitis and asthma.[47]

GARLIC PRESCRIPTION

Dosage: Depends on the protocol, usually 700 mg twice daily.
Contraindications: Do not use garlic supplements with blood thinners, such as warfarin.

QUERCETIN

The bioflavonoid quercetin is found in many plant foods. Just how much you get in your diet, and from what, depends on where you live. In the United States, most of our quercetin comes from onions. In Italy, it's red wine, and in China, tea.[48] Quercetin has generated a lot of interest over the last two decades because of its anticancer potential. Laboratory studies reveal multiple mechanisms by which quercetin can influence cancer cell growth and death. Other studies show that quercetin inhibits tumor growth in animals and that it keeps cancer cells from proliferating in the laboratory. It also interrupts the cell cycle and induces apoptosis.[49] Quercetin increases the amount of a tumor-suppressing protein that regulates the cell cycle and induces cell death.[50,51] Evidence shows that it interferes with signals between cancer cells and so can inhibit growth and initiate cell death.[52] Breast tumors in rats were inhibited by a diet rich in quercetin.[53] Human breast cancer cells showed a variety of antigrowth effects when treated with quercetin.[54] Rats on a quercetin-rich diet had a decrease in the number of breast tumors they developed when exposed to a potent carcinogen.[55] A case-control study using diet history questionnaires revealed that a higher intake of quercetin was associated with reduced risk of stomach cancer.[56] Quercetin also has antiestrogenic properties in laboratory models and these may have a favorable effect on hormone-response breast cancer.[57,58] Quercetin has also improved the effectiveness of adriamycin chemotherapy against adriamycin-resistant cancer cells.[59] Human clinical trials of quercetin for breast cancer have yet to be done, but studies of other types of cancers have shown its promise.

Some controversy surrounds the use of quercetin to treat cancer because it has been shown to be capable of causing DNA mutations. There is no information, however, to suggest that taking quercetin is carcinogenic in people. On the contrary, animal and human studies are encouraging. Studies on rats and rabbits, for instance, have shown it can be consumed even in very large amounts without any harmful effects.[60,61]

There is also some debate over the potential toxicity of quercetin. For example, one study using large intravenous doses of quercetin resulted in kidney damage in some patients. Fortunately, the kidneys recovered when quercetin was stopped. In any event, far lower doses will still provide effectiveness without harming the kidneys. In general, humans seem to tolerate it very well.

Taking quercetin orally, rather than by vein, is gentler on the body, too, but some question whether the body can fully absorb and use quercetin taken this way.[62]

QUERCETIN PRESCRIPTION

> *Dosage:* 1000 mg twice daily.
> *Contraindications:* None known.

Goal 3: Prevent Mutation

Antioxidants prevent damage from free radicals, which are unstable molecules produced by oxidation that can damage cells, including their DNA. Besides preventing the early cell mutations that initiate breast cancer, antioxidant vitamins also prevent further mutation in breast cancer tumors already present.

The most commonly prescribed antioxidant vitamins are vitamin A, beta-carotene, vitamin C, and vitamin E. Melatonin, another antioxidant, has been shown to help suppress breast cancer tumors in humans.

Ronnie took the natural forms of vitamins A, C, and E as well as melatonin (for its antioxidant properties, its immunomodulatory effect, and
the relief it brings for sleep problems).

Goal 4: Inhibit Blood Vessel Growth in Tumors

Tumors require the formation of additional blood vessels (angiogenesis) in order to grow. Without blood to deliver nutrients, the cells die, so
interfering with blood vessel growth in tumors is an excellent cancer-
fighting strategy. Several animal and laboratory studies provide evidence that soy, the omega-3 fatty acid docosahexaeonoic acid (DHA),
and selenium all inhibit that new blood vessel development.[63-67] Shark
cartilage and bovine cartilage have been heavily promoted as ways to
decrease blood vessel growth into a tumor. The data are insufficient to
support that claim, in my view, especially since confirmatory clinical
trials failed to show a benefit in advanced cancer. I don't recommend
either form of cartilage, at least not until better data emerge.

Vitamin D reduced angiogenesis in test-tube studies with breast cancer cells and in mice.[68]

Goal 5: Enhance Immune Function

This area gets a bit tricky, because we seem to live with the popular
notion that cancer patients need their immune systems fixed. A lot of
my patients come in asking me to "stimulate their immune systems."
This is, at best, an oversimplification that rings of "nutriceutical" marketing materials for unevaluated therapies. Enhancing a patient's general immune system function has long been a favorite approach, but in
breast cancer patients, it doesn't necessarily improve the body's ability
to fight a tumor.[69] On the other hand, women with breast cancer do
have somewhat depressed immune function—at least by some measures.[70] Still, it has not yet been proved that stimulating the immune
system can lower the chance of recurrence or progression of breast
cancer. In fact, many studies show no such effect,[71] though others,
described later in this section, do. In my opinion, general immune
therapy can be beneficial, but it is necessary only for those whose
immune panels show specific deficiencies. Examples of nonspecific

immune stimulation include nutritional medicines such as inositol hexaphosphate, or cytokines such as interleukin-2. Three immune-modulating therapies have the best evidence: melatonin, *Coriolus versicolor,* and aerobic exercise.

MELATONIN

Melatonin is a hormone used to maintain your body clock and your sleep/wake cycle—your circadian rhythms. Some scientists believe that low levels of melatonin put women at risk for breast cancer, but the results of studies are mixed. Some studies have, in fact, associated lower blood melatonin levels with breast cancer; but others have shown the opposite correlation: higher levels associated with increased risk.

Melatonin is often used at dosages from 3 to 5 milligrams per day (lower than what most cancer patients use) for jet lag, insomnia, and other sleep cycle disturbances. It has also been reported to lower total cholesterol and low-density lipoprotein levels in rats, and various theories connect low levels of melatonin to multiple sclerosis, sudden infant death syndrome, coronary heart disease, epilepsy, and postmenopausal osteoporosis. It is also a powerful antioxidant and powerful scavenger (quencher) of free radicals,[72] which may offer some anti-cancer protection. Our interest here, though, is in its ability to inhibit cancer by immune stimulation.

Many types of cancer, including breast cancer, have responded to melatonin, and melatonin has antitumor activity as well as immune system effects. It's been shown in the laboratory to inhibit the proliferation and reduce the invasiveness of tumor cells in general, and breast cancer cells—especially estrogen-sensitive ones—in particular (estrogen-insensitive breast tumor cells do not seem to respond in some studies).[73,74] In fact, melatonin may work to stop cell growth that is mediated through estrogen stimulation.[75] Melatonin can increase the cell growth– inhibitory effect of tamoxifen, a common antiestrogen used in breast cancer.[76]

Some studies use melatonin given by vein—dosing every 12 hours seems to be most effective—but animal studies show that melatonin taken by mouth also has cancer-fighting properties. For example, oral doses of melatonin suppressed spontaneous mammary tumors in mice genetically engineered to be at high risk for mammary cancer.[77]

Melatonin may also be a powerful adjunct to mainstream medical treatment. Take, for example, an Italian study of eighty patients with advanced cancer of different types in which half were given chemotherapy and melatonin, and half received chemotherapy alone. In the melatonin group, 19% had a complete regression of cancer, compared with 3% of the group receiving only chemotherapy. Survival after one year was also higher in the patients who received melatonin.[78] The same researchers also studied the effects of taking melatonin with standard chemotherapy, compared with chemotherapy plus placebo, and found that the melatonin group had less suppression of bone marrow function and neuropathy.[79] The same team evaluated melatonin in women with advanced breast cancer who were not responding to tamoxifen hormonal therapy and were then given melatonin to add to their regimen, and 29% then had a partial remission, lasting an average of eight months.[80]

Melatonin is safe if taken at the correct time: before bed at night. It does interact with some drugs, though usually by boosting their effects. That's just one more reason you should always tell your doctor about any medication you take, including supplements and natural medicines.

Melatonin is also useful in women with breast cancer who have trouble sleeping. Melatonin has been reasonably well studied for its effectiveness as a sleep aid, so it may be used at the lower doses for that alone—and perhaps you'll get some cancer-fighting effects, too. Or, if you have the kind of estrogen-sensitive breast cancer that is most likely to benefit from taking melatonin, you may get better sleep as a positive side effect of the higher doses. There is some evidence that nighttime secretion of melatonin in the brain is increased by sleeping in very dark rooms.

MELATONIN PRESCRIPTION

> *Dosage:* 20–40 mg at bedtime. Start with 5 mg and gradually build up over 1–2 weeks. (If you feel groggy in the morning, decrease dose by 5 mg.)
>
> *Contraindications:* Do not take if you also have an autoimmune disease.

PSK

Extracted from the Asian mushroom *Coriolus versicolor*, PSK has been shown to stimulate the immune system in both animals and humans. It has been used in Japan to treat cancer for twenty years. In one Japanese study, patients with advanced breast cancer receiving PSK in addition to chemotherapy had a ten-year survival rate of 81%, compared with 65% for those getting only chemotherapy.[81] Another study of 278 patients with Stage II breast cancer (not estrogen-sensitive) produced similar results: the five-year survival rate for the group getting PSK plus chemotherapy was 96%, compared with 81% of those receiving chemotherapy alone.[82] However, researchers found no significant difference in the five-year survival rates when patients with Stage II breast cancer (estrogen-sensitive) who combined PSK with tamoxifen were compared with those who used only tamoxifen.[83]

I'm among the many naturopathic physicians who recommend PSK for cancer patients, although only a few studies regarding its efficacy have been published. The existing evidence is a strong indication of its promise, and while we must wait for more definitive results, at least we know now that the treatment is safe.

PSK Prescription

Dosage: 600–1200 mg twice a day.
Contraindications: None known.

Aerobic Exercise

You won't find a safer and more effective way of improving your immune system function than exercise! Aerobic exercise increases the activity of natural killer (NK) white blood cells, which recognize and destroy abnormal cells, including malignant cells. Some but not all studies have shown an association of a lower risk of metastatic recurrence with higher levels of NK cell activity.[84] In a study of women with breast cancer who took up moderate exercise, NK cell activity increased.[85]

Exercise may produce a myriad of benefits, but if nothing else, exercise will make you *feel* better. In one study, quality of life was significantly higher for forty-two women with breast cancer who exercised than for twenty-nine women who did not.[86]

One of my patients who went through chemotherapy with minimal side effects told me her secret. She said that every morning at six A.M., no matter how she felt and regardless of the weather, she met her best friend and went on a brisk three-mile walk. This made the difference, she said. It's good advice.

For other, more athletic women I recommend twenty minutes a day of rigorous aerobic exercise.

The melatonin Ronnie was taking was also a powerful support for her immune system. She also took maitake mushroom extract to bolster her immune system. She was exercising and taking the supplements when a follow-up test of her immune system was completed. Because it wasn't quite up to par, I added a four-week course of PSK to her immune regimen. The principle is that an optimal immune system reduces the risk of recurrence.

I believe the future holds a lot of promise in the area of immune therapies, and labs and medical centers all over the country are at work on a wide range of techniques. In contrast to the general immune therapies discussed in this section so far, contemporary cancer immunology research focuses on specific immune recognition—acting on a particular antigen as the polio vaccine does, for example, rather than on strengthening the immune system as a whole, which is a much more nebulous undertaking.

Specific immune recognition is perhaps the most rapidly developing field in all of cancer research. Significant work is under way for patients with all stages of breast cancer. Scientists are looking at specific immune recognition approaches to breast cancer alone and in conjunction with surgery, radiation, and chemotherapy. So far, however, no immunotherapy meets the current standard of care for women with breast cancer. No studies (at least no reproducible studies) have demonstrated that immunotherapy causes regression of active cancer or prolongs remissions or survival. Several randomized studies of vaccines used after a response to chemotherapy for advanced breast cancer are under way to see if they can prolong remissions induced by chemotherapy.

Goal 6: Decrease Effect of Estrogen on Tumor

CALCIUM GLUCARATE

D-gluraric acid, also known as D-saccharic acid or glucosaccharic acid, is a simple sugar made in small amounts by mammals, including humans. We also get it in our diets from fruits and vegetables, including broccoli, carrots, spinach, apples, and potatoes. Oranges are a particularly rich source. Calcium glucarate, a D-gluraric acid–containing supplement, may be useful in both preventing and treating breast cancer.

Animal studies suggest that calcium glucarate can help detoxify the body, eliminating harmful chemicals and excess hormones—including estrogen. It appears to block an enzyme that reactivates toxins previously neutralized by the liver, thus D-glucarate may promote efficient waste elimination.[87]

Clinical trials formally examining the benefit of glucarate in breast cancer are ongoing, and none has yet been published. Therefore, therapeutic doses for humans have not yet been established, and though glucarate appears to be nontoxic, complete information on any potential harm is lacking. Because of the absence of clearer data, I have not prescribed calcium glucarate to my patients.

Goal 7: Remove Initiators and Promoters of Malignancy

It is almost impossible to know why any given woman gets, or doesn't get, breast cancer. But I try to identify possible causes when I can, in order to remove them if at all possible, in line with the core naturopathic principle of removing the initiating cause of disease. In this section, I'll look at some of the most convincing general hypotheses about contributors to breast cancer risk for what we can learn about breast cancer prevention—and prevention of recurrences.

PESTICIDES

Pesticide exposure may be one of the factors responsible for the increasing rates of breast cancer in industrialized countries.[88–90] Controversial scientific evidence links organochlorine pesticides (e.g., DDT) and polychlorinated biphenyls (PCBs), both widespread in the environment, to breast cancer, probably because of their estrogenic properties. One study showed higher concentrations of DDT and PCBs in breast tissue in women with breast cancer than in a control group of women with benign breast biopsies.[91] Another found an association between levels of the DDT by-product DDE in the blood with an increase in risk of breast cancer.[92]

There is still a reasonable dispute among experts about the degree of correlation, let alone causal connection, between these chemicals and breast cancer, but there is sufficient evidence to suggest that women with detectable levels of them in their blood—indicating that an amount five times higher is lodged in their fat tissue[93]—have an additional risk factor for cancer. So I test my patients' blood for pesticides and PCBs, using an excellent clinical toxicology lab for the tests. For patients with detectable levels in their blood, I recommend naturopathic tissue cleansing (see below). I retest them afterward to make sure the pesticide levels have been cleared. The best window of opportunity for this procedure to make a real difference is most likely in the early stages of breast cancer.

DETOXIFICATION

Naturopathic ways to cleanse the body's tissues, where toxins build up, include juice fasting, sweating, and colonic irrigation. For my more athletic patients, I highly recommend a form of hatha yoga done at sauna temperatures (Bikram's yoga). These methods clear the gastrointestinal system and the epithelial cells of the skin. There have been no systematic studies of the effect of these methods on breast cancer patients, but they all have a long tradition of usefulness. Dr. Walter Crinnion's work is also instructive. He's been using these methods to treat cancer for many years, and conducted a ten-year review of cases wherein patients with various disorders, including cancer, underwent his comprehensive naturopathic depuration protocol, which included aerobic exercise in a thermal chamber, constitutional hydrotherapy (contrasting hot and cold towel hydrotherapy), colonic irrigation, homeopathy, body therapies such as massage and chiropractic, and nutritional supplementation. They followed this regimen five days a week for three to six weeks. Patients rated their results on a five-point scale from "worse" through "no change" to "great." Overall, 83% of patients rated their results as "good" or "great." Of eight cancer patients, two (both of whom had late-stage metastatic disease) reported "no change," two saw "good" improvement, and four reported "great" results.[94] Unfortunately, the report gives no information about clinical or survival outcomes in these cancer patients. Until better data are published, I recommend to most patients a three-day juice fast twice a year and Bikram's yoga three times a week to optimize health.

HYPOTHYROIDISM AND BREAST CANCER

Not only is good thyroid function necessary for good general health, but suboptimal thyroid function may increase the risks for breast cancer and its recurrence. Lower-than-normal levels of the thyroid hormone thyroxine and longer duration of ovulation correlate with increased risk of breast cancer.[95] Another study linked enlarged thyroid glands with breast tumor staging.[96] Hypothyroidism is of particular concern in a woman with an estrogen-dependent tumor in the breast because it may increase the number of estrogen receptors.[97]

Most naturopathic physicians do a routine thyroid blood test, and it is particularly important that breast cancer patients make sure they get one and discuss thyroid hormone supplementation with their doctor.

Ronnie's mother had survived a cancer years earlier and had just been diagnosed with a different cancer. Her aunt had died an awful death from breast cancer when she and Ronnie were both young. That event was the one that most affected Ronnie emotionally, but several other family members also struggled with breast cancer over the years. I suspected some inherited component to Ronnie's cancer—or just an effect from a shared environment for such a long time. Either way, these were causes that could not be removed.

Because Ronnie's insurance would not cover the cost of serum pesticide testing, she did not have this test performed.

I did check Ronnie's thyroid. I do it as a matter of course, but I was especially concerned in Ronnie's case because she was so fatigued—a typical experience in hypothryoidism. I didn't find anything abnormal, so we could rule that out as a factor in her cancer and move on to finding the most effective approaches for her.

Goal 8: Provide Nutritional Support Aimed at Cancer Prevention

The nutritional approaches that decrease the risk of developing cancer according to epidemiological studies are not necessarily effective in treating breast cancer once a tumor has been diagnosed. But because supplements may also help in reducing the mutations of the existing breast cancer and so decrease the aggressiveness of the tumor, I, like most naturopathic physicians, prescribe antioxidant vitamins, soy, and essential fatty acids to my patients. This section discusses a select group of nutritional supplements that are a key part of any breast cancer treatment plan.

VITAMIN A/BETA-CAROTENE

Vitamin A is critical in regulating the proliferation and differentiation of cells.[98] Very high doses (350,000 to 500,000 IU) have been shown to augment the effects of chemotherapy in women with metastatic breast cancer.[99]

However, vitamin A is potentially teratogenic (can cause fetal malformations), though at what level has yet to be precisely established. Therefore, vitamin A supplementation must be less than 10,000 IU or avoided completely during pregnancy. Very high doses can also be toxic, though the symptoms go away once one stops ingesting the vitamin, and recovery is nearly always complete. These two concerns are why beta-carotene, found in green and yellow vegetables and fruits, and which the body turns into vitamin A as needed, is more practical for daily use.

Many studies report that a diet high in vegetables containing beta-carotene is associated with a lower risk of breast cancer.[100–103] More narrowly focused studies have correlated a low intake of carotene with increased breast cancer risk in postmenopausal women.[104] Beta-carotene may also be useful in preventing the recurrence of cancer. In a pilot study of fifteen cancer patients receiving beta-carotene and canthaxanthin (a red-pigmented carotenoid), the patients went longer than expected without recurrence after a tumor was surgically removed.[105,106]

Smokers may need to be cautious in using beta-carotene, as studies have shown smokers taking it to have a slightly increased risk of lung cancer and heart disease.[107–109] In general, beta-carotene should probably not be supplemented in high doses in smokers until studies are done to define who may benefit and what are the proper doses and treatment durations.[110]

I prescribe for my breast cancer patients high-dose vitamin A for short intense treatment periods and moderate doses of natural beta-carotene for maintenance supplementation. Purified beta-carotene is five or six times more available to the body than that from vegetables.[111]

VITAMIN A PRESCRIPTION

Dosage: 25,000 to 100,000 IU per day for two to four weeks at a time.
Contraindications: Not to be used during pregnancy or in women with liver disease.

BETA-CAROTENE PRESCRIPTION

Dosage: 50,000 to 300,000 IU per day.
Contraindications: Smokers should not take supplemental beta-carotene.

VITAMIN E

Vitamin E levels are lower in breast cancer patients than in healthy persons,[112] and vitamin E succinate has been shown to induce apoptosis in breast cancer cells.[113]

VITAMIN E PRESCRIPTION

Dosage: 400 to 1600 IU per day (succinate form is preferred).
Contraindications: Should be used with caution by people with blood clotting disorders or those taking blood thinners.

VITAMIN C

Vitamin C in very large doses is one of the most commonly used alternative therapies for cancer, but the science does not yet exist to support that. I don't know of any published studies on the anticancer activity of vitamin C in breast cancer specifically, though one is definitely in order. So I don't prescribe the megadoses, though I do think that at moderate levels it is a useful part of an "antioxidant cocktail."

VITAMIN C PRESCRIPTION

Dosage: 500 to 1000 milligrams daily.
Contraindications: None.

OMEGA-3 ESSENTIAL FATTY ACIDS

Extensive data from hundreds of published papers have shown the anticancer effects of omega-3 polyunsaturated fatty acids, like those in fish oil. To give you just one example: a clinical trial of EPA (eicosapentaenoic acid) and DHA (docosahexaenoic acid) in fish oil, used with vitamin E, showed that cancer patients who took the supplements survived significantly longer.[114]

The American diet in general is deficient in omega-3 fatty acids, so I recommend supplements to my breast cancer patients. I also recommend cold-water ocean fish such as salmon, cod, and halibut as an excellent source of protein. To ensure an adequate amount of omega-3 fatty acids, I prescribe 1 tablespoon of cod liver oil daily.

OMEGA-3 ESSENTIAL FATTY ACIDS PRESCRIPTION

Dosage: 1 gram daily of EPA and DHA combined. You get that
in 1 tablespoon of high-quality fish oil, like cod liver oil.
Contraindications: None.

SOY ISOFLAVONOIDS

Epidemiological studies suggest that a diet high in soy reduces one's risk of breast cancer,[115] though the mechanism by which it works is not yet entirely clear. Soy contains plant substances called phytoestrogens, which can mimic estrogens and bind to estrogen receptors in human breast cancer cells.[116] They are adaptogenic—that is, they have different, even opposite, effects under different circumstances. They can either boost or block estrogen, depending on their location in the body and the hormonal milieu.[117,118]

Soy phytoestrogens are called isoflavones. One of them, genistein, can block estrogen and so has a potent antiproliferative influence on breast cancer cells. On the other hand, several studies show that both genistein and daidzein, another prominent soy isoflavone, are estrogenic: they bind to estrogen receptors and exert effects similar to those of the body's own estrogen. For this reason, I share some of the concerns that soy isoflavones can have proliferative effects, just the way estrogen does, but it may possibly have some degree of antiestrogen effect as well.

The question of using soy isoflavones in breast cancer patients seems to be getting more confusing, and we'll need more information before the answer is clear. In the meantime, I take a conservative approach with my patients, recommending tofu, tempeh, soymilk, and soy cheese as major protein sources but recommending *against* using soy supplements.

ISOFLAVONES PRESCRIPTION

Dosage: Whole soy foods daily.
Contraindications: None.

FLAXSEED

Flaxseed is rich in lignans, another type of phytoestrogen that has been associated with a decreased risk of breast cancer as well as other diseases. Lignans are also found in cereals, legumes, vegetables, seeds, nuts, fruits, berries, tea, coffee, and wine.[119] Flaxseed has by far the most lignans, so it has been used extensively in experimental studies.[120] Like soy isoflavones, lignans appear to be both weakly estrogenic and antiestrogenic.[121–123]

There are several possibilities for how lignans protect against cancer, including breast cancer. They affect human sex hormones, inhibiting estrogen, for example.[124–128] They also inhibit breast cancer growth. One study showed that breast cancer patients secrete lower levels of lignans in their urine than do healthy women, suggesting that lignan deficiency could be associated with, or lead to, an increased risk of cancer.[129]

Diets rich in lignans (and flavonoids) help reduce estrogen-dependent breast cancer.[130] One study in rats showed a 47% reduction in the number of breast tumors in the rats that were fed a flaxseed extract.[131] In rats with induced breast tumors, supplements of any of three forms of lignans resulted in a 50% reduction of tumor size. The numbers and sizes of new tumors were lowest in rats taking the supplements, suggesting that lignans may be effective against all stages of tumor promotion.[132]

I recommend lignans in ground flaxseed as a good source of fiber and for their potential benefits in reducing breast cancer recurrence.

FLAXSEED PRESCRIPTION

Dosage: 1 tablespoon of ground organically grown flaxseeds daily, sprinkled on cereal or salad, or in juice or a smoothie.
Contraindications: None.

As I've mentioned, Ronnie took an antioxidant cocktail daily, including vitamins A, C, and E, along with melatonin. She also took immune-supporting cod liver oil, in part for the omega-3 essential fatty acids it is so rich in.

Ronnie ate lots of soy products and used ground flaxseeds as a condiment on her cereal.

Goal 9: Help Patient Access the "Healer Within"

The mind and the body are intimately connected. One result is that our thoughts and emotions affect our immune systems. The clinical course of breast cancer is influenced by psychosocial factors and the way we respond to stress. Psychosocial stressors not adequately handled are associated with weakening of the immune system. Denial, avoidance, and suppression of one's own basic needs and emotions all seem to lower the natural resistance to carcinogens.[133] A study of sixty-one Stage I and Stage II breast cancer patients found that higher natural killer cell activity could be predicted from perceived emotional support from a spouse or significant other, perceived social support from one's doctor, and social support that was actively sought.[134]

Interpersonal relationships play a part in determining the end of the story for women with breast cancer, as specific studies show. Stress can also be a factor in causing breast cancer. One study measuring life change and stress over a three-year period for ninety-nine women with breast cancer, and ninety-nine control subjects matched by age and residence, showed that participants with stress scores in the highest quartile were nearly five times as likely to develop breast cancer as those with scores in the lowest quartile.[135] A key study by David Spiegel, M.D., showed that participating in a support group significantly increased survival rates in women with metastatic breast cancer.[136]

I urge all my patients to make changes that will bring into their lives more serenity, love, joy, and support from family, friends, and co-workers, and to follow their spiritual paths.

From the beginning, Ronnie had confidence and faith in the effectiveness of naturopathic methods as well as confidence in her excellent oncologist, and I think that too was a factor in her positive outcome. I firmly believe in using what has been scientifically validated, but I also know that the more the patient believes that her treatment of any kind—mainstream or CAM—will work, the more likely it is to do just that. Her conviction in the ability of her body to heal itself, and her hard-won conviction in her ability to choose what was best for her, helped ensure that she'd maximize the benefits of whatever treatments she chose.

Ronnie told me that she'd struggled with depression all her life, and of course getting breast cancer didn't help that any. Low-level anxiety, too, had long plagued her, and her anxiety about her cancer was now significant. When she was first diagnosed, Ronnie saw a psychiatrist, who wrote her a prescription to help her manage her anxiety. But she didn't really want to add yet another pharmacological medication. The B vitamins I recommended have the benefit of working as antidepressants as well.

I also encouraged her to relax about making the right decisions about her treatment. She was spending hours on the Internet and in the library, putting a great deal of pressure on herself to discover her "cure," not wanting to miss some magic bullet. But even for me, all the literature on CAM is confusing enough to be crazy-making—and that's *after* you sort out the marketing hype from the science. Ronnie had a naturo-pathic physician and an oncologist working with her, and she needed to trust them to do their jobs: providing her with state-of-the-art informa-tion on effective therapies. Ronnie needed to conserve her energy and let go of some of her stress. The ability to do so, though it wasn't imme-diate, was one positive thing Ronnie managed to extract from the experi-ence of having breast cancer.

Ronnie also worked with a spiritual advisor, and she developed com-forting and empowering rituals for herself. She told me that even when she was really sick from her treatments, when she could hardly even eat or sleep, she would think of just lying in her bed as being alone with God. She found that to be a powerful way to cut away all the layers, all the superficial stuff in her life, and get down to the only things that really mattered. It forced her to go more inside herself, she said, and she was pleased with what she discovered there. The crucial insight she arrived at was that the whole breast cancer experience was not about death but about life.

Every evening, Ronnie would light a candle. Some days that was all she could manage. On other days she used the flickering light as a focus for a kind of informal meditation she described to me as mainly slow, relaxed, deep breathing mixed with prayer. When she had the energy, she would do the tai chi she had learned from a good friend who teaches tai chi. Moving meditation was the most meaningful to her.

One of my favorite stories told by Ronnie is of how she handled losing her hair during chemotherapy. She had decided to take all that she was going through and embrace it as an opportunity for transformation. Hair loss was very hard—as it always is—but it was also clearly sym-bolic, especially within her new framework. When it started to happen in earnest, she pulled out much of her hair herself and then enlisted her husband to shave the rest off. Then she burned it. "The adriamycin was burning me from the inside; now I was burning my hair on the out-side," she told me. "It was my opportunity to purge my body of all the old stories, neuroses, and anxiety."

One of the first things Ronnie did after receiving her diagnosis was to call every person she knew who was at all religious and ask all of them to pray for her. Jewish, Catholic, Buddhist—it didn't matter to Ronnie. She had tremendous faith in the power of prayer, no matter what flavor it was, and she was already familiar with some of the studies demonstrating its clinical effects. She credits that as an important component of her healing.

Ronnie had long been active in her religious community, but she developed the spiritual side of herself through her breast cancer experience. That not only helped her on her path to healing but also gave her a lasting gift to carry throughout her life. "I saw almost miraculous things happen," she told me. "But I realized those things are always happening; we're just too busy to notice." From the depths of the experience she'd been dreading most of her life, Ronnie actually increased her hopefulness about life in general. This is one of the very best aspects of practicing medicine: being the witness and sometimes the midwife to transformation.

Goal 10: Minimize Side Effects of Conventional Oncologic Treatments

Over the course of my career I have found several natural medicines to be useful in mitigating some of the side effects of conventional therapy. While not all of the methods described below have been evaluated in controlled clinical trials, they have proven themselves over the years by clinical observation.

The point in your menstrual cycle at which you have surgery—whether biopsy, mastectomy, or anything in between—might affect the outcome, but this still engenders controversy. Some studies have suggested that the best time is during the luteal phase: from day 14 until your period begins. In three out of four reports from major cancer treatment centers, the risk of recurrent cancer and/or death increased five to six times after ten years for women who had surgery during days 7 to 14 of their cycle.[137] In another study of 112 premenopausal women who had breast cancer surgery, patients with estrogen-sensitive tumors who underwent surgery in the later, luteal phase of their cycle had a significantly better survival rate than did women with tumors that weren't estrogen-sensitive. After surgery in the earlier follicular phase (from menstrual flow to ovulation, days 1 to 14 of the cycle), whether or not the tumor was estrogen-sensitive made no difference in overall survival. The women with the best prognosis were those whose estrogen-sensitive tumors were removed on days

0 to 2 and 13 to 32. But even women with tumors not sensitive to estrogen that were taken out during the luteal phase had better results than those who had surgery in the follicular phase.[138] An analysis of many reports about the five- to fifteen-year disease-free survival of premenopausal breast cancer patients (a total of over 5000 women) tracked whether they had surgery in the luteal or follicular phase (day 1 to 15). The luteal group had an overall mean 5% benefit in lowering recurrence rates compared with the follicular group. Given all this, I recommend that my patients have surgery in the second half of their cycle (days 15 to 28).

When surgery disrupts malignant tissue, it may allow cancer cells to enter the bloodstream or lymphatic system, so I prescribe modified citrus pectin (1 teaspoon in juice twice daily) to help prevent adhesion of micrometastases (see Goal 1).

Ronnie's surgery was in fact at the recommended point in her cycle, though that happened by chance—she didn't know to request it at the time. Ronnie started naturopathic care after surgery. To prepare her body for, and speed recovery from, surgery, Ronnie took natural vitamins (A, C, and E), zinc, silymarin (an active component of *silybum marianum,* or milk thistle), and homeopathic arnica. They helped her handle the side effects and heal quickly. She also took the modified citrus pectin, as described above. Typically, my patients using this or a similar combination do very well through their surgery. Several patients have told me that their surgeons commented on how few complications they had and how fast they healed up.

Chemotherapy and Radiation

ANTIOXIDANTS

Whether or not antioxidants are safe to take during chemotherapy and radiation is one of the most controversial issues facing women with breast cancer. Some oncologists tell their patients to stop all antioxidants, including vitamins, during chemotherapy and radiation. The theory is that chemotherapy and radiation kill cancer cells mainly by making cell-damaging free radicals, so antioxidants, which protect against the actions of free radicals, could actually inhibit the drugs and radiation from having their full effect. The bulk of the scientific data, however, suggests counterintuitively that antioxidants, including vitamins C, E, and A and CoQ10, actually improve the efficacy of chemotherapy (in laboratory experiments). Vitamin C works that way in animal studies as well, but small clinical trials of vitamin C for advanced cancer were negative.[139]

As I've already explained, Ronnie took a mix of antioxidants as I recommend to most breast cancer patients (beta-carotene 100,000 IU/day, vitamin C 2000 mg/day, vitamin E succinate 800 IU/day). But I did have her stop taking them during—as well as just before and just after—each chemotherapy and radiation treatment. Scientific evidence indicates it would be safe—and some even suggests that the antioxidants enhance the effect of the other treatments—but there's enough evidence warranting concern for me to want to play it safe. When in doubt, leave it out—that's my motto.

Protecting the Heart

CoQ10 has been shown to prevent heart damage caused by the chemotherapy agent adriamycin. I prescribe 200 milligrams twice a day to all of my breast cancer patients for its purported anticancer activity as well as its ability to protect the heart. I also suggest it to women getting Herceptin, which can also damage the heart. So far, however, there has not been a study to validate that CoQ10 can prevent that specific side effect of Herceptin.

The CoQ10 Ronnie took offered protection for her heart, as the adriamycin in her chemotherapy is known to cause heart tissue damage in many patients, so Ronnie didn't have to choose between the health of her heart and the health of her breast.

CoQ10 Prescription

Dosage: 200 milligrams twice daily.
Contraindications: None known.

Protecting the Mucosal Lining

The amino acid glutamine protects the gastrointestinal lining from the effects of chemotherapy.[140,141]

GLUTAMINE PRESCRIPTION

Dosage: 1000 milligrams twice a day.
Contraindications: None known.

MOUTH SORES

For women who develop painful mouth sores with chemotherapy, the simple trick of applying vitamin E directly onto the sores helps them heal quickly.

MENOPAUSAL SYMPTOMS

Vitamin E and dietary soy may help reduce hot flashes. All evidence points to the safety of using either or both.

If that combination isn't effective enough, I recommend the herb black cohosh *(Cimicifuga racemosa)*, another phytoestrogen, to my breast cancer patients with menopausal symptoms caused by chemotherapy or tamoxifen. Studies show that black cohosh reduces menopausal symptoms and, in the laboratory, does not stimulate breast cancer cell proliferation.[142–144] In fact, it can even inhibit proliferation in estrogen-sensitive tumors, particularly in combination with tamoxifen.[145]

Black cohosh is one of the few phytoestrogens that has been tested for safety, and all results point to its being an appropriate treatment. Other phytoestrogens, such as *Glycyrrhiza* (licorice) and angelica (dong quai), are potentially harmful, especially in women with estrogen-sensitive tumors. Until I see data proving their safety, I recommend *against* using them if you have breast cancer.

I also do not recommend the most common mainstream approach to menopause—hormone replacement therapy—for women with breast cancer that is sensitive to estrogen. There is controversy over the use of natural estrogen and/or natural progesterone for women with a history of breast cancer, and some argue that using a combination of natural hormones can actually inhibit the proliferation of breast cancer cells. In my opinion, however, the data are insufficient at this point to prove that the benefits are greater than the risks, and I don't use any hormone therapy with my patients with breast cancer.

Chemotherapy caused Ronnie to go into menopause, and she started having hot flashes. Black cohosh eased them. Now that she was menopausal, even just a little early, she needed to pay more attention to the health of her bones. For that she took a combination of calcium, magnesium, vitamin D, and boron, which she continues religiously to this day.

Black Cohosh Prescription

Dosage: 20 milligrams twice a day, with meals.
Contraindications: None known.

Vitamin E Succinate

Dosage: 400 to 800 IU twice daily.
Contraindications: Avoid if blood clotting disorder is present or if you are currently taking blood-thinning medication.

Peripheral Neuropathy

In some women, chemotherapy with Taxol or Taxotere produces numbness and tingling in the toes, feet, and fingers—a phenomenon known as peripheral neuropathy. I recommend vitamin B_{12} and cod liver oil to my patients with peripheral neuropathy. The omega-3 fatty acids that are so rich in cod liver oil have been shown to ease peripheral neuropathy in diabetic patients,[146,147] and I've seen it help women during chemotherapy as well. If that doesn't do the trick, I recommend a six-week course of weekly acupuncture treatments.

Throughout her course of chemotherapy, Ronnie came in every week for an intramuscular injection of vitamin B_{12} (so it would be better absorbed than orally), which lessened the peripheral neuropathy she experienced with Taxol. She also took a B-complex supplement orally.

Vitamin B_{12} Prescription

Dosage: 1000 micrograms by intramuscular injection.
Contraindications: None.

COD LIVER OIL/OMEGA-3 PRESCRIPTION

Dosage: 1 tablespoon daily.
Contraindications: None.

CONSTIPATION

Constipation is a risk factor for less than optimal health in *anyone*, and certainly for women with breast cancer. Without regular daily elimination of waste, bacterial toxins, exogenous chemicals, and hormonal by-products may be reabsorbed into the body rather than excreted. A nutritious high-fiber diet with plenty of water and regular exercise are often enough to correct the problem. My favorite treatment is a daily serving of the muesli described below.

Like many women undergoing chemotherapy, Ronnie developed a problem with constipation. Dr. Milliman's muesli recipe helped her enormously.

Dr. Milliman's Muesli

My mentor, Bruce Milliman, N.D., long ago developed a recipe for highly nutritious breakfast muesli that is also an effective treatment for mild constipation.

Using organic products whenever possible, in a large paper bag, mix:

1 lb rolled oats	¼ lb sunflower seeds
½ lb oat bran	¼ lb almonds
½ lb lecithin granules	¼ lb wheat germ
¼ lb ground flaxseed	⅛ lb ground milk thistle seeds
¼ lb dried currants	

Store in a plastic bag or other air-tight container in the refrigerator. To serve, soak ½ cup muesli at least 30 minutes in fruit juice diluted with water. Add 3 to 4 ounces of nonfat, organic, live-culture yogurt, along with fruit (berries, chopped apple or pear, etc.). It can also be served warm by soaking for ten minutes in boiling water.

Ronnie had chemotherapy with adriamycin and cytoxan, then four weeks of Taxol and six weeks of radiation. Throughout the process she struggled with fatigue, and I recommended Siberian ginseng *(Eleuthrococcus)* to help restore vigor. She also suffered from insomnia, as many breast cancer patients do, and melatonin helped her get restorative rest. She found that taking cod liver oil, which is also helpful for the immune system, relieved the severely dry skin that resulted from chemotherapy. She used the herbal medicine bromelain to prevent the formation of scar tissue, a side effect of radiation.

Perhaps the biggest help during the chemotherapy process for Ronnie, however, was vitamin B_{12}, which she took by injection for best absorption to help her bone marrow make new healthy red and white blood cells. That's important to the immune system generally, but it can serve a specific purpose as well. According to standard chemotherapy protocol, a patient's white blood cell count must be at least 2000. The normal count is between 4000 and 10,000, but it generally decreases during chemotherapy. A common treatment for this among oncologists is a shot of Neupogen, a hormone that stimulates the white cells to be produced by the bone marrow.

As Ronnie prepared for a treatment, her count was only 2000, so her oncologist gave her the Neupogen. The only side effect he mentioned was a little soreness at the injection site, but it made Ronnie extremely nauseated and made her joints ache so much that she feared she had developed rheumatoid arthritis on top of everything else. She didn't like the experience, to say the least, but her white blood cell count did shoot up to 17,800 in less than twenty-four hours.

Ronnie happened to be in my office just before her next chemotherapy treatment. With a white blood cell count of about 2700, she was definitely not looking forward to having to use the Neupogen again. She was also uneasy about the huge magnitude of the increase in white blood cell counts it caused. I suggested a vitamin B_{12} shot instead, and the next day her count was up to 4000—enough to allow her to proceed with chemotherapy without the Neupogen.

Ronnie then talked her oncologist into getting the vitamin B_{12} shots for her remaining treatments. This was a special order, since he didn't generally use B_{12}, and she had to promise to come back for Neupogen if the B_{12} didn't work. As it turned out, she never had to resort to Neupogen again. Ronnie had to pay out of pocket for the vitamin, as it wasn't covered by insurance, but fortunately each shot was under $20, compared with about $300 per dose of Neupogen.

All things considered, Ronnie got through her treatment very well. She lost her hair, she was exhausted, and it was a struggle to keep up being a soccer mom, but she managed to pull it all together with help from her wonderfully supportive husband, who accompanied her to many of her appointments; her family, friends, and community; and her own strong center, which she discovered on the journey.

Ronnie is just about two years after her diagnosis as I write this. There's been no sign of recurrence—most of which happen in the first two years—and she is doing very well. After all her treatments were over, her natural killer cells were low, and I had her take inositol hexaphosphate for a year until her blood tests showed she was back to average levels. I also recommended periodic juice fasts and sweats, starting six months after the end of treatment, to help clean out any toxins remaining in her body from the treatment.

She still takes vitamin C, vitamin E, selenium, CoQ10, calcium, and cod liver oil. She uses a lot of flaxseed and soy in her diet and has switched from coffee to green tea. She was always careful about what she put into her body, eating organic food whenever possible. Now she binges less often on sugar and drinks less alcohol. She eats more of the salmon she loves, along with other fish like tuna and halibut, for the healthy omega-3 fatty acids these fish contain. She's begun to exercise more than she ever did before her diagnosis (though it was a long time after her treatment ended before she really felt like it), mostly with a group that meets twice a week for a three-mile walk followed by stretching and weight lifting.

Not only has Ronnie gotten back to how she was before her diagnosis, with no lasting harm done by the rough treatments she'd been through—she's made her life and health better than before. In addition to new lifestyle choices that bring benefits for overall health and well-being, I've witnessed in her an incredible transformation as she's found her inner strength. Her experience has brought a wonderful change in her outlook on life, her ability to cope, and her spiritual depth. She's almost a different woman from when I first saw her. Whereas she was self-deprecating and extremely anxious at our first appointment, now I see a powerful, self-affirming woman.

No one should have to go through what Ronnie did to get to that place. But if you have to make the trip, you may as well get something good out of it. Naturopathic medicine at its best can make your path smoother and support you in taking full advantage of the light at the end of the tunnel.

Acknowledgments

Dr. Cheryl Grosshans, a recent graduate of the naturopathic medical program at Bastyr University who began working with me in 1997, has helped me collect, read, and review hundreds of scientific papers on natural medicines for breast cancer. Over the past three years she has become more than just my student; she is also a trusted and valued colleague in our work to screen and evaluate promising CAM therapies for breast cancer. Dr. Jennifer Lush and Dr. Michelle Robeson are also recently graduated naturopathic practitioners from Bastyr University who have been working with us to develop this chapter. I'd also like to thank Davis Lamson, N.D., for his advice on breast cancer treatment principles and therapies, and Michele Bivins for her expert assistance in manuscript preparation.

Resources

Websites

AMERICAN ASSOCIATION OF NATUROPATHIC PHYSICIANS (AANP)
www.aanp.org
(for help in finding an N.D. near you)

BASTYR UNIVERSITY
www.bastyr.edu

NCCAM
www.nccam.nih.gov

DEPARTMENT OF DEFENSE BREAST CANCER RESEARCH PROGRAM
www.darpa.mil

RALPH MOSS, PH.D.
www.ralphmoss.com

CANHELP
www.canhelp.com

Books

AUSTIN, S, AND HITCHCOCK, C. *Breast Cancer—What You Should Know (But May Not Be Told)*. Rocklin, CA: Prima Publishing, 1994.

MOSS, R. *Antioxidants Against Cancer*. Brooklyn, NY: Equinox Press, 2000.

PIZZORNO, J, AND MURRAY, M. *Textbook of Natural Medicine*, 2nd ed. New York: Churchill Livingstone, 1999.

Specialized Clinical Laboratories

ACCU-CHEM LABORATORIES
800-451-0116
www.accuchemlabs.com

GREAT SMOKIES DIAGNOSTIC LABORATORY
www.gsdl.com

CHAPTER ELEVEN

Meditation

Jon Kabat-Zinn, Ph.D.; Ann Ohm Massion, M.D.; James R. Hébert, M.S.P.H., Sc.D.; and Elana Rosenbaum, M.S., M.S.W.

JON KABAT-ZINN, PH.D., is founding executive director of the Center for Mindfulness in Medicine, Health Care, and Society at the University of Massachusetts Medical School. He is also founder and former director of the Stress Reduction Clinic, which celebrated its twentieth anniversary in September 1999. He was professor of medicine in the Department of Medicine, Division of Preventive and Behavioral Medicine, until he retired in 2001. He is the author of two bestselling books: *Full Catastrophe Living: Using the Wisdom of Your Body and Mind to Face Stress, Pain and Illness* (Delta, 1991) and *Wherever You Go, There You Are: Mindfulness Meditation in Everyday Life* (Hyperion, 1994). Dr. Kabat-Zinn received his Ph.D. in molecular biology from MIT in 1971. His research since 1979 has focused on mind-body interactions for healing and on the clinical applications of mindfulness meditation training. His work in the Stress Reduction Clinic was featured in Bill Moyers's PBS special, *Healing and the Mind,* and in the book of the same title.

ANN OHM MASSION, M.D., has been assistant professor of psychiatry at the University of Massachusetts Medical School and UMass Memorial Health Care since 1988. She received her M.D. from Mayo Medical School in 1984. Her clinical subspecialty is in anxiety disorders, with a particular interest in spiritual approaches to psychiatry and medicine. Since 1987, she has been doing research in two areas, anxiety disorders and mind-body approaches to healing.

JAMES R. HÉBERT, M.S.P.H., SC.D., is professor and chair of the Department of Epidemiology and Biostatistics at the Norman J. Arnold School of Public Health of the University of South Carolina in Columbia. Prior to that position, he was professor of medicine and epidemiology at the University of Massachusetts Medical School. He currently directs a number of research projects related mainly to the role of diet in the development and progression of breast and prostate cancers.

ELANA ROSENBAUM, M.S., M.S.W., is a cancer survivor who integrates her many years as a psychotherapist with mindfulness meditation. She was a senior instructor in Mindfulness-Based Stress Reduction (MBSR) at the University of Massachusetts Medical Center for almost twenty years, where she also introduced meditation to patients on the bone marrow transplant unit. She currently conducts retreats and support groups for cancer patients. She also provides training and consultation to health care providers and organizations related to mind-body therapies for cancer patients.

Michael Lerner of the Commonweal Cancer Self Help Program once said that receiving a cancer diagnosis is like being a soldier dropped unexpectedly into a jungle war zone without a map, compass, or training. If you've been in that particular jungle, you'll know exactly what he means. Suddenly you are plunged into an unfamiliar universe of doctors, tests, and hospitals. You are forced to make complex, confusing, and critically important choices, often without enough guidance from a medical establishment that is strongly focused on treating disease aggressively at any cost. And in the midst of it all, in all likelihood you may be experiencing waves of intense and conflicting emotions that make it even more difficult to cope: shock, isolation, depression, fear, bewilderment, self-pity, anger, bitterness, and helplessness.

The practice of meditation can be extremely useful in helping you ground yourself in the depths of your being and in what is most important to you. It can help in making greater sense of your situation as it unfolds, and then charting a course of action. Meditation can be invaluable as a complement to medical care, psychotherapy (if warranted), and social support from family and friends. It provides a powerful psychological framework as well as specific methods for facing and working through emotional turmoil, pain, and suffering. Meditation can provide comfort, meaning, and direction in a time of high stress and uncertainty. In the process, it can help you connect with what is deepest and most nourishing in yourself, and mobilize the full range of resources—inner and outer—available to you.

In an earlier era of medicine, some patients no doubt were able to find and make use of meditation through the religious and spiritual worlds with which it had traditionally been associated. In the past twenty years, meditative practices have become much more accessible and understandable to people as meditation came to be employed in a wide range of different ways with medical patients, including women with breast cancer, in hospitals, medical centers, and clinics throughout the United States. One widespread approach is known as Mindfulness-Based Stress Reduction (MBSR). MBSR is an intensive training in mindfulness meditation and its application to daily living designed for medical patients, including breast cancer patients. MBSR was first delivered to medical patients in 1979 in the Stress Reduction Clinic at the University of Massachusetts Medical Center, one of the first hospital-based mind-body clinics in the country. MBSR is currently in use in more than two hundred clinics and hospitals across the country and around the world.

In this chapter we shall discuss the ways in which meditation in general, and mindfulness in particular, can help women grapple with the physical, psychological, and spiritual dimensions of breast cancer and its aftermath. We will also look at what current research findings reveal about meditation's effectiveness and the ways it may work.

What Is Meditation?

Meditation is many things to many people, but at the heart of anyone's practice is *the intentional self-regulation of attention.* In other words, meditation is simply a way to pay attention on purpose, in the present moment, and nonjudgmentally. Meditation develops greater concentration and awareness as you focus systematically and purposefully on particular aspects of your experience, be they inner or outer, as they are unfolding. There are two general categories of meditation practices: *concentration* and *mindfulness.* Concentration methods cultivate attention focused on one point. They may include the use of mantras (repeating sounds or phrases) as in Transcendental Meditation (TM), koans (phrases or questions in the Zen tradition that are aimed at breaking free of conceptual thought), and the breath. Whatever the vehicle, in concentration practices, the object of attention is used as a single, unvarying focus of attention, and any deviation in the mind away from it is seen as a distraction from which one returns as quickly as possible. Concentration practices can bring about profound states of calmness, inner stillness, and nonreactivity of mind.

By comparison, mindfulness methods may start with a single object of attention to cultivate concentration and stability of mind, but then go on to expand the field of awareness to include a potentially vast range of objects of attention that change from moment to moment. Mindfulness practices aim to cultivate an intentionally nonreactive, nonjudgmental, moment-to-moment awareness of a changing field of objects. The essence of mindfulness is universal, having to do simply with the cultivation and refinement of our ability to be present and awake in our lives. However, from the historical and cultural perspective, mindfulness received its most articulate and developed expressions within the Buddhist tradition, in particular the Vipassana, Soto Zen, and Dzogchen traditions.

In mindfulness practice, rather than becoming absorbed or shutting out the world, you pay attention to the full range of whatever is present in your unfolding experience, no matter where you find yourself in any moment. For this reason, mindfulness is very practical and compelling for people with busy, engaged lives—including those who are dealing with a life-threatening illness like breast cancer and all its accompanying emotional turbulence. Mindfulness helps one face and embrace all aspects of life with increasing degrees of equanimity, wisdom, and self-compassion. These qualities develop naturally as the practitioner spends time each day in periods of intentional silence and nondoing (formal meditation practice), with the focus on present-moment experience as it unfolds, and then as she carries that moment-to-moment awareness into various aspects of daily living (informal meditation practice).

Mindfulness meditation is much more than a technique. It is best thought of as a way of life, a way of being and seeing, a slight but fundamental shift from being caught up in and carried away by the automaticity of our thoughts and feelings, to being aware of them, and being more grounded in awareness itself. Mindfulness invites us to literally come to our senses through focusing on the body and on bodily sensations such as those associated with breathing, and thereby come to be more in touch with and more appreciative of what is deepest and most fundamental in our lives. It emphasizes living life more fully by being in touch with the present moment, which is actually the only moment in which we are ever alive, and, through awareness, learning to accept and honor and work with the full range of our emotions and thoughts without becoming imprisoned by them. In meditation, we don't try to reframe or, most important, "fix" anything, not even particular unwanted or unhelpful thoughts or feelings, or patterns of thoughts and feelings, the way we might in psychotherapy. Instead, whatever appears in our awareness is simply noted without judgment as an "event" in the field of our consciousness in that moment. Over time, our thoughts, feelings, perceptions, and the entire way we carry ourselves in our lives and in relation to our challenges and stresses may change, but not because we set out to change anything—rather, because we embarked on coming home into ourselves, and taking up residence in the body and in our life with awareness and kindness toward ourselves, as we are, moment by moment. Herein lies the healing and transformative power of mindfulness.

Odes to Meditation

All cultures acknowledge and, to varying degrees, value the human capacity to relate consciously to the present moment, and the potentially transformative power it holds for seeing clearly and living with authenticity. In the popular imagination we associate meditation with Eastern cultures, but mindfulness has a venerable, if briefer and less well known, history in the West as well. Take, for example, the words of Sir William Osler,[1] one of the founders of modern medicine. He extolled "the practice of living for the day only, and for the day's work" rather than becoming distracted and derailed by preoccupations with future and past concerns, however enticing or overwhelming. He seems to have discovered, in his own life and work as a physician, the discipline of mindfulness practice in daily living and the value of cultivating equanimity. He urged his students to follow it as "a way of life."[2] Henry David Thoreau extolled the virtues of what he called "the bloom of the present moment" as the major theme of *Walden*.[3] Many great Western poets have captured the power of inner stillness and silence characteristic of present-moment awareness. T. S. Eliot characterized it unforgettably, as "A condition of complete simplicity / Costing not less than everything."[4] The great German poet Rainer Maria Rilke articulated it beautifully in words that perhaps have special meaning for women coping with breast cancer or any potentially life-threatening illness: "I am the rest between two notes / which are somehow always in discord / because death's note wants to climb over— / but in the dark interval, reconciled / they stay here trembling. / And the song goes on, beautiful."[5]

Letting Go of Goals: The Meditation Paradox

Meditation is often mistakenly thought of as a technique that aims at achieving a specific, highly pleasant "meditative state" akin to deep relaxation. But meditation is different from relaxation techniques in both methods and objectives. Its overall orientation is one of nonstriving and nondoing. Other strategies, such as visualization or guided imagery, have targeted goals; usually, the practitioner is simply trying to relax or to cope with some specific condition. In mindfulness meditation, there is no attempt to achieve anything other than awareness through the systematic deployment of moment-to-moment attention. It is about experiencing whatever is present in the moment: allowing sensations, thoughts, and feelings to be as they are, without having to hold onto them or push them away. This is very different from trying to change the present and future—in trying to create relaxation, for example, or reduce pain or anxiety. The only objective is simply to remain aware of whatever is happening in any moment. Specific goals like wanting to feel better, different, more relaxed, or less reactive should be observed as thoughts and desires and held lightly in awareness, but with an overall sense of nonattachment. We are not trying to get anywhere at all, or improve ourselves, or even heal, but for once, perhaps, we are just allowing ourselves, if only for a brief interval by the clock, to be as we are, exactly where we are, and tasting that peace, stillness, and wholeness lie right in this very moment in a very real way, outside of clock time.

As we have seen, mindfulness meditation is a way of being: a way to attend to the full range of one's experience, whether pleasant, unpleasant, or neutral. Thus, we practice meditation for its own sake, every day if possible, not to get anywhere else, but for the sake of being awake to life itself, in this moment. This is a radical departure from most of our other activities, which tend to be very goal-oriented, and from other forms of stress reduction or therapy, which are often practiced only as needed, in an attempt to relieve or cope with a particular condition or mood. Meditation does not set out to create change. Change may come in its wake, and indeed it often does. But getting somewhere is never the goal. Being here and knowing yourself as complete and whole, right here, right now, in any moment, is a more apt description of this "nonactivity."

Because of this radical orientation, meditation teaching and practice can seem somewhat paradoxical. In a medical setting, you are most likely to be referred by a health professional for specific reasons and in order to achieve specific personal goals. The most common reasons patients give for pursuing meditation are stress relief, anxiety reduction, relaxation, pain reduction, greater clarity in decision making, inner peace, and strengthening the ability to cope. Yet, patients are told early on in MBSR training that the best way to "get somewhere" is to not try to get anywhere at all but just to be where they already are, with awareness. Particular goals and objectives are recognized simply as thought formations, no different from any other thoughts in the field of awareness.

This doesn't mean that people don't achieve their intentionally targeted goals through meditation. They often do. But "progress," or development in your practice, is best measured by giving yourself over wholeheartedly to the process itself through continued regular practice, and seeing whether, over time, the practice itself doesn't come to feel profoundly, even perhaps mysteriously, nourishing and meaningful, and by whether you begin to experience a greater sense of well-being, a sense of empowerment and coherence in facing the full spectrum of life experience.

Why Meditation Practice for Women with Breast Cancer?

Meditation is useful for anyone coping with cancer precisely because it is fundamentally concerned with the here and now. In addition to helping you deal with stress and pain, both physical and emotional, dwelling in the present moment can slow your perception of the passage of time and enhance your appreciation of each moment of living. In the midst of profound doubt, fear, and confusion, you may not know what path to take—and there may, in fact, be no way to know. At such a time, knowing how to be still without having to make anything happen, go away, or change is extremely valuable. The disciplined practice of residing in stillness, even for short periods, leads, in time, to new ways of seeing, new pathways for knowing, and new choices for action that might not have been seen but for the stillness itself.

Mindfulness practice involves an element of constant self-inquiry, promoted not through thinking but through sustained awareness and continual, coherent questioning about what one is actually experiencing. Reports from clinical studies as well as personal experiences show that regular practice over the long term can enhance your ability to perceive yourself and your place in the world with acuity, precision, and acceptance. This greater awareness and familiarity with the entire field of your own experience—and particularly your ability to recognize thoughts as thoughts, and feelings as feelings—brings composure, inner stillness, a sense of personal power and authority, and, paradoxically, greater nonattachment and selflessness. All this can help a breast cancer patient cope with the high levels of stress and uncertainty that come with a cancer diagnosis. At the same time, it cultivates wisdom and the capacity to see and act based on your direct experience of connectedness to others and to the world. It points toward compassion as well, including, most important, self-compassion.

Dealing with Pain and Suffering

Mindfulness encourages a willingness to look deeply into any and all emotional states and life circumstances, even negative or scary ones, simply because they are already present and a part of your experience. If pain and suffering suddenly become part of your life, they thus become appropriate to embrace with mindful awareness. Whatever your situation or condition, from the perspective of mindfulness, it is "workable" if you are willing to work with it by holding it gently in awareness.

Pain and *suffering* are often used as interchangeable terms, but from the perspective of mindfulness they are quite different. *Pain* describes basic sensory input, whether physical or emotional, that is perceived as hurtful. *Suffering,* on the other hand, describes an emotional interpretation of that input. In response to any level of pain, we have a choice of many responses: from extreme suffering with very little stimulus, to minimal suffering even in the face of severely traumatic events or stimuli. In mindfulness practice, pain and suffering can be held in awareness and seen with greater patience, clarity, and intimacy, which can provide insight into new ways of understanding and coping with one's situation.

For women with breast cancer, *meditation* can complement the use of *medication* when needed for the control of pain. Meditation calls on you to look deeply and nonjudgmentally into the experience of pain as bare sensation, even if it is only for a few moments at a time at first. As you practice more, you can gradually lengthen the time you attempt to observe the sensations with nonattachment. When you are in pain, this might mean directing your attention to a particular region of the body and coupling it with a sense of the breath moving into and out of that region, observing any changes in sensations from moment to moment. (The body scan, described later in this chapter, can be helpful in this regard.) In this way you might find that thoughts and feelings about pain, such as "this is killing me" or "I don't know if I can stand this," are in fact different from the actual hurtful sensations, like burning, shooting, squeezing, tearing, and aching. And if you ask yourself, "Is this killing me right now, in this very moment?" the answer is almost always no. It is thinking about the duration, meaning, or intensity of the pain that produces most of the suffering. This one realization can reduce both emotional distress and suffering from physical pain.

Elana

In mindfulness, any situation, however painful, can become your teacher—even cancer. In illness, a willingness to look and listen to the actuality of your experience can significantly transform its meaning. Our colleague and co-author Elana Rosenbaum, an MBSR instructor who is now a long-term cancer survivor (non-Hodgkin's lymphoma), writes eloquently about her experiences:

> *I am tired. I tire easily. Yet, I am committed to fanning the flame of my spirit, and I find that this requires true wisdom—sachel (common sense in Hebrew), as my mother would say. It means that tonight I can't go out to be with my friends, even to meditate. Instead, I must rest to recover from the emotions of the day so I can rise tomorrow and be refreshed. I do not like making this decision to stay home, even though it is "wise." But I know that I must listen to my body, not necessarily to live longer but because my fatigue doesn't allow me to be fully present with anyone or anything except the feelings of heavy eyelids and the effort to stay awake. I am committed to being wherever I am as fully and as honestly as possible. I do not like acknowledging limitations or facing my vulnerability. I do not like choosing rest over activity. Yet, I have learned that to maintain my equilibrium, I must be ruthlessly honest with myself and admit when I have to "stop." This is new to me and confronts any shred of omnipotence I might once have held. I may not be my body, but my body does certainly affect my mental and emotional state, and I MUST pay attention.*
>
> *I find that my meditation practice colors my belief system. I am consciously aware now that every moment is a precious moment. This means I walk the tightrope between wanting every moment to be "special" and simply dropping into a space where every moment, be it going to the bathroom or paying a bill, is special. To be fully in the moment, here, not lost in the thought of a wish or a "should," is my challenge, and I find it necessary to be a warrior through the jungle of my self. . . .*
>
> *And as I open to these thoughts, these fears, these illusions of control, these wishes for things to be different, I also open to a deep sense of peace and appreciation of life itself. I receive succor from nature. I have celebrated snowfall and rain. I feel the wind on my cheek and appreciate my warm coat, the solace of my home, and my husband, friends, and colleagues. I feel more deeply connected not only to myself but to others and the universe around.*
>
> *As I teach my classes, my eyes frequently tear up as I am awed by the simple acts of courage I hear and observe again and again in people who*

*are in pain, who struggle to eat or walk, or brush their hair. We practice
meditation together and share and laugh, crying and questioning
together, "Why me?" And in response, it is easier to tolerate and
understand, "Why not me?" We sit quietly together in deep appreciation
of each other and our daily bravery as we come to class and go about the
routines of the day, choosing to live and face our suffering, our enemy, my
enemy, ourselves as we are, human, and imperfect. And in confronting
the truth of ourselves/myself, pain and imperfections become acceptable,
even beautiful, for to allow my humanness is to be free, and to be naked
in my imperfections allows for a perfection that is life affirming, and I
can feel whole regardless of what the CAT scan shows or the statistics say,
and I can begin to truly believe that I am perfect and the pain, the anger,
the negative mind states are as transitory as the bloom of the violet or the
weather in New England. This allows me to go on and to be able to open
up to receive light and love, bringing with it caring and compassion to
myself and all others.*

These personal reflections remind us that meditation involves a grace-
ful sense of accepting the totality of your experience as it is, rather than
forced or mechanical attempts to achieve particular ends—even relaxation, insight, or greater well-being. In fact, it is out of that accepting
embrace that relaxation, insight, and well-being are most likely to come
by themselves. That's the wonderful paradox of mindfulness practice.

Three Dimensions of Meditation

With a simultaneously gentle yet very firm touch, meditation works on
three interrelated and universal aspects of our experience as human
beings:

■ A direct, moment-to-moment sense of connection between your
body and your sense of self. Here meditation serves as a way of "inhabiting" the body with varying degrees of mindfulness, wisdom, compassion (for yourself), and self-acceptance. For a woman with breast
cancer, this dimension might include the painful realization that one's
health and well-being can no longer be taken for granted—followed by

a commitment to work with that situation mindfully and intentionally, no matter how turbulent and tumultuous one's thoughts, emotions, and body sensations may be at times.

▪ An understanding, through self-observation, of the ways in which sensations, impulses, thoughts, feelings, and meaning emerge in coherent patterns that can be seen and held in awareness. For the woman with breast cancer, this might involve admitting that the disease has shattered one's sense of predictability and control, but recognizing that it does not represent a total loss or shattering of one's being by any stretch of the imagination, although it may feel that way at times. Meditation opens up a range of options for perceiving, understanding, and responding to the situation in new ways. As a consequence, she may reach a new degree of mastery and wisdom in facing and comprehending her experience, and charting a course for herself that comes from the depths of her heart's longing.

▪ A sense of belonging, of connectedness, of being in community in the largest sense. While you might understandably think of meditation as something you do alone, apart from the rest of the world, actually it is a way of being in the world both as your individual self and, simultaneously, as an integral part of a larger whole. A friend of Jon's who attended his MBSR classes at the hospital shared his experience of this.

Martin

Martin, a professor at a prestigious university, commented one day that having leukemia and wanting to prepare for a bone marrow transplant had brought him into what he called "this community of the afflicted" where he felt more at home, in a funny way, than with his colleagues in faculty meetings. Pain and life-threatening illness often create that kind of feeling of distance, of inhabiting all of a sudden a separate reality. When we are willing to explore these feelings through mindfulness and acceptance, new openings often occur. In Martin's case, he was struck by a remarkable insight while riding on the subway one day. He saw with utter clarity that the people sitting on either side of him might very well be suffering every bit as deeply as he was. He realized that in this way, the "community of the afflicted" could extend virtually to everybody and went far beyond his own personal problems, preoccupations, and fears. What started as a feeling of separation blossomed into a deeper feeling of inclusion and unity, from which he took considerable satisfaction.

Such a spontaneous experience of mindfulness and insight signals a turning point in one's practice, as mindfulness emerges from the formal setting of meditation and becomes a way of life.

Is Meditation for You?

Meditation practice is a rigorous and demanding discipline. You will need to devote some time every day to formal practice, as well as to the equally challenging task of incorporating it into your everyday life.

Learning meditation under crisis conditions—such as immediately after a breast cancer diagnosis—may be difficult. In fact, it isn't always advisable. At our clinic, our relationship with a breast cancer patient begins with an evaluation interview aimed partly at gauging the appropriateness of the program at that particular time for that particular person and at the potential costs and benefits of participation. Sometimes it is best to wait to begin learning meditation until a little while after receiving the diagnosis. Some people find meditation most helpful after their treatments have ended and they are trying to return to normal activities as a "survivor" and to adopt a lifestyle that promotes optimal health and reduces cancer risk. However, meditation helps many people in dealing with the side effects of treatment and in overcoming the sense of loss of control and mastery over their lives.

Even patients in hospice or receiving hospice care at home benefit from meditation, using it for relief of physical pain, and with emotional pain and suffering. Of course, meditation works best when it is integrated into a comprehensive care plan. It is an excellent adjunct in explorations about death and dying and feelings of loss. Many dying patients find that the calmness and silence of meditation bring profound feelings of acceptance, well-being, and inner peace. On the other end of the spectrum, healthy women at higher genetic risk for breast cancer may be drawn to meditation to reduce environmental and lifestyle risk and to control anxiety.

If you think you'd like to begin meditating, ask your health care practitioner about programs that teach meditation and about the specific approach that seems most appropriate for you. Your meditation instructor may be able to help you gauge whether the timing is right. If possible, particularly at the outset, take a class or work with a group so that you'll have ongoing support and opportunities for clarification and refinement in the early stages of practice.

There is currently no formal certification of meditation teachers for MBSR or any other approach. As the field develops, some kind of certification will probably emerge. In the meantime, you have to rely on word of mouth and on your own perception of instructors and their appropriateness, sincerity, and competency. Even if you get a referral from your health care provider, be sure to take your own impressions and experiences into account in deciding whether or not to work with a particular person. Start from the premise that instructors should be personally grounded in the practice of meditation themselves, with years of experience with daily practice. You wouldn't want teachers asking you to do something they do not actually do themselves— something they do not understand through direct experience. For a list of MBSR programs we know about, see www.umassmed.edu/cfm.

The MBSR Clinic

Participants are referred by their doctors to our Mindfulness-Based Stress Reduction Clinic at the University of Massachusetts Medical Center, and meet with an instructor for two and a half hours once a week. In the sixth week, in addition to the weekly class, everyone attends a day-long silent meditation retreat over the weekend.

Classes generally contain about thirty people with a wide range of chronic medical conditions, including cancer, cardiac disease, hypertension, gastrointestinal problems, chronic pain, and differing levels of disability. With such a heterogeneous group, the approach tends to emphasize what the participants have in common—like the fact that everybody has a body, that everybody is breathing, that everybody's mind goes through periods of agitation and periods of calmness, the fact that everybody is dealing with the stress of their particular condition, and that we all suffer at times from physical and emotional pain, including anxiety and depression, and that we all have profound inner resources for learning to deal more effectively with our fear and suffering. Thus, the focus is primarily on what is right with people and on pouring energy and attention into those domains, rather than on what is wrong. This approach complements the more conventional medical dimensions of each person's treatment. In the Stress Reduction Clinic program, regardless of their diagnosis, everyone is thus able to share experiences of being aware of their thoughts and emotions, work and family life, health and illness in ways that offer new dimensions of both insight and action. This approach allows the participants to come to see themselves more strongly and more accurately as a whole and unique person beyond their identity as "patients."

Many women with breast cancer have participated in the Stress Reduction Clinic's program over the years. At one point, we took part in a study of women with breast cancer in which they went through the eight-week program with all the other patients, but which also added a component more specifically directed toward breast cancer: what we called wrap-around sessions (one before and five after the eight-week program), exclusively for the women in the study.[6] Such an approach can extend and deepen the MBSR experience and provide additional social support and community for individuals dealing with specific illnesses. However, meditation training through MBSR is not meant to take the place of a breast cancer support group. Many women who join our program also participate in such support groups. Although we have not done so to date, MBSR could certainly be adopted specifically for a group made up entirely of women with breast cancer.

Prior to enrollment in the program, a clinic staff member meets with every prospective participant individually to discuss her medical history, her reason for coming to the program, and her motivation. We provide a brief description of the program and its requirements (class attendance and at-home practice). We also gather information to help us keep track of individual and group outcomes. At the end of the program, each person meets with her instructor for an hour to discuss her experiences and develop strategies for continuing with what she has learned. Participants can request additional one-on-one time during the course so that private matters can be discussed outside the group.

Meditation Practice, Step by Step

One of the challenges of trying to describe meditation is that it can seem so mysterious and vague. But while the rewards of meditation are profound, it is really a simple process.

Following are descriptions of the basic types of meditation taught at our Stress Reduction Clinic. They consist of sitting meditation, practiced in straight-backed chairs or on the floor; a body scan meditation, practiced lying down; and mindful hatha yoga, which involves a range of body postures. We often add walking meditation to the mix. This mix of practices, with varying degrees of movement and stillness and different ways to focus attention, helps us reach a broad range of individuals with different personalities, abilities, and degrees of mobility.

Awareness-of-Breathing (Sitting) Meditation

Sit quietly or lie down in a place where you will not be disturbed. If sitting, sit erect but not stiff, in a posture that embodies dignity. If lying down, lie on your back, if possible, on a comfortable padded surface (bed or floor) with a pillow under your knees and your head supported. Allow the eyes to gently close, if that feels comfortable. Otherwise, leave them half open and focused on one point. Bring your attention to the feeling of the breath flowing in and out of your body, moment by moment and breath by breath, without forcing the breath in any way. You can focus on it at the nostrils or at your abdomen, where you can feel the expanding of the belly on each inhalation and the receding of your belly on each exhalation.

Simply stay in touch with the feeling of the breath and/or the belly moving, as if your mind were surfing on the waves of the breath. As best you can, stay with the feeling of the wave of the breath for the full duration of the inhalation and the exhalation, allowing yourself to just dwell here, moment by moment, following the breath as it comes in and as it goes out. Each time you notice your mind has wandered off the breath, which it will certainly do many times, simply note where it has gone (i.e., observe what is on your mind in this moment without pursuing it or rejecting it). Then, without judging it in any way, let go of whatever captured your attention, and gently but firmly bring attention back to your nostrils or your belly and to this breath, whether it is now coming in or going out. If your mind wanders off the breath twenty times, then each time, as soon as you are aware of it, you can note where it is, let go, and come back to the breath.

A period of formal practice might last from ten to forty-five minutes. At least at first, guided meditation (by instructor or audiotape) will be helpful, particularly for longer sessions. You might want to try it at least once, right now or after you finish this chapter, to give yourself a concrete experience of what it can be like. However, the real benefit comes from practicing every day, whether you feel like it or not, and whether you enjoy the experience or not. The important point is for all that time to be just for you, a time for being rather than doing, a time of awareness that is open and spacious, and generous enough toward yourself to allow any and all inner or outer experiences to arise and simply be observed with attention without reaction or judgment as they come, linger, and go in the field of your awareness.

The other mindfulness meditation techniques are extensions or variations of this basic practice and should be done with the same orientation to the present moment described above.

The Body Scan Meditation

Lie on your back, if possible, on a comfortable surface, which can be your bed, but remembering that the body scan is about "falling awake," not falling asleep, an occupational hazard of doing a lying-down meditation. Staying continuously aware of your breath as best you can, gently and slowly direct your attention to the various sensations in different parts of your body in a systematic order, starting from the toes of the left foot, proceeding up the left leg, over to the right foot, up the right leg, through the torso, the arms from fingertips to shoulders, then the neck and finally the head. The idea is to "inhabit" each region of your body with full awareness as best you can, feeling what is there to be felt, and also being aware of your thoughts, emotions, and judgments about particular regions. These too are simply cradled in loving awareness as you move into each region, dwelling with it for a while, and then moving on to the next region. In this way, we are bringing loving attention to the body and to ourselves and our body image and experience in ways that help reclaim our sense of wholeness and honor the sense of loss and grieving that may have come from the experience of the disease or from the treatments you may have had to undergo.

Mindful Hatha Yoga

Hatha Yoga is an ancient Indian tradition of meditation in motion developed over thousands of years. The word *yoga* is Sanskrit, meaning "yoke." It points to the unity of body and mind, soul and spirit, the individual and the larger world. That unity is recognized and its power tapped through the practice itself. Mindful yoga involves standing, sitting, and lying on the floor in a variety of postures while cultivating the same moment-to-moment, nonjudgmental awareness as in sitting meditation and the body scan. It can be extremely gentle or quite vigorous and demanding, depending on how it is taught and practiced. One chapter doesn't allow for teaching the full range of postures, but it shouldn't be difficult to find a class, videotape, instructor, book, or magazine to learn from. Look for hatha yoga classes that emphasize using the breath and slow, gentle movements.

Cultivate moment-to-moment awareness of sensations and an overall sense of the body as a whole as you practice. Each posture also has metaphorical significance that can be felt through the body. For instance, the "mountain" and the "warrior" are both standing poses that embody a sense of rootedness, steadfastness, dignity, and strength in the face of ever-changing life challenges.

Walking Meditation

To use walking as a formal meditation practice, do it slowly. Focus on moment-to-moment awareness of the lifting, moving, and placing of each foot; the shifting of the weight over the forward foot; the breath moving in the body; and a sense of the body as a whole moving. When your mind wanders, note where your attention has gone and intentionally let it go and return your focus to the breath and the other elements of walking already mentioned. Be as embodied as possible in your walking, whether it is during a period of formal practice, or just walking down the street or down the aisles of a supermarket.

Putting It All Together

In our clinic classes, extended stretches of silence during the periods of formal meditation practice are interspersed with short periods of guidance and periodic reminders to stay focused on the breath or return to it if the mind has wandered away. We also spend a lot of time discussing the participants' experiences with meditation at home that week, and the ways it did or did not influence their everyday lives. We assign "homework" each week; participants agree to practice a mix of these methods at least six days per week for forty-five minutes at a time, using audiotapes for guidance. This discipline is extremely important if the practices are to take root in one's life and be adequate to the degree of stress and suffering that our patients are usually facing. Again, one does not have to like the practice, or even feel particularly relaxed—but just doing it for eight weeks in this way tends to develop greater calmness and insight and stability of mind.

In addition to the formal practices, we assign informal mindfulness practices each week, and we encourage people to create their own ways to sustain mindfulness during the course of each day. Informal practices include awareness of different aspects of daily life experience such as breathing, walking, driving, cooking, eating, cleaning, ironing, showering, talking, listening, working, parenting, and playing. That also includes awareness of your emotional states, thoughts, and perceptions during daily activities, along with bringing awareness to particularly stressful situations and one's options for responding to them mindfully rather than reacting to them automatically.

We often introduce meditation and mindfulness through an "eating meditation" exercise at the very beginning of the course: eating one raisin. Each person eats a single raisin very slowly, so as to really be present with the seeing, feeling, tasting, chewing, and swallowing. The point is to focus attention on an ordinary everyday experience to such a degree that it becomes a universe of novel experience. It isn't truly novel, of course—we just never truly tuned in to it before. People frequently tell us that their eating habits have changed as a result of this one exercise!

Other informal meditation exercises we use include drawings; puzzles; communication exercises based on the martial art of aikido; observing the weather and activity in the street from the window of the classroom; theater exercises involving fast, slow, and chaotic walking; and slow backward walking with eyes closed. These exercises produce multisensory experiences in which mindfulness can be used to illustrate, identify, and break out of a broad range of conditioned patterns of perception and behavior.

Courtney

Courtney began mindfulness meditation after an accident left her with chronic pain, several years before her diagnosis of breast cancer when she was not yet forty. She found that it helped her pain and improved her overall well-being. Her daily practice waxed and waned, but every year she went on two long meditation retreats.

As grounded as she was, when her doctor gave her the news, Courtney was really "blown away." "I lived a life that was not supposed to give you cancer," she says. Both her parents had died of cancer by the time Courtney was graduating from college. She was obsessed with maintaining perfect health through her twenties and early thirties, and in fact was never even really ill. As she puts it: "I was on hyper-alert my whole adult life.

"I was terrified when I heard 'breast cancer.' I could hardly hear my treatment choices. It was just so scary. My father died only two months after he was diagnosed, and my mother lived just four months after hers. Cancer meant death to me." Courtney also stopped meditating: "I was too afraid to see what was in my mind. I knew I was just going to think about dying."

Courtney didn't sleep for a week after her diagnosis. Finally one day she decided to go back to her meditation practice. She lay down on the floor late one morning—and after only a few minutes, fell asleep. "That's when I really knew how much I needed it!" she says. She started to meditate at night (though she'd always done it in the mornings before) and found she could sleep a lot better afterward.

Meditation also helped her through treatment. "Staying in the present was the thing that saved me," she says. "When chemo got tough, it was important to not dwell on dying, thinking about the past, my mom and dad's suffering—and just deal with being nauseated today and what to do about that.

"Meditation helps you tolerate what your mind will do. Your mind will do it anyway. But what my mind was doing didn't control me. Treatment is bad enough. Your mind going crazy makes it that much worse."

For Courtney, the biggest benefits of mindfulness actually came after her treatment was over. Through treatment she had developed a thyroid condition and was depressed, out of energy, and gaining weight. She also was very much afraid of finishing treatment—what if some cancer cells were still hanging around, and she had nothing to fight them with? "I got scared because I was no longer fighting the beast. I had this warrior energy—and then no more battles."

At this point, Courtney came to the eight-week program at the clinic. She renewed her commitment to meditation practice and made it a priority. The group support helped her stay with it. She also learned the body scan, which really helped her. "Between preop chemo, surgery, then radiation, I'd been living with this monster for months," she explains. "Treatment was so intrusive and put me in such a vulnerable position, I had to get out of my body somehow. By the time it was over, I felt like I was walking next to my body and couldn't quite get back in, or get comfortable. Doing the body scan, saying to myself, 'You can be in this part of the body whether or not it has betrayed you,' and just being with that body part, made a real difference. I used it a lot with the neuropathy in my foot, for example. Now I can experience my body as whole again. It got me back in my own body."

By the end of the program, Courtney reported that she was as calm as she wanted to be. For a while, any ache or pain would have her convinced the cancer was back, and she felt a low-level background anxiety about recurrence. Those impulses haven't gone away, but with mindfulness they no longer throw Courtney off her stride. "When I meditate I take note of every thought and emotion that comes up, and let them fly by. I try to let them go through without reacting to them. By now they slide through my mind like it's made of Teflon!

"I believe a calm mind cultivates a calm body—and the other way around, too. They feed off each other," Courtney says. To maintain that calmness in herself, Courtney meditates fifteen to forty-five minutes each morning or evening—"both, if I'm lucky!" She practices with a group once a week and takes two long retreats a year, as well as an occasional weekend or day-long workshop.

Like many other breast cancer patients who meditate, Courtney finds that her life has changed dramatically. "I see time differently now," she says. "I refuse to waste it." She also describes a kinder, gentler manner toward herself and other people, where there used to be a kind of painful edge. Most of all, she's simply living in the present. "In the moment, I always know I'm not dying of cancer right now. The only thing worse than cancer is thinking you are dying of cancer when you are not! What you do with your mind matters."

What Research Says about Meditation

Without a doubt, meditation helps people like Courtney cope with serious illness. But does science support the proposition that meditation actually offers medical benefits?

Very few studies focusing on meditation and cancer have been reported in the literature. Only two randomized, controlled trials have looked at meditation as the sole psychosocial intervention in patients with cancer. The first of these focused on MBSR in relation to mood and symptoms of stress.[7] The intervention was similar to the UMass program, consisting of a weekly MBSR group lasting 1.5 hours for 7 weeks plus meditation practice at home. Ninety patients, representing a range of types and stages of cancer, were enrolled. Those patients randomized to MBSR showed a significant reduction in overall mood disturbance and an increase in vigor compared to those in the control group. The meditation group also had fewer overall stress symptoms, fewer cardiopulmonary and gastrointestinal symptoms, and less emotional irritability, depression, and cognitive disorganization by the end of the study than the control group.

Analyses of our study of breast cancer patients (n = 178) undergoing MBSR plus the wrap-around sessions are in progress. A positive effect of this program on psychosocial outcomes in the MBSR participants has already been confirmed. Following the program, we observed increases in levels of active-cognitive coping, a large decrease in level of overall "emotional over-control," an increase in spirituality, and reduced depression and helpless/hopeless thinking in comparison to the control group. At twelve months' follow-up, the MBSR group continued to show a significant improvement beyond that of the other comparison groups in the study (a dietary intervention group and a usual care group) on several psychosocial measures.[8]

Recently, we completed a small uncontrolled study of a combined intensive dietary and MBSR intervention in men with prostate cancer who had undergone prostatectomies and still showed rising PSA (Prostate-Specific Antigen, an indicator of metastasis under these conditions) levels. We observed a slowing of the rate of increase in PSA in these men over the course of the study. Before the program, the mean PSA level was doubling every 6.5 months, while after the intervention, it was doubling every 17.7 months.[9] Results from these studies of meditation with cancer patients are promising, but point to the need for more rigorously designed and executed studies that will inform us about the role of MBSR alone and in concert with other lifestyle interventions.

Despite the small number of published studies at this time on meditation in general and, more specifically, for cancer patients, MBSR has been shown over the years to bring benefits to patients with a broad range of chronic medical conditions, including chronic pain[10-13] and anxiety disorders.[14,15] Women with breast cancer experience more than their share of pain and anxiety, so the results in these areas support meditation for patients with breast cancer, as well as supporting the value of meditation more generally. Meditation has repeatedly been shown to yield both short- and long-term reductions in physical and psychological symptoms, and to enhance psychological well-being in general.

In an unpublished study from the Stress Reduction Clinic, we found that personality traits generally considered unchanging in adulthood—psychological hardiness and sense of coherence—actually increase significantly in many MBSR participants. Follow-ups over three years show that these positive changes last. This helps to confirm that MBSR has the potential to transform outlook and coping capacity in patients with serious medical conditions like breast cancer.

Several other studies of cancer patients have shown the benefits of practices that have much in common with meditation. These include decreases in psychological distress from progressive muscle relaxation and guided imagery; decreases in anxiety and depression with muscle relaxation, hypnosis, cognitive therapy, and biofeedback;[16,17] and improved mood and decreased symptoms and distress with coping skills training, mental imagery, and relaxation (compared with a support group alone).[18] An even more substantial body of evidence proves the usefulness of similar strategies in reducing treatment side effects and pain in cancer.[19-33]

Meditation and similar "self-regulatory" strategies like those mentioned above can affect the immune system, a major factor in the ultimate outcome of malignant diseases like breast cancer. These practices have been shown to augment the immune system by enhancing natural killer white blood cell activity[34-42] and may therefore play an important role in prevention and treatment. Meditation can also affect melatonin levels. Melatonin is an antioxidant, has cancer cell growth inhibitory properties, and helps modulate the immune system.[43-45] In a pilot study, melatonin metabolites in urine—indicating melatonin levels in the body—were significantly higher in healthy women who meditated regularly than in those who did not meditate.[46]

More and better studies are needed to pinpoint exactly how meditation affects the body, especially how it works in breast cancer. There's still a lot to learn about meditation and similar techniques and their relationships to the genetic, molecular, and cellular mechanisms underlying cancer—and healing.

Can Meditation Ever Hurt?

Though meditation is almost always of benefit, not everyone responds positively. Some published case reports and studies report negative effects, including increased tension, anxiety, depression, and confusion.[47] For example, in one study of participants in an intensive silent mindfulness meditation retreat (which some took for two weeks and others for three months), some of these negative effects were reported. But almost everyone also reported strong positive effects. The design of the study makes it hard to differentiate between normal emotional turbulence and serious psychiatric disturbance. It may be that problems stemmed from the context, setting, and cultural and ideological slant given to the meditation practice, or from a mismatch between a person and a practice, and not from the meditation itself.

Our experience with over thirteen thousand patients at the clinic suggests that negative reactions to meditation are very rare, but that some people may experience anxiety while practicing meditation,[48] most often people who have already struggled with anxiety. Almost always, this effect dissipates as the person becomes more experienced with meditation.

In any event, meditation isn't always a pleasant experience. Difficult thoughts and emotions certainly surface as a normal part of being human, and that is certainly the case during meditation. Mindfulness is about welcoming whatever arises in the present moment and holding it gently in awareness without trying to fix it, escape it, pursue it, or deny it. However, if you find you are experiencing an inordinate amount of difficulty with meditation, it may be wise for you to also work with a counselor or therapist, as many of our patients do. You might also explore taking a slightly different tack in your practice. Perhaps in the early stages, more emphasis on practicing mindful yoga or tai chi, with shorter periods of sitting meditation, might be more congenial than extended body scans or intensive sitting. Of course, it is very helpful to have the support of a class or group and to work with a skilled instructor, rather than entirely on your own.

Meditation: A Turning Point

Regular meditation practice is, in itself, a major lifestyle change for most women. It can also lead to other significant changes, like quitting smoking, reducing alcohol use, and improving dietary habits. This is largely because meditating can increase self-efficacy,[49] which is intimately intertwined with self-esteem and the confidence in yourself that you can make real changes in your life. The feeling that you can affect things and bring about change allows you to take charge of your behaviors and make active choices about them. Beyond that, learning meditation means learning how to take better care of yourself as a complement to what the health care system can do for you. Following this line of thinking to its logical end, by changing health-related behaviors, meditation might theoretically influence the course of cancer both directly and indirectly—and even more certainly provide preventative effects.

The use of meditation in cancer therapy has yet to be scientifically tested adequately in clinical trials. But its value as a form of stress reduction and as a time-tested way of calming the mind and body and developing clarity, insight, acceptance, and equanimity recommend it as a commonsense adjunct to other forms of treatment. Meditation can have a profound influence on quality of life for a woman living with breast cancer. It can help her feel a greater commitment and sense of partnership with her health care team while she undergoes medical procedures and treatments, and foster a strong sense of engagement in life. It is a practical complement to standard medical therapies and a pathway to the kind of personal growth that can come through crisis.

Sherry

Sherry started getting annual mammograms when she was only thirty-five (years before it is generally recommended), after an even younger woman she worked with died of breast cancer. Ten years later, she found a lump herself that mammography never picked up. By the time she convinced her doctors to perform a biopsy, the lump was found to be malignant, and she had it removed. It measured 4 centimeters, twenty-four out of twenty-five nodes were positive, and it had spread into tissues beyond the nodes. She was told that her prognosis wasn't good. Now, five years later, she sometimes wonders: did all that radiation cause (or encourage) her cancer? And wasn't it unnecessary anyway, if it couldn't even diagnose her breast cancer early—or at all?

This kind of thinking has plagued many women with breast cancer, and it could be enough to cause long-term anxiety or depression.

Sherry was protected, however. She learned how to observe these kinds of thoughts when they come up, note the emotions that come with them, and differentiate between the two—then let them all go.

"I don't beat myself up anymore," she says. "I know I did the best I could with the information I had. I'd do it differently now. But I lived as I had to live, given where I was. I've moved into the present moment. I don't go off like a firecracker every time something hits my emotion anymore. It's a much better way to live."

That's the kind of perspective we hear over and over again from participants in the MBSR program—people who have learned that if they are not going to be sheltered from the storm, they may as well be the calm at the eye of it.

Sherry says that mindfulness is what got her through the breast cancer whirlwind. "Faced with that kind of fear, and looking at what I thought for a while was a death sentence, I realized for the first time that now is all we have. And it is a wonderful place to live. For a cancer patient or survivor, there is no greater gift. It is a gift to know how precious life is, and a gift to be regularly aware of that. It is so easy to slip into spiritual numbness. But with cancer breathing over your shoulder, you can't be numb."

The difficult times are not over. New aches and pains make her fear a recurrence. She worries about her young children and the anxiety they feel about her illness. She recently lost a friend to breast cancer, and decided to have a prophylactic mastectomy of her other breast. Mindfulness helps her cope with the stress. "Even though it's been over five years since I was diagnosed, I still deal with breast cancer on a daily basis," she says. "I don't know what I'd do without meditation."

Sherry doesn't do much formal sitting meditation. She has fibromyalgia (painful muscle and joints) and finds it very uncomfortable to stay still. For her, mindfulness has become more of a mindset: a constant daily stopping, and coming back to the moment. "I can still hear my instructor's voice saying, 'When you stir the soup, just stir the soup.'

"She also talked about the difference between reacting and responding. That's another gift meditation has given me: the ability to put some space between me and an automatic, visceral reaction, and the ability to take time to take a breath—and then respond."

Sherry does use the body scan once or twice a day. It helps her to manage her pain from the fibromyalgia and from lymphedema, and to get to sleep. In addition, Sherry discovered that after the trauma of diagnosis and treatment, she was shut off from her own body, angry at its betrayal—on top of the raw fact that she was now missing a breast. The body scan helped her heal into her wholeness again.

"It helps with the whole process of aging. I've got aches and pains I didn't before. Inside I sometimes still feel twenty-two, but I'm decades beyond that now. Physically there are some things I can no longer do. Meditation puts it all in perspective. Somehow, it makes it OK. You miss what you miss. You love what you love. You go on."

Like many breast cancer survivors, Sherry says the disease changed her life and her outlook on life. But the change really came because having breast cancer brought her to mindfulness. "What I won from cancer was the rest of my life," she says, "thanks mostly to meditation.

"It changed me dramatically. People's reactions to me have changed dramatically. People tell me, 'You seem so peaceful,' 'You seem so calm,' 'Don't you ever get upset or angry?' 'What do I have to do to feel like you feel?' That tells me something real happened.

"Before I was diagnosed, I was a workaholic. And my focus was there, more so than on my family. I thought I was being a good parent, and I thought I needed to be a good provider, but life was proceeding at breakneck pace. We got everything done, but at warp speed. Everything was orchestrated—it needed to be. We had little time to breathe.

"Cancer stopped me in my tracks. It had to. I was back at work ten days after my mastectomy, still trying to do it all. I think I still would be, but for meditation. It is a wonderful way to slow down. When I took time to stop and look at what I was doing—to really experience my life, my kids, what we needed, what our lives looked like—suddenly it all seemed very different to me. I switched my job to part time, but you know how that goes: part-time pay, full-time hours. So I left altogether. I do some consulting now. I spend time with my kids. When they are older, I'd like to go back to work. But they are happier this way. This is what they need right now. This is what I need right now.

"I used to have these huge fits of temper. When you're moving that fast, when you have that many balls in the air, things never go right. It's constant frustration and anger. It is hard to imagine feeling that now. I still get angry sometimes. I can still blow up at my kids for leaving dirty clothes all over the house when I've asked them a thousand times to just throw them in the hamper. But mostly I feel content. Peaceful.

"It wasn't easy at first. Especially right after diagnosis, the minute you stop being so busy, terror is the first thing that comes up: I have a disease that might kill me! But until you can let that kind of emotional noise go and be, to the extent you can, quiet, calm, still—really stop—you can't effectively deal with your situation."

In any event, meditation does not deliver some kind of constant state of bliss. You have to take the bad with the good. Sherry has a favorite story that illustrates the point.

Her mother died shortly before Sherry was diagnosed with breast cancer. Not long before she died, Sherry took her mother, who loved movies and especially cartoons, to see a re-release of *Bambi*. The theater was mostly empty, but just in front of them were a young woman and her daughter, who looked about five years old. At the pivotal scene, in which Bambi's mother is shot by hunters and Bambi is running away terrified, the little girl started to cry. Her mother tried to soothe her, reassuring her that it was just a movie. The girl cried harder. The mother tried harder to calm her down, clearly beside herself. Suddenly the girl just stopped, turned to her mother, and said, "It's OK to cry, Mom. This is the sad part."

Meditation teaches us what this girl understood—what we all knew to begin with but forgot somewhere along the way as innate wisdom was socialized out of us. Cry in the sad part. Laugh in the happy part. There will be both.

Resources

For information on MBSR programs at the clinic, professional training opportunities, and guided mindfulness meditation audiotapes, contact

THE CENTER FOR MINDFULNESS
UMass Medical Center
Worcester, MA 01655-0267

508-856-2656
fax: 508-856-1977
www.umassmed.edu/cfm
www.mindfulnesstapes.com *(guided mindfulness meditation practice tapes by Jon Kabat-Zinn, including the body scan, sitting meditation, and mindful hatha yoga)*
www.retreats2renew.com *(guided meditation CDs by Elana Rosenbaum, especially for people with cancer)*

Recommended Reading

BECK, C. *Nothing Special*. San Francisco: HarperCollins, 1993.

BECK, C. *Everyday Zen*. San Francisco: HarperCollins, 1989.

COHEN, D. *Finding a Joyful Life in the Heart of Pain*. Boston: Shambhala, 2000.

EPSTEIN, M. *Thoughts Without a Thinker*. New York: Basic Books, 1995: 146–147.

GOLDSTEIN, J., KORNFIELD, J. *Seeking the Heart of Wisdom*. Boston: Shambhala, 1987.

GUNARATANA, H. *Mindfulness in Plain English*. Boston: Wisdom, 1991.

HAHN, TN. *The Miracle of Mindfulness*. Boston: Beacon, 1976.

KABAT-ZINN, J. *Full Catastrophe Living: Using the Wisdom of Your Body and Mind to Face Stress, Pain, and Illness*. New York: Delacorte, 1990.

KABAT-ZINN, J. *Wherever You Go, There You Are: Mindfulness Meditation in Everyday Life*. New York: Hyperion, 1994.

KABAT-ZINN, M., KABAT-ZINN, J. *Everyday Blessings: The Inner Work of Mindful Parenting*. New York: Hyperion, 1997.

KAPLEAU, P. *The Three Pillars of Zen*. Boston: Beacon, 1967:53.

KORNFIELD, J. *A Path with Heart*. New York: Bantam, 1993.

KRISHNAMURTI, J. *Think on These Things*. New York: Harper & Row, 1964.

LERNER, M. *Choice in Cancer: Integrating the Best of Conventional and Alternative Approaches to Cancer.* Cambridge, Mass.: MIT Press, 1994.

LEVINE, S. *A Gradual Awakening.* New York: Doubleday, 1979.

LEVINE, S. *Who Dies?* Garden City, N.Y.: Doubleday, 1982.

LEVINE, S. *Healing into Life and Death.* Garden City, N.Y.: Doubleday, 1987.

McLEOD, K. *Wake Up to Your Life.* San Francisco: HarperSanFrancisco: 2001

ROSENBERG, L. *Breath by Breath.* Boston: Shambhala, 1998.

ROSENBERG, L. *Living in the Light of Death.* Boston: Shambhala, 2000.

SALZBERG, S. *Lovingkindness.* Boston: Shambhala, 1995.

SANTORELLI, S. *Heal Thy Self: Lessons on Mindfulness in Medicine.* New York: Bell Tower, 1999.

SOYGAL RINPOCHE. *The Tibetan Book of Living and Dying.* San Francisco: HarperSanFrancisco, 1992.

SUZUKI, S. *Zen Mind, Beginner's Mind.* New York: Weatherall, 1970.

THERA, N. *The Heart of Buddhist Meditation.* New York: Weiser, 1962.

TOLLE, E. *The Power of Now.* Novato, Calif.: New World Library, 1999.

TOOMBS, K. *The Meaning of Illness.* Boston: Kluwer, 1993.

CHAPTER TWELVE

Directed Prayer and Conscious Intention: Demonstrating the Power of Distant Healing

Marilyn Schlitz, Ph.D.; and Nola Lewis, M.S.

MARILYN SCHLITZ, PH.D., is the director of research at the Institute of Noetic Sciences and senior scientist at the California Pacific Medical Center in San Francisco. Dr. Schlitz serves on the Editorial Board of Alternative Therapies and on the Board of Directors of Esalen Institute and the Institute of Noetic Sciences, is on the Scientific Program Committee for the Tucson Center for Consciousness Studies, and has been a member of the Advisory Council for both the Office of Alternative Medicine and the National Center for Complementary and Alternative Medicine at the National Institutes of Health. Dr. Schlitz has conducted research and published more than one hundred articles in the areas of mind-body medicine and consciousness studies.

NOLA LEWIS, M.S., is a researcher and writer with broad experience in translating scientific information into popular language. Through her work as research program manager at the Institute of Noetic Sciences, Ms. Lewis is conversant with cutting-edge scientific developments in the field of consciousness research, including mind-body medicine. She is co-author of *The Heart of Healing* (Turner Publishing, 1993) and served as research coordinator for a six-hour television series of the same name, contributing toward the structure of the series and its content. She is also a creative writer and member of Writers on the Edge, a San Francisco–based performance troupe specializing in theater based on life stories. For more than twenty years, she has been a practitioner of spiritual mind healing, and is a certified clinical hypnotherapist. She is also a breast cancer patient.

People who face serious illness value their time in a new, more urgent way, and do not wish to waste it. If you are in treatment for breast cancer,

you no doubt understand this very well. Like many women at this junc-
ture, you may be feeling a greater-than-ever longing for a spiritual connection in your life. Illness often represents a spiritual turning point for
patients, leading them to seek out new sources of comfort, strength, and
purpose.

It's too bad that conventional medical or surgical treatments, while
necessary for treating the disease, do little or nothing to address this
inner longing. The medical establishment is simply not equipped to
help patients acquire a sense of spiritual well-being. Even many alternative therapies don't offer the kinds of immediate support women
need at this stage to strengthen themselves emotionally and spiritually.
Fortunately, this hasn't stopped a majority of them from seeking and
finding help anyway. What is astonishing is that until recently, no one
has paid any attention to how they're doing it. The answer, in a word, is
prayer.

"Stay Strong, Fight Cancer," advised a recent article in a major health
magazine. The article went on to describe five promising complementary therapies for patients to use along with conventional medicine:
imagery, herbs, diet, exercise, and acupuncture. Prayer, or any form of
mental healing, didn't even make the list. Yet, in the first six months
after diagnosis, prayer is the one form of alternative therapy chosen
most often by women with breast cancer.[1] When breast cancer patients
in a 1999 study were given a list of eighteen possible alternative therapies, 85% indicated an interest in prayer, and 76% reported using it in
response to the cancer diagnosis and treatment.

There's no question that for a great many women, prayer has tremendous personal value and is a much-needed source of courage and
strength. In another study of religious and spiritual coping strategies
among women newly diagnosed with breast cancer,[2] subjects reported
that their religious and spiritual faith provided distinct benefits, most
notably the emotional support necessary to deal with their breast cancer
(91%), social support (70%), and the ability to make meaning in their
everyday life (64%), particularly during their cancer experience.

None of this, however, proves that prayer actually helps people to heal
from a physical disease. Indeed, because prayer is so difficult to study, it's
simply been easier to dismiss reports of spiritual healing as a lot of wishful thinking. While anecdotal evidence has long appeared to support the

idea that intentional or directed prayer can be beneficial to people who are ill, there were no sound methods for studying the phenomenon in a scientific way.

This is changing. While it is too early to offer any firm conclusions, various studies of the effects of prayer—particularly prayer aimed at "distant healing" (praying from afar for someone who is ill)—suggest some remarkable possibilities. In this chapter, we will discuss several studies whose results are eye-opening, to say the least. They have enormous implications for breast cancer patients—and for everyone. The set of clinical experiments we describe here will show that although we don't yet understand why, benevolent human intention, or prayer, can positively influence the life experience of people with serious illnesses. Regardless of whether a "natural" explanation is found for these events, the outcome is significant and challenges our conventional worldviews. Later in this chapter, we'll offer practical suggestions and exercises for the breast cancer patient who would like to incorporate these practices into her treatment in a focused and deliberate way.

First, what is distant healing? And what do we know about the kinds of conscious intentions or prayers that are the basis for it?

Distant Healing and the Prayer Experience

Distant (or nonlocal) healing may be defined as a conscious act of the mind, intended to benefit the physical and/or emotional well-being of another person. It includes deliberate thoughts, wishes, feelings, images, intentions, meditation, rituals, or prayers. Thus, the term encompasses prayer as well as psychic healing, spiritual healing, shamanism, animism, and remote attention (the ability of one person to affect the physiology of another). Those who engage in distant healing often share the conviction that their practice goes beyond "mental" processes and into contact with ineffable spiritual realms. As we begin to explore the evidence for distant healing, a useful first step is to examine what we mean by prayer as a form of distant healing intention.

The work of researcher Margaret Poloma sheds light on the nature of prayer, who prays, and what the inner experience is like for that person.[3-5] A survey conducted by Poloma in 1985, and a subsequent series of Gallup polls,[6-8] have helped clarify the prayer habits of Americans and flesh out our understanding of what prayer is like "from the inside." The surveys found that most Americans pray, and the majority say they pray daily. Nearly half of those who pray don't have a special time set aside for the activity, and often it is performed right along with other activities, such as housework, jogging, or driving. For those who pray with others, the most frequent setting is a church.

While early research on prayer provided data about how often people pray, it gave little information about the content or effectiveness of prayer practice. Poloma's observations on the nature of prayer and the experience of those who pray are based on Western culture, specifically American culture. Most of her respondents were Christian. Although many of the world's spiritual traditions are now found within the United States, we don't know whether these categories also apply to them, and whether surveys of other cultures would result in similar or identical categories of prayer. This is an important question relative to spiritual traditions that do not address a personal God—for example, Taoism and Buddhism.

It is clear, however, that prayer is a near-universal practice found within all the major religions of the world. In many ways, prayer and healing intention serve as a source of comfort, connection, and well-being across cultures worldwide, whether it is the shaman interceding on behalf of a client or tribe, the Pope lifting his arms above St. Peter's Square to bless the throngs gathered to celebrate mass, the rabbi reading a ritual prayer, or the individual woman sitting quietly in her bedroom calling upon God for help.

Poloma's personal experience had taught her that prayer means different things to different people. She became interested in finding ways to measure the distinct types of common prayer and to assess the way different pray-ers experience intimacy with the divine. An analysis of the responses to her survey revealed four different forms of prayer.

Colloquial prayer is a conversation with God—like a letter to a trusted friend, personal and self-revealing. It's the kind of praying people often do along with another activity, like jogging or washing the dishes. In it, the pray-er asks for guidance, blessing, and forgiveness. Its aim is not particularly to establish a "divine connection"—rather, it's a way to vent anxiety, as you might do with another human being.

Petitionary or intercessory prayer, as it is often called, asks God for help. A petitionary prayer may ask for specific, concrete personal needs to be met, either for oneself or for others (e.g., a student praying, "Lord, help me pass this exam," or a parent praying, "Please God, let my child's fever go down right now"). Or it may ask for the fulfillment of more general spiritual needs—for example, the alleviation of world suffering.

Ritual prayer, the third of Poloma's four categories, consists of reading prayers from a prayer book or reciting prayers that have been committed to memory—for example, saying the rosary or reciting the Lord's Prayer.

Meditative prayer is qualitatively different from the first three categories and is the focus of our greatest interest because it appears to be connected to distant healing. Colloquial, petitionary, and ritual prayer are all verbal prayers, which could be described as one-way conversations with God. The prayers take place through the medium of words, whether spoken audibly or internally. Meditative prayer takes a different stance: a stance of listening. It is a prayer of being, rather than of doing; it is felt, rather than spoken. In meditative prayer, the praying individual awaits the presence of God as a felt experience. Such prayers call for the pray-er to "be still and know," to "practice the presence" of God. It asks for an intimate dialogue with God, rather than the monologue common to the other forms. And it may be wordless. To attain this inner state, the prayer focuses on the deity (as opposed to the self and its needs) and develops a stillness that allows for an inner response. Most people who pray use this form occasionally.

The Healing Implications of "Feeling Close to God"

Margaret Poloma found that all those who prayed described feeling close to God, and those who prayed more frequently felt more closeness. Participants in her survey said they experienced a profound sense of peace and well-being, felt divinely inspired, and received deep spiritual insight from prayer.

Her results show that all forms of prayer give rise to this feeling in some measure. Poloma also found that those who pray combine different types of prayer in response to the needs of the moment. So which form of prayer (if any) was most responsible for their feelings of "close-ness to God"? To answer this intriguing question, Poloma subjected her data to statistical analysis and found that of all four types of prayer, only meditative prayer was consistently related to feeling close to God. This is an important finding, since most clinical studies of prayer have focused on petitionary or intercessory prayer. When people's experience of prayer intimacy was analyzed, she also found that meditative prayer led to the experience of closeness to God in a way the other forms did not.

Does feeling close to God affect one's day-to-day life? People who pray often indicate a higher degree of life satisfaction, general happiness, and existential well-being, even when other factors (income, sex, education, race, and so on) have been taken into account.[9] As a breast cancer patient you may find that feelings of intimacy with a source larger than yourself may very well help enhance your quality of life, and nurture a sense of empowerment after the trauma of diagnosis. As you face the uncertain road ahead, spirituality, prayer, and a feeling of meaningful connection with a deep inner presence may provide important resources on your healing journey.

The Importance of Spirituality to Health

Spiritual aspects of medical care are not typically a part of the medical school curriculum. But physicians would be well advised to learn more about the relationship between religion and health for purely medical reasons.

Levin and associates have gathered over two hundred studies that touch on this relationship.[10] In one such study, for example, investigators at Dartmouth Medical School found that one of the best predictors of survival for patients after heart surgery was the extent to which they drew comfort and strength from religious faith.[11] Those who did not find solace in this way died three times more often than those who did. And patients recovering from hip fractures who considered God a source of strength had less depression and could walk farther on discharge than those who did not.[12] Attending religious services raises the levels of some immune measures and alters the levels of others, even when other factors that could affect them are accounted for.

Taken together, these results suggest that while the mechanism remains unknown, attending religious services results in healthier immune systems.[13] This points toward an important role for religious belief in relation to physical health. Since many studies have now found that religious belief and practice have a positive effect on physical and mental health,[14] medical educators have begun to recognize the need to translate these important findings into practice, introducing more compassionate caregiving into the medical school curriculum.

Thus far, we have seen that prayer is important because people use it widely and because it enhances their quality of life. Prayer has also been shown to correlate with improved health in people recovering from life-threatening illnesses. To anyone who believes that a patient's frame of mind can play a role in recovery from illness, this makes sense. But do we know whether the powers of prayer have anything more than a psychological explanation?

Distant Healing in the Laboratory

Over the past half century, researchers have developed techniques for measuring whether distant healing can have an effect on living systems.[15-18] The typical goal of these experiments has been to influence a form of plant, animal, or human life in a way that can be objectively measured. The best experiments use careful, controlled designs that rule out the possibility of physical manipulation, suggestion, and expectancy on the part of the subject.

Before we describe some of these studies, a few words of explanation. There is no precise job description for a "healer" and no universal agreement about what constitutes one. We may question whether healing abilities are a rare gift bestowed on certain individuals, or whether everyone is capable of cultivating them. Some of the healers referred to in the studies below work in a professional capacity, and some do not. All, however, identified themselves as actively engaged in some kind of religious or spiritual practice.

As for the human subjects of the experiments, while they knew they were participating in a study and were aware of its nature, none knew whether they belonged to the test group or the control group. Any placebo effect at work would apply to both groups equally and does not explain why the results would differ between the two groups.

Praying for Signs of Vitality

In the first major research category of experiments, a healer seeks to lessen a harmful process or condition in a target organism. In other words, through conscious intention alone, the healer aims to improve the organism's vitality or decrease its morbidity. The following studies give dramatic evidence that this is possible.

A classic study was conducted by biologist Bernard Grad, a pioneer in the field. Grad watered seeds with saline solution that either had been prayed over by a healer, or not. In a careful, double-blind design, he found that the seeds watered with healer-treated saline were more likely to sprout and grow successfully.[19] Another biologist, Carroll Nash, reported that the growth rate of bacteria could be influenced by conscious intention in controlled double-blind studies.[20]

Some studies within this category involved an attempt to influence the course of a naturally occurring disease or condition. For example, healers have successfully reduced the growth of cancerous tumors in laboratory animals, compared to tumor growth rates in control animals with no interventions from healers.[21]

Other experiments have attempted to affect the course of an artificially induced disease or condition. For example, in a series of studies using mice, Grad and his colleagues[22] found that skin wounds healed more rapidly when treated by healers who laid their hands on them. Grad, a traditionally trained biologist, worked with several exceptional healers—Justa Smith, Oscar Estebany, Olga Worrall, and others—over many years. The experiments carefully controlled for possible influences, such as extra warmth from the hands. Grad's pioneering work also showed that goiters induced in mice could be inhibited by these healers, even when they acted indirectly by treating cotton balls and placing them in the cage with the mice.[23]

Healers also apparently have been able to increase the recovery rate of wounds imposed on the skin of human volunteers.[24] Statistical analysis typically shows that the rate of wound healing in the treatment group is significantly higher than that in a control group that is otherwise similar but receives no distant healing treatment.

Distant Healing's Effect on Human Physiology

With even more dramatic results, numerous studies have addressed the question whether physiological activity in humans might be susceptible to distant healing. One series of experiments measured electrodermal activity (EDA) fluctuations—the same factors measured in lie detector tests. Because these EDA fluctuations are involuntary, are easy to measure, and reveal much about the activity of the nervous system, they're extremely useful and relevant to the area of healing research. Studies using these measures give us a consistent series of results that can be analyzed in comparison with one another.

Beginning in the 1970s, William Braud and Marilyn Schlitz conducted a series of experiments in which skin resistance was measured in the target person while an "influencer" in a separate room attempted to interact with the distant person by means of calming or activating thoughts, images, and intentions.[25,26]

While the specific details of the experiments differed slightly, the general method across studies had one person generate specific intentions toward another person, whose nervous system was simultaneously measured to detect unusual activity. Throughout the experiment, the two persons occupied separate, isolated rooms, and all conventional communication between them was eliminated to ensure that the results were truly attributable to distant intention.

Simple physiological measures across thirty studies showed a highly significant and characteristic variation during periods when the subject was being "prayed for" by the influencer, compared with randomly interspersed control periods. Researchers at many other institutions have now replicated these studies. With a high level of consistent findings from different laboratories, it is extremely unlikely that the results are due to some systematic methodological flaws. While the effect sizes are small, they are comparable to (or, in some cases, eight times larger than) those reported in some recent medical studies that have been heralded as medical breakthroughs.[27,28]

Scientific Investigation of Prayer and Distant Healing in Clinical Studies

But what is the clinical relevance of these experiments? Can prayer and distant healing be expected to play a positive role in medical treatment?

To date, only a few scientific studies have addressed the question whether prayer can affect the physical course of events in individual patients. But they provide encouraging evidence that intercessory prayer and distant healing can improve medical outcomes in people suffering from a diverse range of medical conditions, including arthritis, cardiac problems, hernia surgery—and even advanced AIDS.

A seminal study by cardiologist Randolph C. Byrd[29] led the way in this applied research. Nearly a dozen years ago, Dr. Byrd, then at San Francisco General Hospital, conducted a randomized, double-blind, prospective study to assess the effects of intercessory prayer on health outcomes in 393 patients admitted to the coronary care unit. Each patient was randomly assigned to a "prayed for" or "control" condition; otherwise, they all received comparable medical treatment. The healers chosen were "born again" Christians, defined by Byrd as people with an active Christian life manifested by daily devotional prayer and an active fellowship with a local church. Each prayed daily for a specific outcome: rapid recovery, prevention of complications and death, and any other areas they believed helpful to the patient.

The prayers seem to have helped. Members of the group that received healing prayer were five times less likely to require antibiotics and three times less likely to develop pulmonary edema. In addition, fewer of them died than in the control group, and none of the prayed-for group required endotracheal intubation, whereas twelve in the "unremembered" group did.

While these results are intriguing, the study is not definitive. Byrd did not, for example, assess the psychological health of those entering the study. Thus, it is possible that the two groups were different in this regard, which could affect the study's interpretation. Nonetheless, the results of this well-known study have been quoted from pulpits to podiums, and hailed enthusiastically as proof that "prayer really works."

Given the spiritual, social, and scientific relevance of Byrd's findings, it is surprising that it took another dozen years for other researchers to conduct a replication study, which is needed to ensure that the original results were correct. However, Dr. Harris,[30] working with 999 patients admitted to the coronary care unit of his hospital, also found that the medical course of his patients was better in those who were prayed for. This study, unlike Byrd's, used distant healers from a variety of Christian traditions (35% were listed as nondenominational, 27% as Episcopalian, and the remainder as either Protestant or Roman Catholic). Harris also chose a more global score to assess the outcome of this prayer on coronary recovery. Like Byrd, Harris concluded that his patients benefited significantly from the intercessory prayer they received.

Taken together, these two studies provide strong evidence that the intention of people engaged in healing prayer can affect the physical well-being of people at a distance. A third study on the effects of distant healing prayer in heart patients is now under way under the direction of cardiologist Mitch Krucoff of Duke University Medical Center. Dr. Krucoff was a volunteer in a spiritually based hospital in rural India. There he observed that despite sometimes primitive facilities (he said it was the only place where he had ever seen bare feet in an operating room) and poor prognoses, the patients appeared relaxed and calm, filled with a sense of well-being. What creates a "healing space" such as the one he experienced? And if that same atmosphere were translated back to a state-of-the-art hospital in the United States, would the combination of modern medical care and attention to spiritual well-being help patients more than medical care alone?

Krucoff and his colleagues set about answering these important questions. They began a study that used techniques called noetic interventions. These are interventions that have physiologic or spiritual effects without the use of a drug, device, or surgical procedure. The researchers set out to determine whether prayer by strangers might influence the medical outcome of patients in a coronary angioplasty laboratory. In a pilot study, the subjects all received standard medical care. In addition, they were randomly assigned to either a control group or a test group that received prayer (again, offered by a highly varied group of prayer agents and groups) or a type of noetic treatment—either touch, stress relaxation, or imagery. (Those in the control group did not receive any noetic treatment.) In the pilot study, those prayed for had the best outcomes of any group: 50% to 100% better than those in the control group. A new and much larger study is now under way that builds on these early results in a population large enough to enable firm statistical conclusions to be drawn.[31]

Another study of distant healing, reported in the *Western Journal of Medicine* by Fred Sicher and his colleagues,[32] looked at the effects of intercessory (petitionary) prayer on patients with advanced AIDS. The choice of healers in this study was interesting. Since we do not know whether one form of distant healing is likelier than another to promote physical healing, the researchers engaged a wide range of self-identified healing practitioners, representing many different healing and spiritual traditions. They reasoned that by combining efforts in this way, they would be more likely to see an effect than if they focused on a single type of practice, which might one day be found ineffectual. Healers received a photo of their distant subject, the last name and first initial, and sometimes the T-cell count (immunologically active white blood cells). Six months later, the treatment subjects had acquired significantly fewer new AIDS-defining illnesses, had lower illness severity, and required fewer doctor visits, fewer hospitalizations, and fewer days of hospitalization. Their mood was also improved, compared with the control group.

A replication study is now under way that is being funded by the National Center for Complementary and Alternative Medicine (NCCAM), the center established by the National Institutes of Health to study the effectiveness of nonmedical healing methods. In addition to replicating the earlier results, the new study seeks to answer another important question: Can ordinary people be taught how to do distant healing in a way that benefits medically ill people? The original study used self-identified healers from a wide variety of traditions. However, critics have argued that despite these important results, distant healing has limited value because so few people are capable of doing it. But is this assumption correct? To test this assumption directly, the new study will train nurses involved in the care of study subjects to offer distant healing on behalf of their patients.

One study has been published that did not find support for the effectiveness of distant healing. F. Scott Walker[33] investigated the effects of nondirected intercessory prayer ("May the spirit of love replace the spirit of alcohol in their life") as an adjunct to standard treatment in patients entering programs for alcohol abuse or dependence. He found that no clinical benefit could be demonstrated under the treatment conditions. Walker's study emphasizes the need for sensitivity to the possible differences between different groups of people. For example, it raises questions about whether alcoholic persons are somehow less receptive to distant healing, either because of the effects of long-term alcohol use or because of psychological or social factors.

Nevertheless, the results of a wide range of clinically based scientific studies suggest that prayer and distant healing have measurable effects that may be of benefit to seriously ill people.

Distant Healing and the Breast Cancer Patient

Just how do prayer and distant healing work? The explanation is unclear. One theory is that natural physical laws are at work. Many people believe that the human organism is surrounded and permeated by a natural energy field, or "biofield"—described as qi in China, or prana in India. Oscar Estebany, one of the healers who participated in Bernard Grad's laboratory experiments, describes it as an ocean of energy, which we live within and depend upon for survival. Under conditions of ill health, he says, some defect occurs in contact with this bioenergetic cosmos. The role of the healer is then to act as a link between the atmospheric energy and the patient to normalize this essential rapport.[34] Such subtle fields have yet to be measured; however, a recent pilot study showed that gamma radiation surrounding a subject fluctuated in response to the healing efforts of polarity therapists.[35]

Of course, most people who pray do so out of faith that God exists and hears their prayers. If God or another "supernatural" force is at work here, then by definition it is beyond the range of science. In this realm, the source of healing is inherently inaccessible and unknowable, although it responds to the healing intention flowing through prayer.

Critics of the data on distant healing suggest that results of these early studies are unreliable and that "all will be explained" later on through better, more precise experiments.[36,37] At present, we simply do not know enough to reach any firm conclusions. It is equally possible that distant healing research will lead us to revise the assumptions that guide modern medicine itself. Can human beings actually change reality through consciousness alone? New findings about the power of prayer have the potential to transform the way we think about our relationship to the physical world.

Conclusions

In this chapter, we have presented considerable evidence showing that certain individuals, operating at a distance under controlled conditions, can positively affect a wide range of living systems, including plants, microbes, animals, and human beings.

When we consider the effects of distant healing on persons with a wide range of diseases, the results are encouraging. To date, none of these studies specifically addresses whether distant healing can help the breast cancer patient with the question of survival. However, it has been shown that women who rely on religious and spiritual practices for coping find that they receive emotional and social support through this practice, which also enhances their ability to make meaning within their everyday lives. These are important benefits.

In her book *Kitchen Table Wisdom*, Dr. Rachel Remen observes, "An unanswered question is a fine traveling companion. It sharpens your eye for the road." For the breast cancer patient reading this book, we hope that these findings—and the questions remaining to be answered—will serve as helpful companions on your journey.

Exercises: Prayer, Distant Healing, and You

Whether you pray every day or never give it a thought, you may decide after reading this chapter that you'd like to deepen your spiritual experience or invite the healing intentions of others into your life. If so, here are some suggestions. These exercises are based on my understanding of spiritual mind healing, derived from many years of teaching and practice.

While in this chapter we have put the greatest focus on meditative prayer, in fact all forms of prayer are illuminating. A mix of approaches may prove to be more productive than any one approach exclusively, so give them all a try.

—NOLA LEWIS

Experiencing Prayer

COLLOQUIAL PRAYER: HAVING A TALK WITH GOD

Here's an exercise I learned during a class that focused on using positive intention. We were asked to think about a current situation in our lives and to write everything negative we could think about it on one side of the page. We were then asked to respond to each of these complaints on the other side of the page, as though we were a close friend who could see all these negatives as positives. For example, if on one side of the page you had complained about your sister, "She's moody and difficult," your "friend" might respond by saying, "She's very sensitive and has great depth of emotion."

When I did this exercise, the results were immediate and astonishing. I was able to change my point of view about a situation that had once troubled me. I found that by changing my consciousness about a particular relationship, I was able to affect the nature of that relationship.

In a related exercise, write a "letter to God" as though to a friend who has known you since childhood. You won't need to go into minute detail, but you can assume that the reader is familiar with your background. Your friend's intentions toward you are unconditionally benevolent. Name your life concerns and tell your friend what worries you, what you are learning, and how you feel. Know that your friend will listen receptively to anything you want to tell. Seal the letter, date the envelope, and put it in a safe place.

QUESTIONS FOR REFLECTION

How did you feel after writing the letter? While writing it, what picture did you have of the recipient—was your "friend" male or female, young or old? Notice what happens in your life in the next few days, particularly whether you have dreams that reflect in any way the content of your letter. In six weeks' time, open and reread your letter. Have things changed? Do you feel differently about anything you wrote? Now write a follow-up letter, taking note of the changes that have occurred.

This exercise helps us frame our concept of God in a friendly, benevolent, and completely loving way, which might be a very different image from the one we were raised with.

Petitionary Prayer: Asking for What You Want

Asking God for something goes against the grain for many people, particularly those who are well educated and accustomed to being in control of their lives. You might feel silly or embarrassed asking God for help, but this one time, give yourself permission to do it.

For this exercise, find a quiet place, and reflect on something that would make your life happier. Ask for something recognizable to you: something personal and meaningful but concrete. (If you ask for world peace, how will you know your answer?) Perhaps it's a new car, or a raise, or to write the Great American Novel. Turn your attention inward, and address the stillness. Tell that silence what you would like. Be honest, and state your desire simply. When you are finished, make a conscious choice to release all thought about this experience, as though it were a seed planted in good soil.

Questions for Reflection

In a month's time, revisit your desire. What has changed? Do you still want what you said you did a month ago? Has anything happened that corresponds to your wish, or that changes it? Often I find a process of unfolding that is akin to peeling an onion. I may have begun with a particular desire, but as I go deeper I find that what I really wanted was something else—often something less tangible. For example, you might start out thinking you want a new car, and later realize that what you really want is the freedom that the car represents.

RITUAL PRAYER: THE RHYTHM OF THE SPIRIT

I grew up in an evangelical Protestant church that was not overly fond of ritual. When I went away to college, I found myself deeply attracted to the color, the meaning, and the beauty conveyed through ritual in a nearby Catholic church. I came to love the rhythm and repetition in the words I heard, even though I could not understand Latin. But the elements of ritual prayer are found in many other spiritual contexts as well—for example, repetition of mantras or affirmations.

For this exercise, find a short phrase with a spiritual dimension or one that elicits a spiritual feeling in you. It may be drawn from a scriptural verse, a story about a religious figure or inspiring person, or a deeply held personal value. It should be short, simple, and evocative. For example, "Love guides me." "Gandhi's peace in me." Hold this phrase within your mind when you awaken in the morning and when you go to bed at night. During the daytime, repeat it over and over to yourself—while you are driving, waiting for an appointment, preparing dinner. Do not try to have "deep thoughts" about your phrase; simply repeat it for the next week.

QUESTIONS FOR REFLECTION

Did you find that after the first day or two, the phrase arose spontaneously during your daily life? What feelings did you notice? Were you calmer than usual, less likely to respond irritably to minor inconveniences? Did you enjoy the repetitiveness and rhythm of your chosen phrase? If you did, consider continuing the practice with the same or a different phrase.

MEDITATIVE PRAYER: A STATE OF INNER UNION

Meditative prayer is at the heart of many healing traditions and is present in all other forms of prayer in some measure. If you've ever felt "at one with the universe" in a beautiful natural setting, you've experienced it. It is based not on doing but on being. The outer identity quiets and recedes as we become open to inner experience. "Thy will be done" summarizes this form of prayer.

Meditative prayer can be approached as a four-step process, which I've outlined below. First, be sure that you are comfortable and will not be interrupted for whatever time you select for your meditation. Twenty minutes is often good for beginners. Tell yourself that you will meditate for that length of time. Timers and alarms are often jarring, and you might like to see whether you can meditate for a given period of time through intention alone.

In preparation, sit down in a relaxed position, with spine straight and eyes closed. You may sit on a chair or a pillow, with legs straight or crossed "lotus-style" as you like. Many meditators like to light a candle or use some other ritual that helps separate this time from ordinary time. It's also helpful to establish a pattern for your meditation, using the same place at the same time every day. But all of these are less important than the intention to make yourself available to the meditation.

Step 1: Relaxing Awareness of the Outer Environment

With your eyes closed, take a deep breath in, and as you slowly release it gently become aware of the world around you and its sounds. As you settle into this awareness, let your whole body relax as you affirm statements like the following (choose your own):

I release all attention to my outer world.
My environment is comfortable, safe, secure.
I can allow my attention to move more deeply inside.
With each breath, I go deeper and deeper.
I am fully at peace with my world.
I allow my awareness to move deeper and deeper inside.

If your mind disagrees (e.g., "How can I relax when . . ."), don't argue. Just repeat the affirmation until you feel a sense of peacefulness.

Step 2: Relaxing Awareness of the Physical Body

As you breathe in deeply, move your awareness through your body, again with the intention of allowing yourself to go deeper with affirmations like the following:

I release all attention to my physical body.
I am free to move deeper within.
My body serves me perfectly.
This meditation relaxes and renews my body.
For this time, I can relax and allow my awareness to go deeper and
  deeper.

STEP 3: RELAXING AWARENESS OF THE MENTAL BODY

Continue to breathe deeply as you move beyond your surface mind,
which deals with the outer conditions of your life and helps to make
logical decisions.

I relax my mind.
I bless my mind for all the ways it helps me make good decisions and
  move through life.
Right now, my mind is free to relax, to be at peace.
I am calm and content, knowing I am perfectly cared for.
I allow my awareness to move beyond my surface mind into deeper
  levels of awareness.
My attention is free to move deeper and deeper within.

STEP 4: MOVING THROUGH FEELINGS AND EMOTIONS

Often as we relax and breathe deeply, we become aware of things we
may not have paid attention to in our more outwardly focused states.
They may surface as we continue to go deeper. Again, the point is to
allow, not argue. Yes, that feeling may be there, but right now my intention is to meditate.

I am now aware of my beautiful feeling nature and all it brings to
  my life.
I allow my feeling nature to relax and be at peace.
My feelings are a wonderful source of information to guide my life.
I can return to my feelings later. Right now, I intend to meditate.
As I relax my feelings, I go deeper and deeper into peace and whole-
  ness.

I am deeply at peace inside.

I allow myself to relax, setting aside all outer concerns and focusing my attention inward.

There are many ways to describe the inner experience of meditation, but each meditator (and each meditation) is unique. It's important not to judge and not to expect your own meditation to be like someone else's. Focus on allowing your experience to unfold, rather than expecting to follow some anticipated pattern. Some sample affirmations:

I allow myself to enter a state of contentment, unity, wholeness.

I merge with love at the core of my being.

I am whole, complete, perfect now.

I am deeply at peace.

I am one with all that is good.

All is well within me. I am at peace.

At the end of the time you have set for your meditation, reverse the steps by gently disengaging yourself and reentering each state of awareness (feelings, outer mind, physical body, environment). Affirm that the deep inner experience of meditation blends with and enriches each state as you move back into ordinary awareness. Acknowledge that you are completely alert, aware, and present to each level of your being. Then open your eyes, and return to ordinary reality.

Four Ways to Apply Distant Healing in Your Life

1. Find a distant healing (DH) or "prayer partner," and work together to help each other deepen your practice. This could be anyone—a friend, a relation, another breast cancer patient. It should be someone who shares your commitment to use intention for healing. The other person does not need to share your particular problem, but it may be helpful if he or she does. Make an agreement that you will work for each other regularly. Decide how you will pray or focus your distant healing intention, and how you will recognize a positive result. The DH should be mutual; that is, you will work for that person, and the other per-

son will do the same for you. Set up a way to follow through: "Let's talk once a week (or take a walk together) to see how things are going." During your check-in, discuss frankly anything that comes up in your distant healing time. Look for ways your experience changes through this practice. Learning how to recognize answers is an important skill. Each answer helps deepen faith and commitment to practice.

2. Discuss the idea of prayer and healing intention with your breast cancer support group leader. If you belong to a support circle for those with breast cancer, this is an ideal place to bring up the issue for group discussion.

3. Make an appointment with someone from your spiritual tradition—rabbi, minister, spiritual teacher. Learn all you can about the practice of prayer and healing intention, and how it is viewed within your own tradition. Ask him or her to pray for and with you.

4. Create a healing circle. You may find that other women (and men) share your desire for a deeper experience of using DH. Set a time when you can be together to talk, share an article you may have read, or explore one of the many spiritual books on DH and prayer or a more popular book on the subject (Larry Dossey's many books come to mind).

CHAPTER THIRTEEN

A Mind-Body-Spirit Model for Cancer Support Groups

Elisabeth Targ, M.D.; and Ellen G. Levine, Ph.D., M.P.H.

ELISABETH TARG, M.D., is director of the Complementary Medicine Research Institute at California Pacific Medical School, assistant clinical professor of psychiatry at the University of California, San Francisco, and a Fellow of the Institute of Noetic Sciences. She holds an award from the National Institute of Healthcare Research for her curriculum for training psychiatry residents in the area of spirituality and psychiatry. She is principal investigator of a large Department of Defense–funded project for the study of the role of spiritual exploration and lifestyle change for women with breast cancer. She has received two major research grants from the NIH for her clinical research in the medical application of prayer and distant healing.

ELLEN G. LEVINE, PH.D., M.P.H., is a clinical psychologist and epidemiologist. She serves as the director of psychosocial oncology research at California Pacific Medical Center (CPMC) and was the co–principal investigator and research director of the Breast Cancer Personal Support and Lifestyle Intervention Trial, a collaborative trial between CPMC and University of California, San Francisco. She has extensive training and experience in medical psychology and behavioral medicine, and has worked with cancer patients clinically and in research settings for more than twenty years. She has research experience in cancer, quality of life, and spirituality. She has received a grant from the Breast Cancer Research Program of the University of California to study coping and stress among adolescent boys and girls whose mothers have breast cancer. In 1994 and 1997 she received grants enabling her to develop and conduct a pilot for a spiritual support group for women with metastatic breast cancer and a complementary medicine retreat for low-income (mostly minority) women with breast cancer.

Judy, a California schoolteacher, had long considered that she might be affected by breast cancer. Her mother and grandmother had both died of the disease. But that hardly prepared her for the diagnosis when it came, just after her fifty-seventh birthday.

"I was terrified," she says, "just terrified. I went into denial."

Cancer is a shock—physically, mentally, and spiritually. And the treatments a woman must undergo for breast cancer often create their own set of physical, mental, and emotional difficulties. During this stressful period, she may confront her own mortality for the first time. She may be afraid of physical pain, social isolation, or the disfigurement of losing a breast. She may feel overwhelmed and confused about her treatment options. It's understandable that many women react to diagnosis of breast cancer with varying degrees of anger, fear, and depression.

While for many patients, the distress of cancer surgery and treatment declines within one year, it has been estimated that up to 30% of women continue to have some disruption in quality of life one year after treatment for breast cancer.[1] One landmark study of 215 cancer patients found that 47% of the participants had significant psychiatric disorders and could have benefited from group or individual therapy.[2]

It's clear that psychotherapy can go a long way toward helping a woman manage the emotional side effects that often accompany breast cancer. In the mid-1980s, a landmark study by David Spiegel, M.D., at Stanford University found that women attending group psychotherapy survived three times longer than women who did not.[3] Most of these therapies emphasize group discussion and encourage problem solving, sharing, and support.

These standard support groups involve the mind and emotions but not the body and spirit. However, innovative new programs are emerging; in addition to standard "talk therapy," they embrace noncognitive approaches such as body movement and expression, artwork, or spiritual exploration. In this chapter, we describe one such program, the Breast Cancer Personal Support/Life-Style Intervention Trial, conducted by the University of California and the California Pacific Medical Center in San Francisco. We helped to develop the program in 1996 and have been associated with it since then in our respective roles as psychiatrist and psychologist/researcher.

While programs like ours are described as *mind-body therapies,* we believe that *mind-body-spirit therapies* is a more accurate term. We discuss here the principles that form the foundation of our program, the specific therapies we practice, and why we believe that programs taking a mind-body-spirit approach offer even greater benefits than traditional support groups for patients who, like Judy, must struggle to cope with the frightening ordeal of cancer and its treatment.

Mind-Body Treatments: A Little Background

It is estimated that up to 72% of cancer patients now use some type of complementary or alternative medicine, mostly as a supplement to conventional therapy.[4-7] Not only are people seeking out these therapies on their own; a growing number of health professionals are recommending various sorts, including mind-body treatments. A recent survey of 772 Northern California HMO physicians found that 16% are using or recommending guided imagery, 48% are prescribing meditation, and 27% are prescribing movement therapies such as yoga, tai chi, or qigong as additional therapy.[8] A study in a Midwest breast cancer clinic found that 85% of women were using spiritual approaches to cope with their illness. Retreat centers that offer mind-body approaches for cancer patients, such as Commonweal Institute in California, have long waiting lists. Anecdotal reports from these programs suggest that in addition to offering some patients a respite from anxiety and depression, they may also provide an introduction to a deeper and more fulfilling life experience.

We shouldn't be surprised that mind-body programs affect people at a very deep level. Practices such as meditation and yoga, for example, were originally developed as spiritual practices for helping people achieve union with the divine and to experience self-transcendence. While in modern studies, meditation has been shown to decrease blood pressure, relieve anxiety, and diminish skin lesions, it was originally designed for a much more profound purpose.

The use of dance, movement, art, imagery, and music in the service of healing also has its roots in spiritual tradition. All these practices have been used by shamanic healers around the globe as well as by teachers from a variety of Western religious traditions. These approaches have been used to help patients face and overcome inner blocks or fears that may impede their healing. In modern settings, some of these techniques, such as imagery, have been used with some success for relaxation or to control physical processes. An interesting and frequent "side effect" of these processes is that patients are able to access their own inner resources in a new and deeper way. This is consistent with survey results indicating that people who use complementary therapies are significantly more likely to state that they have "had a personal transformative experience" and that they "believe their medical treatment should involve mind, body, and spirit."[9]

Most mind-body interventions, such as meditation, yoga, movement, and art therapies, are experiential in nature. When well taught, they can lead the patient toward greater self-awareness and fuller self-expression. They allow patients to take the time to contact their pain, longing, confusion, and strengths with their full attention and full being. The result of this is a richer and more relaxed life experience.

The Role of Spirituality in Cancer

The concept of spirituality is different from religious belief or participation. A simple definition of spirituality is that it encompasses "any activity or thought that embodies the search for experience of something beyond the self."[10] This century has witnessed a dramatic separation of spirituality and medicine. Until very recently, fewer than 5% of psychology training programs contained any discussion of spirituality or religion at all. Compare this with the finding in one national study that 75% of patients want their health care providers to address spiritual issues with them[11] and that 73% of patients rate their spiritual or religious practice to be "very important" in coping with life-threatening or chronic illness.[12]

In our support group, we find it useful to look at three different aspects of spirituality, and we try to cultivate these elements among participants.

Meaning and Purpose

On the concrete level, "meaning and purpose" may refer to one's social identity, job, or culture. Or it could extend to a sense of personal life mission, or participation in a cosmic pattern, dance, or evolution.

Connectedness

This could range from a feeling that one is connected bodily to oneself (as opposed to being numb, dissociated, or "on automatic"), to being bonded with friends or family, to having a direct awareness of how what affects one individual affects others as well.

Subjective Experience of the Sacred

This phrase, coined by psychologist Frances Vaughn, describes the sense of peacefulness, innate joyfulness, or love that is available to most people in occasional quiet moments or in prayer, but which is often expanded or stabilized in long-time meditators or in spiritual adepts. This is the state in which the individual's identity is no longer limited to a personal body, a personal story, or personal feelings. He or she experiences openness and dynamic flow between a sense of small self and larger Self. This is the reverent or awestruck experience of transcendent love described by the Buddha, Jesus, the Hasidic elders, the poet Rumi, William Blake, Ralph Waldo Emerson, and countless modern seekers. The universality and accessibility of this experience are what Harvard researcher Herbert Benson, M.D., points to when, after years of psychophysical research on meditation, he concludes that we are "hard-wired for God."[13]

For many people, a diagnosis of cancer triggers a spiritual crisis. In a religious person this may take the form of anger at God, feeling abandoned by God, or a deep questioning of a previously held faith. The illness directly threatens those abilities, opportunities, or personal features that may have constituted our sense of purpose. A model with breast cancer may feel that she is no longer who she was as a woman. A mother with breast cancer may feel that she can no longer provide for, or be emotionally available to, her children. Any woman with an investment in long-range plans or projects may wonder, "What's the point?"

A woman's sense of connectedness is also directly threatened by breast cancer. She may find that her friends do not share or understand her concerns. A woman who has to take time off from work may find she has lost an important community. People with cancer often feel as if they are in a "different world" from everyone else. Any of these factors can lead to anxiety, numbness, and depression. Once a woman falls into that state of emotional shut-down, her subjective experience of sacredness, connectedness, wholeness, love, and intrinsic meaning may be locked out. In traditional religious language, it is "the dark night of the soul." She loses her sense of meaning, of hope, of being part of a larger whole, and of participation in that larger whole. She has lost what for many is a crucial point of reference: the sense that she personally has intrinsic value, and that whatever happens to her is part of a process greater than her personal story.

We are often asked, "Is your program able to meet the needs of patients with no spiritual interests or orientation?" and "Do you meet the needs of patients with conservative or fundamentalist religious orientation?" The answer to both of these questions is yes. Approximately 30% of patients entering our program stated that they had a previous spiritual or religious practice. The rest did not. There was no difference in satisfaction between the people who did or did not have a spiritual orientation when they entered the program. Only a small number who entered the program had a very conservative religious background, and they were able to make excellent use of the program. As one woman stated, "Imagery made 'the Book' come alive for me." At first, this woman was extremely wary of practices she felt might not be sanctioned by her church. But through imagery, contemplation, and energy-based movement work (qigong), she was able to deepen the experiential basis of her relationship to God. Despite her initial misgivings, her church supported her fully.

The UCSF/CPMC Integrated Program and How It Works

Our program began in 1996, when the U.S. Department of Defense funded a formal head-to-head study to compare standard group psychotherapy for women with breast cancer to a complete mind-body-spirit program. The study set out to address these questions:

1. Would a mind-body-spirit program succeed in decreasing depression and anxiety in women with breast cancer?

2. Could it help restore a sense of spiritual well-being?
3. Would it affect physical outcomes?
4. Would it be more useful for certain types of women than for others?

The trial was carried out at the University of California and the California Pacific Medical Center in San Francisco and was called the Breast Cancer Personal Support/Life-Style Intervention Trial. For the purpose of the study, women with breast cancer were randomly assigned either to participate in a standard weekly group psychotherapy or to come to the twice-weekly Integrated Program, which involved meditation, yoga, dance, art, imagery, contemplative work, and group discussion.

We deliberately set out to create a program that could operate within a medical center and be staffed by the health care providers typically found in a medical center. To help these providers develop the skills needed to run this program, we gave them intensive in-service training and actively encouraged them to pursue outside study. They also took part in several retreats.

The Integrated Program involves groups of six to ten patients who meet twice a week for two and a half hours a day over a three-month period. Each day is divided into two sessions. On the first day, the women practice meditation or contemplative work, followed by a break and then group discussion. On the second day, the time is divided between a "health series" focusing on managing symptoms and lifestyle change, followed by a ninety-minute session of yoga or dance work. The women also have access to an active art therapy program, which is available on a drop-in basis.

The program has been running for three years at a mainstream hospital setting staffed by psychologists, psychiatrists, nurses, social workers, a dance therapist, and an art therapist. While the core program is somewhat time intensive, often it has offered an opportunity for very dramatic lifestyle and attitudinal changes among the hundred women who have participated thus far. We have also conducted a series of follow-up groups for program participants, which meet once a week for ninety minutes. They follow a similar model: the first thirty-minute period is used for a short meditation and experiential exercise, and the following hour is devoted to discussion and support.

Although the study data are not complete, the results from the first three years of the trial have shown that women in the Integrated Program experienced significant improvement in their depression, anxiety, and quality-of-life scores. Compared with those in the standard program, these women also showed greater improvement in both physical and overall well-being. This was measured by their rate of agreement with statements such as these: "I feel alive and joyful at the ordinary things in daily life." "I spend time alone by choice to reflect on my life and purpose." "I spend time in nature to feel more balanced and connected." "My personal relationship with God/Higher Power/Universal Energy gives me a great sense of well-being." "I can listen to others with a loving heart." "I try to forgive others who may have hurt or harmed me in some way." "I see death as a normal process in life." By the end of the intervention, women in the Integrated Program, despite having started with exactly the same level of spiritual orientation (30%) as those in the standard program, showed significantly higher levels of spiritual integration and had incorporated regular spiritual practices such as prayer, meditation, or contemplation into their daily lives.

In the words of one participant, "The program has been a life-transforming experience. I feel more hopeful, more in love with life. No matter what happens as a result of my condition, I will have lived a bigger life because of this program."

The Care Provider–Patient Relationship

For many women, one of the most painful aspects of undergoing treatment for breast cancer is a kind of dehumanization. This is greatly exacerbated by the distancing that occurs between the woman and her medical care providers. In a hospital setting, often a woman is stripped of her identity, skills, background, and story—and tended to in an infantilizing way by providers who rarely acknowledge her identity, her pain, or their own hopes or fears in relation to her illness. She is treated as a "problem" to be solved. One of the primary tenets of the Integrated Program is that staff members practice seeing the participants as whole and complete people—not defective, but living out a transformative life process. Staff members were encouraged to practice the same techniques given to the patients. In their own group sessions, staff members received support and explored the same questions, such as mortality, forgiveness, meaning, sexuality, and anger, that were presented to the program participants.

It is always our role as health care providers to hold in our hearts a sense of hope for the patient, even when the patient has none. This may not necessarily be a hope or belief that the person will physically recover from the effects of breast cancer, but it is a hope that she will find meaning and peace in her life and that she will grow, be happy, love, and be loved. In the Integrated Program treatment, we deliberately avoided setting up a division between "experts" and "patients." Instead, we health care providers were continuously reminded that the program participants were women, just like ourselves, who had encountered a life challenge that we too may encounter. At the orientation to the program, the care providers shared their belief with patients that "all of us have breast cancer. Some of us have it in our bodies; some of us have it in the bodies of our friends, mothers, sisters, and relatives— it affects us all through our community." Our goal has been to encourage the program participants to trust us, and we succeed only if we prove ourselves to be truly trustworthy. This means we must never abandon them; instead, we must skillfully encourage and allow all forms of expression, including anger or disagreement. At the same time we must always provide emotional and physical safety. Trust also means accommodating special needs and disabilities that inevitably occur and, above all, maintaining a vision of hope for the participant.

General Principles of Mind-Body-Spirit Medicine

Hundreds of mind-body or mind-body-spirit interventions are currently taught and used in the United States. Each one is based in some way on the premise that important aspects of healing lie within the patient herself. Yoga, meditation, imagery, art therapy, and movement work are all based on the practice of quieting the mind; becoming aware of feelings, images, and impulses; and examining them through witnessing or self-expression. Traditionally, it has been thought that allowing unconscious tendencies or fears to come into awareness allows us to deliberately release the inner tension that may get in the way of the flow of life energy. Unequivocally, releasing fears and negative tendencies allows us to be more flexible in our responses and freer in our life choices.

Many forms of yoga, meditation, imagery, energy healing, and dance have been trademarked, and some are available only for high fees or from exclusive teachers. We prefer to focus on certain principles rather than on particular techniques, and we have found them to be the foundation of effective mind-body therapy. These principles are

Awareness
Acceptance or relaxation
Intention
Compassion
Perspective

When these principles are incorporated into our work with breast cancer patients, they encourage the three elements of spirituality mentioned earlier: meaning and purpose; connection to the self, community, nature, and the cosmic order; and a subjective experience of the sacred.

The healing potential in this approach seems to stem from a mental, physical, and emotional relaxation that decreases the patient's stress and limits her overidentification with negative life circumstances. As one participant told us, "The program helped me to let go of attachment to my prior job and helped me find a place of serenity and a less stressful life." By going through a process of mindful self-inquiry, the patient learns to deeply experience and attend to her current state of being while simultaneously holding a view of her larger self—a self with meaning, community, and connection to a greater purpose. Below, we look more closely at how we apply these principles in our program.

Types of Healing

The word *heal* comes from the German root *hale*, meaning "to make whole." Certainly, most people with cancer come to a treatment program with the fundamental hope that they will be cured. Nevertheless, healing comes in different forms. Not all women with breast cancer who practice imagery or meditation will survive their illness. Certainly, there is growing evidence of benefits to the immune system from many types of mind-body practices, and many of these practices, such as yoga or good nutrition, will have direct benefits to the body. However, these practices are fundamentally designed to improve a person's state of mind, level of happiness, and spiritual awareness. We can theorize that decreased stress may improve the body's ability to fight cancer. Many people also theorize that illness constitutes a form of communication from the body to the mind of the patient; for example, the idea that "illness is nature's way of telling you to slow down." However, there is currently no evidence for this.

Spiritual Bypassing and New Age Guilt

Breast cancer patients who adopt spiritual practices into their medical treatment should be aware of two important psychological risks. One is called *spiritual bypassing*. This happens when a patient denies or suppresses her true feelings because she believes they are not "spiritual enough." An example would be a woman who says, "I can't be angry about my illness because God gave it to me," or someone who denies obvious frustration, fear, or depression, saying, "I have learned to accept." The fact is that no amount of "acceptance" makes feelings not exist. In fact, our feelings are extraordinary tools of insight and awareness. The task is not to eliminate real feelings but rather to avoid getting so caught up in them that we cannot move forward. Another form of spiritual bypassing occurs when someone uses spiritual practices as a distraction from pain or difficulty, or as a substitute for needed medical treatment. This person may run from one spiritual teacher or healer to the next, insisting that if she is able to only "think good thoughts" she will be cured. In the meantime, she may be avoiding real medical issues.

Another psychological trap some people fall into is what author Larry Dossey has termed New Age guilt.[14] This can occur when a woman begins to blame herself or various perceived inadequacies in her behavior, personality, or spiritual practice for her illness. For example, we have sometimes heard women in our program saying, "I think I got cancer because I was too uptight all my life," "I got cancer because of that job I had last year," or, more commonly, "Other people are telling me I got cancer because I give too much." In our society, there is a tremendous drive to find reasons to explain occurrences. In psychiatry we often find that people would rather blame themselves for something (such as an assault, or the death of a friend) than accept the powerless position that many things occur beyond our control. Women with breast cancer are barraged by New Age literature attributing their symptoms to past lives, to bad thoughts, to unresolved feminine issues, and so on. This can be a source of tremendous pain. There is no evidence to substantiate any of these claims. The data from our study show that women who see "illness as a punishment" show more anxiety, more depression, and lower quality of life.[15] At the same time, we find that women who feel their illness is meant to teach them something experience less anxiety, less depression, and a higher quality of life. These are women who look at their experience as a positive challenge and an opportunity to learn something that may benefit other aspects of their lives. As one woman told us, "It was cancer that caught my attention long enough to make the changes I needed to make anyway."

There's a big difference between the idea that cancer is an experience we can learn from, and the notion that cancer is a direct result of some error or negligence on our part. In dream or imagery work, a woman may experience her cancer as having occurred at the bodily site of an unexpressed emotion. However, it would be a mistake to conclude that she developed cancer because of this unexpressed emotion. Imagery and dream work can be part of a multilevel transpersonal process that offers symbolic wisdom but does not necessarily operate according to the same cause-and-effect rules as ordinary material reality.

Awareness

When we practice awareness, we deliberately turn our attention to our current or immediate experience. We experience through the five senses, and we also have thoughts that may come to us as images, impulses, or sensations. Most schools of meditation include formal training in developing one's awareness of moment-to-moment experience. For the patient, this type of training is especially helpful in managing pain and anxiety. It can help her distinguish between her worries about past or future problems and the actual experience of "right now." For example, we had a patient who would vomit at the mere sight of her doctor's business card. It was a classic conditioned reflex, brought on because she had come to closely associate her doctor (represented by the business card) with the negative experience of chemotherapy and its side effects. In the process, her "right now" experience at the moment she looked at the card became much more unpleasant than it needed to be.

When we are distracted or disassociated from our "right now" experience, our lack of awareness hurts us in several ways. First, it reinforces potentially false beliefs about an experience (e.g., "it was bad before; it will be exactly the same again"). Second, it prevents us from being present to receive the gifts that are there in the moment: having a doctor to talk to, or feeling connected to sources of help such as family, friends, and religion. As the patient/practitioner comes to recognize and accept her "right now" experience, she learns to release fear and develop more awareness and curiosity about what is actually available to her. In this context, people often have important insights and emotional releases as they see how much energy they have been using to avoid feelings and fears.

While this may all sound rather esoteric, practicing awareness or mindfulness has a great deal of relevance to daily life. A simple inventory can tell us something about the degree to which we fully experience our lives. For example, do you eat dinner out of a can while standing in front of the refrigerator? Or do you consciously prepare a healthful meal out of food you select for its ability to support your body in particular ways? Do you know where the food was grown, or does it come waxed and sprayed from a supermarket? Do you know why you eat? Do you set an intention for your own growth, happiness, or contributions to the world as you sit down to nourish yourself? Do you connect yourself to other people or a universal power through prayer before you eat? Do you find a moment of gratitude for the farmers, the truck drivers, your family, or your God? We can ask similar questions with regard to how we exercise. Do you work out on a treadmill while watching TV, or do you consciously attend to the stretch, pain, or strength in your body?

In the Integrated Program we use mindfulness meditation, yoga, imagery, art, and dance/movement work to support the participants' practice of awareness. Meditation will be described in more detail later. In yoga, participants learn to use breath to bring awareness to their bodily sensations and to create enough inner stillness so that they can experience tension and release in their bodies. Much of our movement work has participants focusing on their bodies' own subtle impulses toward movement, and simply allowing that movement to express itself without directing or impeding it. In this way, awareness is very much related to acceptance. Awareness is a practice of looking to see what is there before making any attempt to change it.

Art, imagery, and dance allow a patient to bypass her intellectual and rational mind and directly access a rich emotional and symbolic realm. Approaching these practices with mindfulness often enables patients to connect with deeper healing resources. For example, a patient may get in touch with old anger or trauma that needs to be released, or a fear that is no longer relevant and is holding her back, or a deep and sweet tenderness and self-love that can inspire or soothe her. With these art and movement therapies, it's important that patients don't worry about "failing" or being judged on their "performance." In our program, we encourage participants to cultivate a spirit of exploration and curiosity without judgment.

Acceptance

In the context of cancer, acceptance does not mean giving up. Acceptance has to do with finding meaning, trust, hope, peacefulness, happiness, improved quality of life, and fighting spirit. Women who accept have not surrendered; rather, they feel themselves more in partnership with a meaningful course of events.

A woman with cancer may face multiple losses, pain, uncertainty, an inability to work, mutilating surgeries, and the possibility of death. Acceptance of any one of these "unacceptable" realities requires her to be aware of and acknowledge her fear, depression, and anger. It also requires her to examine and question her personal and cultural beliefs about a particular issue. For example, in modern Western society, death is considered a source of suffering and the end of growth. On the other hand, Eastern perspectives and some Western religious and spiritual traditions see death as a transition to another state of awareness and a time of potential growth and development.

In our groups, women have found it helpful to discuss the basis of their assumptions and beliefs about death, as well as about suffering in general. We discuss the idea that suffering occurs either when we want something we don't have, or when we have something we don't want. Through meditation, movement, art, imagery, and sharing stories, we help women feel and examine the depth of what they are experiencing. Many women have expressed surprise at the peacefulness, expansiveness, and love they feel even while they contemplate such an otherwise frightening idea as their own death. The group provides the safety and context to talk about these issues, which are rarely discussed openly. Conscious stillness and patience seem to allow a sense of something much greater than our usual reactions and judgments in the face of difficulty. These discussions of death have often led to further discussion about the nature of being and the question of reincarnation. Often, especially in our non-Caucasian patients, they lead to a sense of direct connection to their ancestors, mothers, and grandmothers.

Acceptance also plays an important role in forgiveness. In psychology, forgiveness is encouraged because it is seen as relieving distress in the person who does the forgiving. However, patients often struggle with *how* to forgive—especially when someone has done them a severe injury. Rather than magnanimously exonerating someone who has hurt them, we encourage patients to accept that while the situation might not be as they wished, it is still possible to see their own strength and make a loving commitment to their own future well-being.

Intentionality, Prayer, and Healing

Intentionality occurs when we actively and consciously focus on a desired outcome. Practices such as imagery, visualization, affirmations, ritual, prayer, and "energy" or spiritual healing often use intentionality in an overt, participatory, and active way. It is important to note that the patient may or may not explicitly define her intention. An intention may be for disappearance of a cancer, for relief from pain, for understanding, for personal growth, or for alliance with a divine plan—as in the prayer "Thy will be done." In the context of imagery or visualization, the patient may use the mind to create a multisensory inner experience of wellness and vitality. In imagery, as with hypnosis, focused attention is used to address doubts and rational concerns. It also serves to rehearse the healing process.

Affirmations serve a similar purpose. They are positive statements designed to replace the pattern in our minds that tells us to expect a negative outcome. A positive affirmation sets a positive intention that may override the negative reflex of fear and catastrophizing. In the Integrated Program, women work alone and in small groups to create personalized affirmations, which are then read back to them in a ritual way by the group as a whole. When a woman is ill, or if she is approaching surgery or a difficult procedure, she might be invited to stand in the center of the circle and receive the silent or spoken intentions or wishes of the group: "May you know your beauty," "May your body heal," "May the hands of the surgeon be skillful and sure," "May you always be embraced by our love for you."

Intention can help a person define her values and priorities. Psychologist Lawrence LeShan developed an exercise in which he asked, "What if your fairy godmother came to town and could use her magic wand to give you the life you want six months from now?"[16] This exercise helps patients begin to look at their values and their resources, both inner and outer. They might include personal faith, a support system, or money in the bank. With these resources in mind, they begin to shape their intentions in a way that is both realistic and meaningful to them.

A therapist can work with a patient to set deliberate intentions. For example, many patients come to a therapist and say, "I wish I felt better" or "Life is really stressful." The therapist might help the patient to reformulate the statement to be "May I feel better" or "May my life be peaceful and full of meaning." This type of statement is very similar not only to the techniques used in cognitive therapy but also to prayer.

It states, but it also surrenders the wish. It allows for the possibility that not only the small or local self may be involved in how events will unfold. An intention does not have to be a project or a plan. We simply make a statement, then let go of our expectations.

For many people, prayers for themselves or others are an active part of daily life. Prayer itself is a broad term with many meanings. Prayers may be explicit requests for help, healing, or solace extended to a higher power or released to a universal life force. Prayer may also be simply a state of relationship with this higher power or force. In the context of this expanded relationship, a person may feel or express devotion, gratitude, love, awe, or simply peaceful surrender. For different people in different cultures, prayers may be tied to certain acts such as lighting a candle, leaving an offering at the ocean, writing on flags held high to the breezes, or speaking into tobacco to be tied in tiny prayer bundles. In our groups, prayers were sometimes sewn into quilt squares, left on a program altar or "memory table," or sometimes spoken aloud to the group.

Many types of mental or spiritual healing techniques incorporate intentionality, including some types of prayer, "energy healing," shamanic healing, laying on of hands, and healing rituals. Research on prayer or distant healing has found that in both animal and clinical populations, intentions set by experienced healers or pray-ers may benefit a patient at a distance, even when he or she does not know such healing efforts are being made. The National Institutes of Health have developed a scientific term for such phenomena: *distant mental influence on biological systems*. To date, there have been more than 135 published studies of controlled laboratory and clinical trials of distant healing effects. More than two-thirds of these trials have shown positive results.

In our own laboratory, we recently published a randomized clinical trial of distant healing for people with AIDS.[17] In this trial, compared with a control group, people with AIDS who received distant healing intentions from healers located all over the country showed fewer new AIDS-defining illnesses, lower illness severity scores, fewer doctor visits, fewer hospitalizations, and improved mood. This occurred even though the patients never met any of the healers involved in the study and did not know whether or not they were receiving the healing efforts. A similar randomized trial studying more than a thousand patients undergoing cardiac surgery and recently published in the *Archives of Internal Medicine*[18] also found a significant benefit of distant healing under blinded conditions. Although very little information is available as to what types of distant healing (prayer, visualization, etc.) might be most effective, the research evidence has found benefits that seem to relate more to the presence of intention rather than to the use of any particular technique.

Compassion and Lovingkindness

Compassion is a word that has replaced the word *love* in many circles because *love* is often confused with dependency or sexuality. Our use of the word *compassion* refers to an open-hearted loving acceptance, which does not bind and has no expectations. *Lovingkindness* extends the idea of compassion to cultivate a loving connection with all of life. Compassion and lovingkindness are innate human capacities, which arise naturally in certain circumstances—for example, when we feel loved by someone else. Our feelings of compassion and lovingkindness may intensify when we contemplate the suffering or the innocence of someone we love. We may also cultivate these feelings by meditating on loving or compassionate intentions. In this practice, one calls to mind another person and silently in the heart holds the intention "May you be happy," "May you feel safe," "May you feel love." This meditation may be extended to the larger community of all beings, or may (sometimes with difficulty) be applied to the self.

In our program, women often notice how much easier it is to extend compassion and lovingkindness to others, and how harsh they usually are to themselves. The lovingkindness practices seem to help women care more for themselves and offer their care toward others from a stronger and more fulfilled center. The women are no longer giving away their love; they are sharing it. Seeing the self from a compassionate perspective can lead to extraordinary growth. When working with patients who feel painful or stuck feelings arising, we ask them, "Could you try holding that feeling with compassion—and just observe what changes?" As one woman observed, "I can see myself as if I were my own beloved child."

In the words of another participant, "Learning to love myself was absolutely the biggest thing I took away from this program. I've always known that was important, but now I understand it in a much more profound way. I think that like a lot of women, I've spent my life serving other people and trying to live up to their expectations. Now I know on a deep, bodily level how important it is to take good care of myself. Because nobody else is going to do it."

Perspective

The perspective of many mind-body therapies and approaches derives from spiritual traditions. For example, yoga and qigong classes often begin or end with discussions of our essential unity with all other beings, of the importance of compassion, of service to others, of belief in life after death, of an intrinsic meaningfulness to all events, or of the concept of life energy running through the body. Words such as *gratitude, surrender, love, compassion, unity, peace,* and *forgiveness* are used frequently in these discussions.

Meditation is also fundamentally a spiritual practice. Meditation instruction emphasizes accepting nature rather than trying to control it and the belief that our usual state of consciousness gives us only a limited view of reality. These teachings deemphasize goal-oriented achievement and acquisition and suggest the opportunity for peacefulness through surrender and acceptance. From this perspective, life becomes a school for continuous learning rather than a task to be completed and mastered. Likewise, the dying process is seen as inevitably an opportunity for transformation and an inspiration to personal growth. Such perspectives are highly subjective, and while they may appear obvious to some people, they are in direct conflict with the material-based, goal-oriented approach of modern medicine.

Group Structure and Format

The mind-body-spirit work we undertake in our program requires intense exploration, which in turn requires trust and courage on the part of participants. We try to provide them with a safe, loving atmosphere and a framework for understanding the experiences they may go through.

After experimenting with different formats for our groups, we've found that the following approach works best:

1. Sit in a circle, to symbolize and facilitate community.
2. Start with a short meditation or reading, ringing a bell, or another means of bringing attention into the room and onto the work.
3. Set aside a fixed period of time for some sort of experiential exercise or educational work.
4. Do a formal "check-in" process wherein all participants have a chance to talk about important feelings or life events.
5. Have a minimum of one hour for general discussion.
6. Do a formal closing with a meditation, short imagery, or a reading.

The time set aside for experiential work is also the time for any formal instruction such as teaching meditation, or introducing a specific theme such as forgiveness, death and dying, or coping with pain. While there are many contemplative exercises for exploring these themes, we have found it helpful to provide a framework for thinking about these issues before plunging in. We have also often found it useful to work in groups of two or three, with one person speaking to the theme while the other(s) serves as witness. Experiential time may also be used for writing, drawing, or movement exercises, or for group activities, such as watching a relevant film clip to serve as a focus for discussion. Themes will emerge out of group discussion, and a creative group leader will be able to find or develop an exercise to explore the roots of whatever is most present for the group. Themes that we always address with breast cancer groups are death and dying, healing, sexuality, femininity, compassion, forgiveness, anger, pain, spirituality, and visions of the future.

Basic Techniques or Therapies

Since we believe that the practices discussed below offer benefits for breast cancer patients, we encourage you to pursue any or all that appeal to you. Many medical centers offer classes in yoga and even qigong for cancer patients. You may also look for classes in your area aimed at the general population. If you currently belong to a support group, you might propose that the group incorporate meditation, movement work, art, or other therapy into your sessions. If practitioners are not readily available through your medical facility, look beyond it. Get on the Internet; check out chat groups and news groups to learn more about these practices and how you can get more involved with them. You can also learn more about meditation from chapter 11.

Meditation

Meditation has been described as "the intentional self-regulation of attention."[19] It has been used as a contemplative and spiritual practice for thousands of years.[20] We have seen that for the woman with cancer, meditation can help her to look at her inward experience in order to enhance self-awareness, make sense of what is happening to her body, and decide upon a course of action. The practice of meditation can "provide deep comfort, meaning, and direction in times of high stress and uncertainty."[21]

There are many forms and schools of meditation. The two most common are mindfulness meditation and concentrative meditation. Mindfulness meditation is most widely known as a result of the work conducted by Jon Kabat-Zinn with chronic pain patients at the University of Massachusetts Medical Center. He teaches patients to practice observing the contents of their minds from a perspective of acceptance, without trying to change or manipulate their thoughts.[22] Mindfulness meditation can build patience, trust, and acceptance of the self and of things as they are.[23] It has also been shown to be useful in controlling cancer pain and reducing suffering.[24–26] This form of meditation is currently taught to people with cancer and other illnesses at the California Pacific Medical Center through the Community Wellness Program at the Institute for Health and Healing. It is also used at sixteen Kaiser hospitals in Northern California, at Commonweal,[27] and at two hundred other hospitals throughout the country. Other types of meditation ᵈ yoga are being taught through the Ornish Heart Disease Reversal ᵐ.[28] One of the few randomized controlled studies of mindfulness meditation with breast cancer patients is being conducted at the University of Massachusetts Medical Center.[29]

Concentrative meditation and relaxation are often used together. Concentrative forms of meditation involve focusing on a particular word, phrase, or object (which may include the breath or a devotional figure). Herbert Benson, M.D., at the Mind-Body Medical Institute, has extensively researched this form of meditation at Harvard University. Benson has named the physical results of this form of meditation the "relaxation response."[30] This form of meditation may help cancer patients develop the skill to still the mind sufficiently for mindfulness meditation; diminish distressing thoughts, thereby lessening anxiety;[31] and focus on a positive image and benefit from the positive attributes associated with that image (e.g., peace, lovingkindness, fearlessness). The lovingkindness practice described earlier is a form of concentrative meditation practice. For some women, mindfulness practice seems too abstract and unstructured. Lovingkindness meditation feels more concrete and structured, which is especially helpful for women who are experiencing a lot of anxiety.

Imagery and Contemplation

Imagery has many possible uses. It can be directed at managing symptoms or at cultivating self-awareness and discovering buried inner attitudes, desires, and creative impulses. Imagery has been widely used with cancer patients, especially for reducing anxiety, fatigue, nausea, and pain.[32-35] Several studies have shown that cancer patients who used imagery had significantly improved psychological outcomes.[36-38] In our program we work with several kinds of imagery. Every group practices developing an image of the cancer and then developing images of the cancer healing or healed. We strongly encourage each woman to fully experience a sense of wellness. Other imagery practices include developing a personal sense of a "safe beautiful place," contacting an inner guide or wisdom figure, and several other imagery sequences in which participants find special gifts or sources of healing. Many women find it helpful to integrate their imagery into their cancer treatment. A patient with a Christian background, for example, used visualization during her radiation therapy to "see the Christlight descending into the radiation machine, and then following a brilliant beam to heal my body." Imagery may be visual, auditory, kinesthetic, or olfactory.

Our program also used several guided contemplations. These are exercises in which participants listen to a script suggesting images, ideas, or sensations of a psychological and spiritual nature. They contemplate a series of statements about the inevitability of death and about the fact that we have with us only our state of mind at the moment of death. Our contemplations also include a practice of forgiveness and of compassion for ourselves and others. This is sometimes done as paired exercise, in which women gaze into each other's eyes as they listen to a script guiding their focus to the fullness of each person. This has often produced intense experiences. Women were able to connect deeply to the strength and the pain in their partners far beyond what words allowed. The eye contact, which at first was uncomfortable for many, became especially healing. As one woman said, "I never looked into someone's soul before." Another woman asked for a copy of the script and tape-recorded it to use with her husband. Many authors have published scripts for such contemplations. We have found it useful to modify the basic script to fit the concerns of a particular group.

Contemplations are always most effective when we begin with a discussion of the topic. For example, the contemplation of death requires that participants prepare themselves by discussing any fears they may have about picturing their own death. In preparation for a forgiveness meditation, we discuss the purposes and mechanisms of forgiveness. For contemplation of compassion and meditation, patients discuss their own resistance to sending loving thoughts to themselves.

Yoga

The word *yoga* means "union," the union of body, mind, and spirit.[39] Physical yogic practices such as gentle stretching and breathing have traditionally been used as preparation for meditation, for the purpose of stilling the mind.[40] Yogic postures and breathing are thought to make the practitioner more self-aware and more available to a "healing energy," which will benefit both emotional and physical well-being.[41] Yoga is also known to improve circulation, improve strength, and promote relaxation. Yoga is often incorporated into mind-body healing retreats to help patients experience the direct relationship between their physical and emotional states.[42]

One advantage of yoga for the woman with cancer is that she may develop more body awareness, which will allow her to respond more appropriately to changes in body sensations and to develop a sense of patience and compassion for her recovering body. In a yoga program within the context of cancer, it is especially important for the patient to understand that the benefit of the posture comes not from perfect performance, but rather from being aware of the limits of comfort. Learning to accept the sensations at one's limit in a pose can sometimes bring more healing than pushing through the pain brought on by the pose.

Dance and Expressive Arts

Arts such as music, dance, drawing, mask-making, or collage allow participants to be creative, to explore, and to express themselves in a context where they feel free and their defenses are relaxed. The goals of dance and movement therapies are to increase flexibility and range of motion (very important for women who have had mastectomies), increase blood flow, foster a sense of belonging to one's body, and enable the women to become more aware of body sensations.

In our groups, women use movement to explore rage, sadness, joy, and community. They have created group dances and movement rituals. In the Dragon Breath Dance, women symbolically put things to which they direct anger in the middle of the circle and use force to get rid of them. These items range from cancer to treatment pain to having too much to manage in their lives. Here the women kick and push with their hands, and breathe fire at these items. In another group dance, women begin with a belly dance and veils and move to a ritual of gathering and scattering. The gathering movements give the women a chance to identify things and qualities they would like to have for themselves, and the scattering represents the things or qualities they would like to spread to their friends, family, or other women with cancer. The dance and movement work enables women to explore their sensuality through belly dance (a favorite), explore emotional and physical polarities, and learn breath work, soothing self-touch, and the art of stillness. Comments have included "The belly dance let me reclaim the power of my pelvis" and "Contact with my partner felt like cookies and milk." In response to a self-touch exercise, one woman noted that she felt "soothed and energized, like having been touched by a wondrous lover." Women often use movement as a way of expressing and responding to painful experience. One participant, for example, used a session to "rock and comfort" the breast she lost to mastectomy. Another stated that the movement work helped her to "mobilize my stagnant anger."

At the beginning of the program, women have an opportunity to lie down on a large sheet of paper and have their body traced. Throughout the remaining twelve weeks, they periodically spend time with markers filling in their body outline. They indicate body stories from the places or parts where they feel confidence and from places or parts that have numbness, wounds, scars, or vulnerability. One of the measures of a balanced body image is whether they can portray both the positive and negative aspects of themselves. One woman commented of her drawing that "the pink around the body shows the wholeness and body connection" that she didn't know she had.

Other art exercises have included making collages representing the self before and after cancer, drawing overleaf images of the participant and of her mother, and drawing the self as a boat or as a tree and then discussing the images. One highly intimate and powerful exercise chosen by about half of the participants was to make plaster casts of their busts, scars, and mastectomy sites. They then decorated these casts with items ranging from flowers to barbed wire.

The movement and expressive arts work typically begins with a quick check-in. A topic is presented to the group, and then the women are invited to create some visual representation of that idea through drawing, collage, or some other means. For example, in one exercise the women depict where they used to be, where they are now, and where they want to be. As with some of the discussion exercises, participants often work in pairs, so that one person serves as a witness to the expression of another.

Council

Sometimes in our groups we substitute a council process for general discussion. In a council process, we present a specific topic or question to the group, such as "Stories of Healing," "Death," "My Anger," or "My Femininity." Rather than talking in a conversational way, group members are invited to pick up a "talking piece," which may be a special stone, a decorated stick, or even an ordinary object like a stapler or a chalkboard eraser. The object helps the speaker focus her attention. The talking piece may be passed clockwise around the circle or placed in the center of the room for participants to pick up when they feel moved to speak. In our program we work with four rules of council derived from *The Way of Council* by Jack Zimmerman and Virginia Coyle.[43] The first is to speak from the heart, of something that really matters. Passion and simplicity are good descriptions of heartfelt speaking. The second is to listen from the heart. This means simply bearing witness to whatever is being spoken. Participants do not interrupt or ask questions of the speaker. There is no attempt to fix or rescue. The third rule is "lean expression." This is a practical consideration. Heartfelt speech has its own eloquence and does not require excessive detail. The fourth rule is spontaneity. Participants are asked not to plan or rehearse what they are going to say. A council process may be followed by general discussion, but often it is helpful to let it resonate quietly with the participants. It may be difficult for some group members, but it always challenges people to take responsibility for their inner feelings and attitudes. It also gives quieter members an equal chance to participate, which strengthens the group.

Good Medicine for All

The practices and perspectives learned in a group often figure directly into the group process. For example, when one participant accidentally hurts another's feelings, there is an opportunity to illustrate forgiveness and make the concept come alive. This approach carries the possibility of taking crises and using them to help the patient move toward a deeper understanding of herself, expanding the scope of her vision and generating hope. The techniques used are less important than the patient's willingness to look inside and accept her feelings without judgment. It also depends on the loving presence of a guide or therapist who can support her unequivocally and help her relax into her own experience.

Through our program, we have witnessed the great extent to which mind-body-spirit therapies enable patients to grow and change even in the midst of the pain and chaos of cancer therapy. For Judy, the teacher quoted earlier, the program not only helped her cope with her fears and anger about having breast cancer, but also marked a turning point in her life.

"It was the experiential aspect of the program that made the difference for me," she says. "I see now that it's not enough just to talk. Through the exercises, and by actually doing meditation, yoga, and dance, I began to understand the connection between the body and the mind in a powerful way. That's what made it so rich. And I've learned the importance of taking time out for myself, whether it be for meditation or exercise or being with other people."

The community formed in a group can provide the patient with a significant source of encouragement, support, and important new perspectives. Although we have described this work here in the context of treatment for cancer, all the therapies and perspectives involved could be of use to people with other illnesses or without an obvious physical disease. Cancer may provide the catalyst, but the integration of mind, body, and spirit is good medicine for any of us who are still occasionally trapped by pain, anxiety, or hopelessness.

Acknowledgments

This work was funded by a generous grant from the United States Department of Defense Materiel Command (Grant No. 17-96-1-6260) to the University of California, San Francisco Medical Center and to the California Pacific Medical Center. We would like to express our appreciation to Dr. Laura Esserman as principal investigator for the New Vision of Breast Care grant, of which this project was a portion; to the clinical staff of the Breast Cancer Personal Support/Life-style Intervention Trial of UCSF and CPMC; Rosalind Benedet, R.N., N.P., Jnani Chapman, R.N.; Janelle Eckhardt, Ph.D. R.N.; Deborah Hamolsky, R.N., Adina Klien, M.A.; Cory Fitzpatrick, Ph.D.; Sian Cotton, Ph.D.; Kristie Dold, B.A.; Michelle Baumgardner, M.S.W.; Sylvine Jerome, M.D.; Carol Kronenwetter, Ph.D.; Diane Neighbor, D.T.R.; Cindy Perlis, M.A.; Megan Rundel, M.A.; Brook Stone, L.C.S.W.; and to Ms. Alison Brady, B.A., for outstanding administrative support.

CHAPTER FOURTEEN

The Charlotte Maxwell Complementary Clinic: A Healing Place for Low-Income Women

Beverly Burns, M.S., L.Ac.; and Linda Wardlaw, Dr.P.H.

BEVERLY BURNS, M.S., L.Ac., is one of the founders and clinical director of the Charlotte Maxwell Complementary Clinic, a health care center dedicated to increasing access to complementary and alternative medicine for low-income women diagnosed with cancer. She has a traditional Chinese medicine practice located in San Francisco, California, that focuses on treating women diagnosed with cancer. In addition, she is an acupuncturist and researcher at the University of California, San Francisco Carol Franc Buck Breast Care Center Complementary and Alternative Medicine Program.

LINDA WARDLAW, DR.P.H., has been on the Board of Directors for the Charlotte Maxwell Complementary Clinic since 1998. She has a doctorate in public health with a special interest in socioeconomic status and health. She has also conducted research on public perception of health risks and on the impact of HIV/AIDS caregiving among friends and family members.

Sally Savitz, a licensed acupuncturist and homeopath, had spent years offering her services to women with cancer, including free services to those who couldn't afford to pay. She knew from experience how much these women could benefit from alternative healing methods. She also knew there were many women in need who faced unique challenges resulting from poverty and lack of access to resources.

In 1989, with the goal of helping many more women than she could reach as an individual, Sally assembled a group of health care providers and other activists to develop plans for a free clinic. The clinic would serve low-income women with cancer by providing a full range of complementary and alternative medicine (CAM) and other services in a private-practice setting.

Sally drew inspiration for the project from the memory of Charlotte Maxwell, a patient who had died of ovarian cancer in 1988. Although Charlotte lost her own battle with cancer, the complementary treatments she turned to in the latter months of her life did much to ease her suffering and improve the quality of life remaining to her. Her dedication to social justice led her to understand the importance of access to high-quality care for those who could not afford to pay for treatment. She expressed the hope that one day, low-income women would be able to receive the outstanding complementary care she had been fortunate enough to receive.

As a result of the effort and expertise of that initial group of volunteers, the Charlotte Maxwell Complementary Clinic (CMCC), a licensed, nonprofit, primary care facility serving low-income women with cancer in the San Francisco Bay Area, was born.

About the Clinic

CMCC provides free services such as acupuncture, homeopathy, massage therapy, visualization, and Chinese and Western herbs. The aim of these therapies is to offer the client relief from the terrible side effects of both the cancer and its treatments, including the pain, nausea, fatigue, and loss of appetite so common among cancer patients. Additionally, CAM treatments can strengthen the immune system and potentially influence long-term prognosis. Current research on CAM treatments is aimed at evaluating their effectiveness when integrated with Western treatments and, in some instances, as stand-alone therapies.

While these treatments will continue to be studied, the benefits of group support and enriched community have already proved to have tremendous value. Those of us who volunteer at the clinic have experienced this firsthand. During the years of planning to develop the policies of CMCC and to obtain licensing from the state, we spent quite a bit of time meeting and getting to know one another. The relationships we developed helped to energize and motivate us, and they provided a foundation for our sense of community.

Currently, the clinic serves only low-income women because they have been so consistently disadvantaged by virtue of gender, race, and socioeconomic status. Low-income women often live and work in areas that place them at risk for higher exposures to carcinogenic substances. Lack of access to timely and sensitive medical care may result in delayed diagnosis of their cancer. The treatment they subsequently receive is likewise often inadequate. Low-income women must often terminate conventional treatments prematurely because the financial burden is too great. Thus, disadvantage is compounded at every step, contributing to a poorer prognosis for long-term survival.

While our clients are diverse, their common denominator is a lack of access to CAM treatment and often a lack of access to conventional treatment as well. In some cases, we have been able to help clients gain better access to care within the Western medical establishment.

From the start, everyone involved with the clinic wanted to help as many women as possible, which made it difficult to decide who should qualify for care. But we also knew our limitations. Complementary treatments are rarely covered under health insurance plans, despite considerable evidence supporting their safety and effectiveness. As a result, few cancer patients are able to benefit from complementary care unless they can afford to pay for treatments and herbs out of pocket. Patients living in poverty, with few or no resources, will certainly be unable to access these healing methods. For this reason, these women are CMCC's priority.

When we first began outreach to the local public hospital, we met with considerable reluctance from health care providers. There were two main reasons for this. CAM treatments were less common then, and many medical practitioners were skeptical about them. In addition, many doubted our commitment to provide these services for free.

At the hospital, we developed a relationship with an oncology nurse named Bill, whose first referral was Brenda. The mother of two young children, Brenda was at risk for not completing her chemotherapy. She could barely make ends meet and was trying hard to continue her job as a clerk at a small business. When she came to CMCC, she received a great deal of support. We helped with emergency funds, particularly for food and utilities. We also educated her about nutrition, cooked for her, and taught her how to prepare better-quality food for herself and her children.

Though Brenda had no previous exposure to CAM therapy, the benefits of participating in her own healing were clear. She repeatedly told her providers, "You're listening to me. Nobody does that!" After Brenda finished her chemotherapy and radiation, Bill called CMCC and told us he'd be sending more patients our way.

Many of the initial clients were women who were already interested in complementary medicine. Another of our early clients was diagnosed very young. Karen earned her living as a massage therapist and had just purchased a new massage table for her practice. Her cancer was extremely aggressive, and Karen was quickly making life decisions. She came to CMCC one day, when we were still borrowing space in an office, and told us she wanted to give her massage table to the clinic. She never received treatment on that table at CMCC, but she was happy to know someone else would be able to receive treatment on it. One of the last things she said was, "CMCC is the only place I go where all of my decisions are listened to. Nobody tells me what to do."

Before they come to CMCC, many clients have experienced only rushed, impersonal health care that gives them no opportunity to ask questions, much less be touched. Even something as basic as privacy may be denied to them. At one of the local public hospitals, for example, patients receive their cancer diagnosis while they are separated from the next patient by only a curtain. Our clients long for personal attention and the opportunity to be heard, and they get it at CMCC.

> They dedicate so much of their hearts and souls to helping women with cancer. They walk with us through our battle. They give such strength, determination, and hope. I always leave the clinic and go home feeling very encouraged and positive, believing I will get well.

Offering Help beyond Health Care

As the clinic's clientele grew, we realized we needed to provide support that went beyond CAM treatment. Because of this, the clinic now offers social work assistance to help the women cope with the myriad of socioeconomic struggles faced by low-income women after a diagnosis of cancer. For instance, housing and transportation difficulties are common among CMCC clients. Referrals for financial and legal assistance are now provided on a regular basis. We also offer transportation services and regular supplies of fresh organic vegetables and bread.

The catalyst for this program came from two different sources. One of CMCC's early clients was an elderly woman, Helen, with breast cancer. Helen was raising her grandson, and during her treatment she found it extremely difficult to shop and cook for him. Initially, she did not mention this to anyone at CMCC. As she developed a friendship with one of the massage therapists who often provided her care, she started talking about her problem. The massage therapist wanted to help. At the same time, some of the volunteers at the clinic had been purchasing food from a weekly organic delivery service. Arrangements were made, and the company began donating boxes of food to CMCC for the clients to take home. For Helen and her grandson, this made a tremendous difference.

Another "angel" who helped the clinic expand its services was Jean, a dedicated social worker who initially volunteered her services for three years! Jean, a cancer survivor herself, works hard to minimize clients' practical and financial hardships so they can devote more of their energy to healing.

Since 1997, the clinic has served as an internship site for students studying to become social workers. These students provide the clinic with vital assistance for case work and community outreach. And the need for these services is constantly growing. In the past year, four women came to CMCC who were homeless during the course of their treatment for breast cancer. This means that during their chemotherapy they returned to a shelter at night but were often on the street during the day. The chance that they would finish their treatment was very low. One of these women, Laura, had two children, in the third and fifth grades. Day-to-day living was extremely challenging for Laura and her family. Eating, getting the kids to school, and having a place to sleep each night were difficult enough, let alone going to treatment. Laura relied heavily on CMCC for emergency food, transportation, and emotional support for herself and her children. Additionally, she used acupuncture, herbs, and massage. Laura told us that no one had touched her in a very long time. On top of that, when she received the chemotherapy, she didn't have any nausea and felt that she was sleeping much better.

CMCC helped two of these homeless women complete their treatment despite incredibly difficult personal circumstances. CMCC's clients often endure great hardship in their lives, which only becomes worse when they are diagnosed with cancer.

A Place to Communicate

One of the most enjoyable aspects of life that has developed at CMCC is the community waiting room. Here food is served, conversation flows, and friendships develop. Out of this experience came the desire of many clients to communicate more with one another, with clinic volunteers, and with the world. Several years ago, a former client started a newsletter to provide clients with a place to express, in their own words, the meaning of cancer in their lives. Through the newsletter, they communicate with one another, with volunteers and staff, and with the community at large.

THE BEST THINGS IN LIFE . . .
by Betty Lawson-Eugene

> I can't remember where or when
>   the thought first came to me:
> There're lots of riches in this world
>   (on this you might agree).
>
> It's easy to forget this fact
>   in times of tragedy,
> At Charlotte Maxwell hopes are born
>   from riches that are free.
>
> In '92 my doctor said:
>   "Prognosis is one year . . .
> Your cancer is inoperable"
>   (Such hopeless words to hear!)

I'm sure it was the prayers by friends,
  and family members too,
That through these prayers I found out
  what some selfless women do.

They volunteer their therapies
  and expertise, for free,
To women who might miss such care,
  could not afford the fee.

These dedicated women
  (Charlotte Maxwell's aims in view)
Are such a credit to her name
  through what they say and do.

At CMCC I have felt
  (through therapies of choice)
The understanding and support
  of women with one voice.

So . . . CMCC women
  we appreciate your sharing
Your deep respect and precious time,
  the richness of your caring.

The Need for Post-treatment Support

JM is in her 50s. She believes she could not have completed chemotherapy without the care she received at CMCC. But now her fears turn to the workplace: "Will I be able to think?" "Will I be able to drive to work?" "Will I have the energy to make it through a workday?"

She is not alone in her fears for the future. Yet, there are virtually no resources available for women once they have completed chemotherapy and/or radiation. For many women, the profound nature of what it means to be a cancer survivor becomes most deeply felt when the visible signs of crisis are waning.

Once the chemotherapy is over, the radiation treatments are completed, and the external signs of trauma such as hair loss are no longer evident, women are encouraged to "put the cancer behind them." This is difficult even for women who are diagnosed and treated early in the course of the disease. The low-income women who come to CMCC for care are often diagnosed in advanced stages of cancer. Most struggle with chronic fatigue, pain, swelling, and other manifestations of cancer treatment that complicate their recovery. CMCC now sees increasing numbers of very young women whose recovery is further complicated by the impact of the cancer and its treatments on child-bearing.[1]

Every month, several CMCC clients complete their course of chemotherapy and/or radiation. In the early years of the clinic, we could continue to see them for several months to assist them in the transition back to work and family roles. However, the number of newly diagnosed women coming to CMCC has increased dramatically. Because we must give them priority for treatment, few if any available slots are open to those who are no longer in active treatment. At any given time, there may be thirty to forty women who must be assigned a lower priority, not because they no longer need our services, but because they have completed chemotherapy and/or radiation.

For women at this stage, the physical and emotional demands of resuming their interrupted roles within the family or at work often lead to profound, lingering fatigue and depression. Among those fortunate enough to have jobs waiting, many find that they are unable to perform their previous tasks because of the complications of cancer and its treatments. Others need to find new work, wondering if and when to disclose their cancer diagnosis. Many are in need of legal or financial advice to address employment-related discrimination, housing, or other problems that plague them on a daily basis. Thus, many clients who have completed their chemotherapy and/or radiation are terribly disappointed to learn that the clinic can no longer offer them the healing and support services that helped sustain them through their conventional treatment.

We know that they could benefit from the treatments we offer. For instance, herbal supplementation could assist them in restoring strength to their immune system and help them cope with the lingering fatigue commonly experienced after cancer treatment. Acupuncture could ease their pain. Massage therapy could reduce the lymphedema so often exacerbated by the resumption of physical tasks. Moreover, the lack of emotional support, the sense of isolation, and their fears of disclosing their cancer history all make it difficult to readjust. Just coming to the clinic and being with other women who know what they are experiencing could provide much-needed help.

The absence of services to women after treatment is a significant gap in the spectrum of support for cancer survivors. It reflects the myth that cancer is not a chronic condition: that physical and emotional health are easily restored once treatment is completed. To address these concerns, CMCC has secured funding for a program for women who have completed conventional treatments. Initially, the program will provide ongoing CAM treatments and support services to CMCC clients. Eventually, if funding is available, other cancer survivors from the community could be seen as well.

The post-treatment program owes its existence to the clients of CMCC who told us how much they needed one. They have articulated their concerns, met with the board of directors, and otherwise worked to push forward post-treatment care as a clinic priority. As important as the program is to clients, it is also gratifying for staff and volunteers to provide a clearly needed service to women they have already come to know and care about.

Some of our clients are newly diagnosed and are weighing their treatment options. Others are in the midst of chemotherapy or radiation treatments. Still others are struggling with recurrent cancer and fears of death. Most have a primary diagnosis of breast cancer or of metastatic disease secondary to breast cancer. They are living evidence of the profound toll that cancer takes on physical and emotional health, on work and family life, on hopes and dreams for the future. Because CAM therapies are effective for both physical and emotional symptoms, CMCC clients are able to receive care that addresses the many levels of distress so common after a cancer diagnosis.

Easing the Transition: Caring for Patients at Home

CMCC recently initiated a home care program for women diagnosed with terminal cancer. In the early days of CMCC, it became apparent that many clients needed help during their transition toward death. Volunteer practitioners would often go into a client's home to provide treatment, but we wanted to do more. We received funding from the Symington Foundation to provide CAM treatment to women who are too weak to come to the clinic for care. Debilitating pain, fatigue, and oxygen starvation effectively prevent the terminally ill from completing life tasks, healing relationships, or simply enjoying the time left to them. CMCC has held specialized training for home care volunteers to prepare them for working with low-income women with terminal cancer. To date, we have served twenty women in the hospice program, providing massage, acupuncture, and herbal medications to ease the symptoms of end-stage cancer. The level of intimacy that develops with this kind of care creates a unique and powerful bond. Most important, it clearly improves the quality of life for clients in their remaining days. This is both clinically significant and emotionally gratifying for the patient, for her family, and for the volunteers who have come to care for the women on a personal as well as a professional level.

Staffing and Operating the Clinic

The clinic is fundamentally a volunteer organization. Over the past decade it has grown from a tiny clinic serving a handful of women one afternoon a week to one that struggles to serve more than 220 women. CMCC owes its existence to the acupuncturists, herbalists, massage therapists, visualization practitioners, homeopaths, and support staff who donate more than $200,000 worth of services each year.

Because volunteers are so central to the clinic's mission of providing CAM at no cost to low-income women, it is essential that we devote considerable time, energy, and resources toward recruiting, training, and sustaining an active core of volunteer practitioners. As part of its outreach strategy, CMCC posts notices for new volunteers in public newsletters and flyers, on the Internet, and in CAM professional settings.

Approximately twenty new volunteers attend each training. They hear presentations on the origins and treatment of cancer and the role of alternative medicine in addressing the disease. The training is designed to enhance understanding of the ways in which sexism and racism, in particular, may work to diminish the health and well-being of low-income women living with cancer.

CMCC volunteers must be not only professionally skilled but culturally sensitive as well. Our clients are low-income women with cancer. Beyond that, they are diverse in age, in race and ethnicity, in sexual orientation, in degree of religiosity, and in many other dimensions of personality and life circumstances. Thus our agency must always work to ensure that our services are provided in an atmosphere of acceptance, advocacy, and genuine entitlement for all women who come through our doors. At any time, the waiting area may hold a lesbian couple, an Asian family, or single women waiting to be seen. Some will want to talk and to share the story of their cancer; others will prefer to keep that information private.

When a woman comes to us for care, she is introduced to the range of treatments and services available to her at CMCC. Each client is prioritized according to her need. The volunteer clinical director and the practitioners of all the different healing modalities attend meetings to discuss each case. The practitioners are encouraged to consult with each other in order to provide the best possible care to each woman at the clinic. They discuss the clients' needs and anything that may have arisen during treatment.

CMCC has initiated a continuing medical education program for acupuncturists, funded by the Susan G. Komen Foundation. The program enables the clinic to improve the quality of care it offers clients, to ensure a source of new volunteers, and to provide caregivers with intensive exposure to the clinical complications of cancer in low-income women.

Participants attend day-long and evening sessions on a variety of issues relevant to traditional Chinese medicine (TCM) and cancer. Current CMCC volunteers, and those willing to commit to a year of volunteer service, may attend at no charge. The topics covered include Western diagnosis and staging, TCM diagnosis and treatment options, drug-herb interactions and contraindications, and immune enhancement. Most important, the very foundation of the course is based on the treatment needs of CMCC's low-income clients, a constituency most often ignored in the course of conventional treatment and research.

In addition to training aimed at care providers, CMCC volunteer Betty Siegal has also developed a program to help clients and volunteers manage lymphedema. This is a significant problem for many women after surgery, one that is often overlooked. Betty has recruited individuals from the community with experience in lymphedema treatment to help clients learn how to treat themselves and seek out additional care.

One form of education the women at CMCC greatly appreciate is nutritional guidance. Healthful recipes are included along with the food bags they receive, and clients may attend seminars about eating to better balance their system according to traditional Chinese medicine theory.

Managing the Clinic's Rapid Growth

When the clinic served a handful of women, it was relatively easy to coordinate care and communicate vital information about each client's situation. As the numbers have risen over time, so too has the complexity of running the clinic. CMCC now has a full-time clinic coordinator as well as a volunteer coordinator. We have come to rely more and more on the computer to schedule and track both clients and volunteers. Making sure clinic shifts are fully staffed, that all appointments are filled, that rooms are assigned, and that herbs are in stock requires considerable time and attention. Nevertheless, it is essential that the full spectrum of CAM treatments is available during every clinic shift. Not only does this ensure optimal care for each client; it also saves her time, money, and energy by cutting down the number of trips she needs to make to the clinic.

The continued growth of the clinic has many benefits and a few drawbacks. On one hand, it is gratifying to see our outreach efforts succeeding and bringing more women to the clinic who can benefit from our services. Yet, steadfast volunteers, who have been around since the clinic's grassroots beginnings, also miss the intimacy of the old days, when there were no paid workers and every volunteer saw every client. Virtually anything related to the clinic was subject to discussion—how, when, who—making the process difficult but ultimately richer for the dialogue. CMCC still works hard to ensure that everything can be discussed, debated, and, hopefully, resolved. But that's a significant challenge now that we have 220 clients, more than one hundred volunteers, four paid staff members, and a board of directors, all holding legitimate concerns and passionate opinions about what CMCC should be.

The Politics of Cancer

The cancer activist community has made tremendous progress in calling attention to the social and political dimensions of a cancer diagnosis. However, the majority of activists are white, middle-class and upper-middle-class women. The critical issues facing low-income women with cancer are simply not the same. Women who cannot afford medical care, who must forgo available screening tests, are often diagnosed in advanced stages of cancer with a poorer prognosis for recovery. Such women may have little energy to devote to a political movement that has not been defined in collaboration with their own community. Thus, a part of the clinic's mission is to create an environment where low-income women with cancer can define the priorities that are relevant to them.

We provide CAM therapies primarily because we believe in their efficacy and safety in treating the side effects of cancer and its treatments. But it is equally vital that our treatment be provided in the context of respect and autonomy. Women do not cause their cancer, and we will do everything we can to prevent a woman from blaming herself for her cancer. We are committed to increasing our individual and collective understanding of cancer, including the societal factors that influence risk. We honor each woman's experience and believe that she alone can speak to the meaning of her cancer diagnosis.

In Western medical research, the degree to which patients adhere to treatment regimens is a significant issue, because the patient's ability to stay on course with treatment may spell the difference between life and death. But we don't believe that patients "fail" treatment. Rather, they are failed by a system that does not recognize the complexity of their everyday lives.

CMCC is a different kind of healing institution in several ways. Perhaps foremost is our commitment toward the integration of both Western and complementary treatments. Furthermore, we work with the premise that cancer is a crisis of body and soul that has profound ramifications in every area of life. Thus, we understand that basic economic and psychosocial needs must be addressed if low-income women are to have the energy and resources to devote to their own healing. Such women have generally been excluded from clinical trials because the difficulty of coping with their daily lives is so much greater. When their more basic needs are addressed, as they are in CMCC's integrative program, they are better able to participate in research studies.

The CMCC Population

The target population for CMCC services is low-income women with cancer living in the nine counties surrounding the San Francisco Bay Area. Women who are receiving cancer care at any of the county hospitals are eligible for services. Likewise, those who are enrolled in California's Medicaid program (Medi-Cal) are eligible. Otherwise, the financial cutoff is 200% of the current federal poverty level.

Outreach for low-income women occurs largely through county hospitals, community clinics, and community-based organizations serving low-income persons. CMCC is especially committed to reaching women as quickly as possible after their initial diagnosis of cancer so that they have the opportunity to include complementary modalities as early as possible in their decision making after diagnosis.

Although CMCC treats women with all cancers, approximately 70% of the women we serve have a diagnosis of breast cancer. In fact, the San Francisco Bay Area has one of the highest rates of breast cancer in the world. Although the majority of diagnosed cases occur among Caucasian women, women of color have the highest mortality rates. Simply put, women of color are much less likely than Caucasian women to be living five years after a diagnosis of breast cancer. Because the prognosis for surviving cancer is significantly less for nonwhite women, CMCC is committed to vigorous outreach to low-income women in communities of color.

In Search of Funding

CMCC, like most community-based organizations, struggles to meet increased demand for services in the midst of rising costs. Community support is vital to the survival of any nonprofit organization. The unrestricted use of individual donations is critical to covering day-to-day operations. Moreover, ensuring that a significant portion of revenue comes from individuals is critical to the clinic's continued legal status as a nonprofit organization.

In fact, CMCC receives many contributions from friends and family members of clients and former clients. They give what they can afford year after year to honor or remember their loved ones and to thank the clinic for the care provided to them. The dollar amounts are not significant, but the level of community endorsement and support they represent is substantial. So it is unfortunate that the critical factor in the legal framework is the amount of money raised, not the number of people donating.

CMCC has often had a difficult time presenting its services in a light that meets the requirements of many granting organizations. Early in the history of the clinic, the services we provide were often considered unnecessary. More recently, with the rise in interest in CAM therapies, we are competing with many organizations that have established Western medical services. As CMCC grows, fund-raising efforts have become more creative to meet the clinic's increasing needs.

CMCC is fully committed to ensuring that the board of directors represents the community we serve. Thus, board outreach is directed toward women with cancer as well as women of color residing in the communities where our clients live. Over time, a significant number of former clients have served as board members, time and health permitting. In addition, we seek participation from CAM practitioners and other health care professionals. As a result, our policies and procedures, and, more importantly, our vision for the future all benefit from a truly participatory process.

Although the organization is committed to this path, there is no doubt that fiscal security comes more slowly than it might if we were to choose board members on the basis of their fund-raising ability.

In the initial planning of CMCC, a discussion arose about accepting fee-for-service clients. While this would have benefited the clinic finan-cially, the idea was rejected out of concerns that it would make treat-ment less available for CMCC's core constituents: low-income women.

The Heart of CMCC

Since it was founded in 1989, the Charlotte Maxwell Complementary Clinic has developed into a unique healing environment, providing treatment to help balance and nurture individual women who rarely have access to personalized, compassionate care.

Many skilled and talented people volunteer their services at CMCC, and many clients have told us that the support they find at the clinic has a healing energy all its own. CMCC is their advocate for recovery, addressing not only their symptoms and side effects but the practical problems, financial burdens, and other difficulties that so often pre-vent low-income women from completing their recommended course of treatment.

For so many of our clients, that support makes all the difference.

As an uninsured, low-income African-American patient, during the entire year of 1999 I underwent eight treatments of chemotherapy, mastectomy, and thirty-three treatments of radiation at a county hospital in Oakland. And during that terrifying ordeal the entire staff and volunteers of Charlotte Maxwell provided me with expert care, counseling, fresh food, and education at no cost. While at the county hospital and at another so-called nonprofit hospital I was always asked how I was going to pay for treatment—basically, that is, how was I going to save my life? Thank the universe, Charlotte Maxwell Complementary Clinic was more interested in fighting to prolong and improve my life during and after my treatments.

I am now back at work again full time. And I credit this organization for building my physical and mental fortitude. I continue to recommend it to every woman friend who is fighting, struggling, surviving, and sometimes not surviving cancer.

CHAPTER FIFTEEN

Evaluating Health Information

Keren Stronach, M.P.H.

KEREN STRONACH, M.P.H., directs the Ida and Joseph Friend Cancer
Resource Center at the University of California, San Francisco and is author
of the book *Survivors' Guide to a Bone Marrow Transplant: What to Expect
and How to Get Through It,* National Bone Marrow Transplant Link, 1997.
She is an active member of the Bay Area Cancer Coalition and the Cancer
Patient Education Network at the National Cancer Institute. She has
participated in a variety of national committees, including the American
Cancer Society's Task Force on Nutrition and Physical Activity and the
National Comprehensive Cancer Center's Committee on Physician Patient
Communication. She leads a support group for young adults with cancer
and has counseled cancer and AIDS patients for over ten years. She serves
on the board of directors of the National Bone Marrow Transplant Link and
the UCSF Mount Zion Auxiliary, has contributed to a variety of
publications, and has spoken in public forums locally and nationally.

Health information can be extremely useful, empowering us to make
important health decisions. However, health information is being continually created and revised, and sifting through it can also be confusing and overwhelming. Adding to the confusion is the fact that
information may be contradictory. In some cases, this happens because
there are different valid approaches to treating a particular condition.
In other cases, the intent or purpose of the author or publisher will
shape how the information is presented, leading the author to present
the information in a more positive light or to present only a narrow
viewpoint. Information can be provided as a public service with the
intention to inform, or it can be produced with the intention of selling
a product or changing an attitude. Thus, its quality and reliability may
vary depending on the source and the intent behind the publication.
Given the proliferation of information available through the Internet,
journals, and other sources, it is important to be able to assess its quality.

Although there is no simple rule for determining the quality of the information you encounter, there are some useful guidelines that can help you determine whether information is credible and accurate.

Is the Source Credible?

Ideally, information in a journal or on the web should have an identifiable source or an author. In considering the credibility of the source, ask yourself whether the particular source you are reading is likely to be fair, objective, and lacking in hidden motives. Take care to examine the credentials of the source to determine whether the author or organization has the required expertise and training to provide the information. If the information is medical, credibility is generally enhanced if it is provided by a medical professional, such as a physician or a nurse, or by a medical institution. Having the publisher's or author's contact information listed in the form of a postal address or phone number can also add to the legitimacy of the information.

Information published by a large organization such as a hospital, a university, a government health agency, or another entity that brings together medically knowledgeable professionals is generally considered credible. Knowing that a publication has undergone peer review by a panel of professionals in the field can also add to the credibility of the information.

In a nutshell, when you are assessing credibility, consider the following:

- Who is publishing the information?
- Who are the authors?
- What are their credentials?
- Do the authors have a hidden agenda?
- Is the information peer reviewed?

Is the Information Accurate?

When you are assessing the accuracy of the information, try to determine whether the information is supported by evidence from scientific studies, other data, or expert opinion. If you are receiving your information from a medical journal, take note of the size and the type of the study. Is the information based on a large or a small study? Read the section on limitations carefully to see whether the authors discuss any limitations or weaknesses of the study. The most reliable evidence comes from randomized controlled studies. However, other types of studies, or the opinions of respected authorities in the field, can also lend validity to the information. If you are receiving information from a secondary source such as an Internet site or a newspaper article, keep in mind that you are relying on another person's interpretation of the data. Is the information based on evidence from a study, on expert opinion, or merely on the opinion of the writer? Although your local newspaper may provide excellent information on certain topics, it lacks the expertise of a cancer journal or a national organization specializing in the field of cancer. If you need to make an important medical decision, substantiate the information you receive through the local paper with information from a physician and other credible sources. Also check to see when the information was published or when the web page was last updated. This is particularly important in the health care field, where information is constantly changing as new discoveries are made.

In a nutshell, when you are assessing accuracy, consider the following:

- Is the information based on scientific evidence?
- Is the information supported by data?
- Is the original source referenced?
- Do other sources substantiate the information?
- Is the information current?

Red Flags

Information that has no identifiable publisher or author should not be relied on, unless it is substantiated by information from other sources that meet the criteria for credibility. If the purpose of the information is primarily to sell a product, there may be a conflict of interest, since the manufacturer may not want to present findings that would discourage you from purchasing the product. If you suspect that the intent is to sell you a product, you should consider getting some additional information from a more neutral source. At other times, the source may not disclose all the information or may have a bias that is more subtle and difficult to detect. Even well-respected medical journals or websites may have a slight bias, depending on their experience. For example, a journal targeting surgeons may not discuss other valid treatment options such as radiation or chemotherapy. Although the information may be accurate, it may have a slight bias because of its particular perspective.

When reading health information, notice the date of publication. Given that health information is constantly changing as new discoveries are made, it is important to make sure that the information is current. If the information is based on a study done several years ago, you should look for more recent information to ensure that the information is still valid. For example, a website that has not been updated recently, or an article that is several years old, may not include information on new promising treatments.

Be skeptical of sensationalist claims of a "secret cure" or a "miraculous result" that no one else has heard about and that is not backed by evidence. Remember to use good judgment when receiving information from forums such as chat rooms and bulletin boards on the Internet. Keep in mind that the experience of one individual does not necessarily apply to you. Although such forums can provide valuable information, there are very few safeguards in place to ensure the credibility or accuracy of the information. Any individual, regardless of expertise or experience, can dispense advice. Information from such forums should be substantiated by more reliable sources of information.

Bad grammar or spelling errors also indicate poor quality control and may indicate cause for caution.

Red flags:

- The information is anonymous.
- There is a conflict of interest.
- The information is one-sided or biased.
- The information is outdated.
- There is a claim of a miracle or secret cure.
- No evidence is cited.
- The grammar is poor and words are misspelled.

It is important to recognize that the search for information can be confusing, even when you find credible sources of information. At times you may find that even reputable sources of information provide conflicting information or recommend different treatments. Such differences of opinion arise when there is no solid evidence regarding the best way to treat a particular condition. In these cases, you may want to consult with several different practitioners to decide the best course of treatment for you. In reviewing information, use your judgment, recognizing that evaluating quality is something of an art. Although very few sources will have all the criteria for credibility and accuracy, familiarizing yourself with these criteria can help you sift through information more critically and will provide important clues that will help you differentiate between good-quality and poor-quality information.

Resources

Audiotapes and CDs

Cancer Guided Imagery
Belleruth Naparstek
800-759-1294
www.touchstarpro.com

Contacting Your Inner Healer:
A Guided Imagery Relaxation Tape
with Action Plan
Neil F. Neimark, M.D., R.E.P.
www.amazon.com

Creative Transformation
Rebecca Herrero, M.S., M.Div.
415-721-1791

Creative Visualization:
Meditations from the Book
Shakti Gawain
800-972-6657
www.nwlib.com

Deep Relaxation/Audio Cassette
Robert Griswold
941-948-1660
www.efflearn.com

Effective Meditations for Health
and Healing
Contemporary Meditation Series
941-948-1660
www.efflearn.com

Effective Meditations for Stress Relief
Contemporary Meditation Series
941-948-1660
www.efflearn.com

For People with Cancer, Guided
Imagery, Health Journeys
www.healthjourneys.com

Guided Imagery and Meditation
Bernie Siegel, M.D.
800-759-1294
www.touchstarpro.com

Healing Images
Bernie Siegel, M.D.
800-759-1294
www.touchstarpro.com

Healing Journey
Marci Archambeault
www.amazon.com

Healing Journey
Emmet Miller
www.cygnus.uwa.edu.au/~gaianet/
  nam/Miller-audios.html

Healing Yourself: A Step by Step . . .
Health through Imagery
Martin Rossman, M.D.
800-726-2070

Health Journeys for People
Experiencing Stress
Belleruth Naparstek
800-800-8661
www.healthjourneys.com

Health Journeys for People
Managing Pain
Belleruth Naparstek
800-800-8661
www.healthjourneys.com

Health Journeys for People
Undergoing Chemotherapy
Belleruth Naparstek
800-800-8661
www.healthjourneys.com

Health Journeys for People with Cancer
Belleruth Naparstek
800-800-8661
www.healthjourneys.com

Heart Zones
Planetary Communications
800-372-3100

How to Meditate
Lawrence LeShan
800-243-1234
www.audioforum.com

The Inner Art of Meditation
Jack Kornfield
800-333-9185
www.soundstrue.com

Kindness to the Body
Cathy Holt, M.P.H.
800-404-9492

Letting Go of Stress
Diana Keck
800-759-1294
www.touchstarpro.com

Meditation for Beginners
Jack Kornfield
800-333-9185
www.soundstrue.com

*Meditations for Enhancing Your
Immune System*
Bernie Siegel, audiotape
800-759-1294
www.touchstarpro.com

Meditations for Everyday Living
Bernie Siegel, M.D.
800-759-1294
www.touchstarpro.com

*Meditations for Finding the Key
to Good Health*
Bernie Siegel, M.D.
800-759-1294
www.touchstarpro.com

Meditations for Peace of Mind
Bernie Siegel, M.D.
800-759-1294
www.touchstarpro.com

Mindfulness Meditation Practice Tapes
Jon Kabat-Zinn
Stress Reduction Tapes, P.O. Box 547
Lexington, MA 02420
www.mindfulnesstapes.com

*The Miracle of Mindfulness:
A Manual on Meditation*
Thich Nhat Hanh
www.amazon.com

Pain Control with EMDR
Mark Grant
www.netstoreusa.com/abbooks/157/
    1572240741.shtml

*Peaceful Body, Quiet Mind: A Healing
Program of Curative Images, Positive
Affirmations, and Serene*
Harriet Sanders
www.amazon.com

Positive Imagery for People with Cancer
Emmet Miller
www.cygnus.uwa.edu.au/~gaianet/
    nam/Miller-audios.html

Prepare for Surgery, Heal Faster
Peggy Huddleston
www.healfaster.com/private.html
orders@healfaster.com

Preparing for Surgery
Henry Bennett, Ph.D.
Patient Comfort Inc.
204 Park Avenue
Madison, NJ 07940
800-213-3223

Relax, Refresh and Be Your Best
Naomi Judith Offner
1176 Belmont Terrace
Vista, CA 92084
760-598-5224 or 800-655-6668
www.gentleyoga.com
naomi@gentleyoga.com

Relaxation and Guided Imagery
Martin Rossman, M.D.
800-726-2070

Roots & Wings
Puja Thomson
914-255-2278
www.rootsnwings.com

Seeds of Peace
Cindy Dern
914-679-8184

Self-Healing: Creating Your Health, Loving Yourself
Louise L. Hay
800-654-5126
www.hayhouse.com

Sounds True
800-333-9185
www.soundstrue.com

Stress (2 tapes)
Belleruth Naparstek
800-759-1294
www.touchstarpro.com

Stress First Aid
Patricia Brennan
www.facingthedawn.com/
   ftdsetsmall.html

Audiovisual Ordering Companies

Conference Recording Service
1308 Gilman
Berkeley, CA 94706
510-527-3600
fax: 510-527-8404

East West Books
800-909-6161
fax: 650-988-9884
www.eastwest.com

Gaia Bookstore
1400 Shattuck Ave.
Berkeley, CA 94709
510-548-4172
fax: 510-548-6134
www.darmer.com/gaia.htm

Jon Kabat-Zinn's Mindfulness Meditation Practice Tapes
Sounds True
800-333-9185
www.mindfulnesstapes.com

TouchStar Productions of Meadville, PA
Barry Bittman, M.D.
800-759-1294
www.ecap-online.org

Yahoo Online Video Shopping
shopping.yahoo.com/video

Videotapes

8 Overcoming Tools: How to Overcome Your Fear of a Diagnosis of Cancer
888-599-1112

A New Vision of Living & Dying
Sogyal Rinpoche
800-256-5262; 415-392-2066
store.yahoo.com/zamamerica

Affirmations for Getting Well Again
Carl Simonton, M.D.
800-459-3424
www.simontoncenter.com/Pages/
  fbooks.htm

Affirmations for Living Beyond Cancer
Bernie Siegel, M.D.
800-759-1294
www.touchstarpro.com

Approaching the 14th Moon: Women
and Health Professionals Discuss
Menopause
Elizabeth Sher
fax: 510-527-1031
www.ivstudios.com

The Art of Meditation
Alan Watts
shopping.yahoo.com/video

Be a Survivor: Your Interactive Guide
to Breast Cancer Treatment
Lange Productions
I.V. Studios, P.O. Box 8123
Berkeley, CA 94707-8123
888-LANGE-88
www.langeproductions.com

Between Us: A First-Aid Kit for Your
Heart & Soul
Mary Katzke, Affinity Films
212-979-6269

Cancer: Just a Word Not a Sentence
Joy Hopkins-Hausman
800-759-1294
www.touchstarpro.com

Choice in Cancer
Michael Lerner, Ph.D.
Commonweal
415-868-0970

Conversations at the Edge:
Healing and the Spirit
Rachel Naomi Remen, M.D.
Commonweal
415-868-0970

Coping with Workplace Issues: A Guide
for Cancer Patients and Their Families
Cerenex Pharmaceutical, a division
  of Glaxo Incorporated

Focus on Healing through Movement
and Dance
Sherry Lebed Davis
800-366-6038
www.mobilityltd.com
shsh@mobilityltd.com

Gentle Yoga for the Physically
Challenged
Margot Kitchen
www.yogacalgary.org/pricelist.html

Healing and the Mind, Volume 1:
The Mystery of Chi
Bill Moyers
shopping.yahoo.com/video

Healing and the Mind, Volume 2:
The Mind Body Connection
Bill Moyers
shopping.yahoo.com/video

Healing and the Mind, Volume 3:
Healing from Within
Bill Moyers
shopping.yahoo.com/video

Healing and the Mind, Volume 4:
The Art of Healing
Bill Moyers
shopping.yahoo.com/video

In Touch for Life: A Wellness Program
for Life after Mastectomy
Mary Nissenson
ICI Pharmaceutical
Wilmington, DE 19897

*Kids Tell Kids What It's Like . . .
When a Family Member Has Cancer*
Cancervive
6500 Wilshire Blvd., Suite 500
Los Angeles, CA 90048
310-203-9232

Living with Cancer
S.F. Regional Cancer Foundation
www.blockbuster.com

*Look Good . . . Feel Better Caring
for Yourself Inside and Out*
CTFA Foundation
800-395-LOOK
www.lookgoodfeelbetter.org

*On with Life: Practical Information
on Living with Advanced Breast Cancer*
NABCO
888-80-NABCO
nabcoinfo@aol.com

*One Move at a Time: Exercise for
Women Recovering from Breast Cancer
Surgery*
Christine Clifford
www.cancerclub.com

*Prepare for Surgery, Heal Faster:
A Guide of Mind-Body Techniques*
Peggy Huddleston
www.healfaster.com/private.html
orders@healfaster.com

Qigong for Health
800-759-1294
www.touchstarpro.com

Relax, Refresh and Be Your Best
Naomi Judith Offner
1176 Belmont Terrace
Vista, CA 92084
760-598-5224 or 800-655-6668
www.gentleyoga.com
naomi@gentleyoga.com

Scenes from a Special Providence
Wellcome Oncology
McCarthy Medical Marketing, Inc.
500 W. 8th St., Suite 100
Vancouver, WA 98660

Therapeutic Touch
Janet Quinn, R.N., Ph.D.
303-449-5790
janetquinn@aol.com

Yoga with Stephanie Foster
800-759-1294
www.touchstarpro.com

*You've Just Been Told You Have Cancer:
Taking Charge after a Diagnosis of
Cancer*
Life Care Concepts, Inc.
457 West 22nd St.
New York, NY 10011
800-401-2233
fax: 212-243-1063
www.cancerresources.com

Videotape Ordering Companies

Explorations
Order videotapes and many other
   yoga-related or cancer-related
   products.
800-720-2114

Yahoo Online Video Shopping
shopping.yahoo.com/video

Journals and Newsletters

*Advances: The Journal
of Mind-Body Health*
advances@fetzer.org

*Alternative and Complementary
Therapy*
Mary Ann Liebert, Inc., Publishers
914-838-3100
www.liebertpub.com

*Alternative Medicine Alert: A
Clinician's Guide to Alternative
Therapies*
American Health Consultants
3525 Piedmont Rd., Building 6,
    Suite 400
Atlanta, GA 30305
800-688-2421
fax: 800-284-3291
www.ahcpub.com
customerservice@ahcpub.com

*Alternative Therapies in
Health and Medicine*
Subscription Department
P.O. Box 615
Holmes, PA 19043-0615
800-345-8112
www.alternative-therapies.com

Common Boundary
301-652-9495
connect@commonboundary.org

*David Sobel's and Robert Ornstein's
Mind/Body Health Newsletter*
800-222-4745

Dr. Andrew Weil's Self Healing
P.O. Box 2061
Marion, OH 43305-2061
800-523-3296 or 888-337-9345
www.drweilselfhealing.com

The Healing Arts Report
800-915-9335

*The Healthy Mind, Healthy Body
Handbook*
David Sobel and Robert Ornstein—
    Center for Health Sciences
800-222-4745

The Integrative Medicine Consult
P.O. Box 1603
Newburgh, NY 12551-1603
617-641-2300
fax: 617-641-2301
www.onemedicine.com
consult@onemedicine.com

Nutrition Action Healthletter
Circulation Department
1875 Connecticut Ave. NW, Suite 300
Washington, DC 20009-5728
fax: 202-265-4954
www.cspinet.org/nah
circ@cspinet.org

*Spirituality and Health: The
Soul/Body Connection*
www.spiritualityhealth.com

*Tufts University Health
and Nutrition Letter*
Subscription Department,
    Tufts University
P.O. Box 420912
Palm Coast, FL 32142-8242
800-274-7581
healthletter.tufts.edu

*University of California, Berkeley
Wellness Letter*
Subscription Department
P.O. Box 420281
Palm Coast, FL 32142-0281
800-829-9170
garnet.berkeley.edu/~sph/
    WellnessLetter
well_ltr@uclink4.berkeley.edu

Alternative Health Websites

Alternative Health News Online
www.altmedicine.com

Alternative Medicine
www.alternativemedicine.com

The Alternative Medicine Home Page
www.pitt.edu/~cbw/altm.html

Alternative Treatments
www.healthy.net/clinic/therapy/
index.html

American Academy
of Medical Acupuncture
www.medicalacupuncture.org

American Botanical Council
P.O. Box 144345
Austin, TX 78714-4345
800-373-7105
fax: 512-926-2345
www.herbalgram.org

Center for Alternative Medicine
Research in Cancer
University of Texas Health Science
Center
P.O. Box 20186, #434
Houston, TX 77225
www.sph.uth.tmc.edu/utcam

Commonweal
P.O Box 316
Bolinas, CA 94924
415-868-0970
www.commonweal.org

Jon Kabat-Zinn's web page
www.umassmed.edu/cfm/life/
zinn.cfm

Medicine Online: Medical
Professionals Directory:
Alternative Health
NIH—National Center for
Complementary & Alternative
Medicine
800-531-1794 or 888-644-6226
www.mol.net or nccam.nih.gov

The Moss Reports
144 St. John's Place
Brooklyn, NY 11217
718-636-4433
fax: 718-636-0186
www.ralphmoss.com

National Center for Complementary
and Alternative Medicine
nccam.nih.gov

NCI CAM Citation Index
nccam.nih.gov/nccam/resources/
cam-ci

Quackwatch
www.quackwatch.com/index.html

Traditional Chinese Medicinal
Therapies
www.acupuncture.com

Breast Cancer Websites

Bosom Buddies Breast Cancer
and Lymphedema Support Group
www.go-icons.com/
bosombuddies.htm

Breast Cancer Compendium
www.microweb.com/clg

Breast Cancer Lighthouse
commtechlab.msu.edu/CTLprojects/
breastcancerlighthouse

Breast Cancer Network
www.breastcancer.net/bcn.html

Breast Cancer.net
breastcancer.net
This news site supplies current information on breast cancer in recent
and archived articles.

The Breast Gene and BRCA1 2 3
Information Directory
www.ncgr.org/gpi/bc_pg_front.html

Breast Reconstruction
www.surgery.uiowa.edu/surgery/
   plastic/brecon.html

Celebrating Life: A Site for African American Women with Breast Cancer
www.celebratinglife.org

Community Breast Health Project (CBHP)
www.med.stanford.edu/CBHP

Doctor's Guide to Breast Cancer Information
www.pslgroup.com/
   breastcancer.htm
Provides general news and alerts, discussion groups, and related sites for physicians, patients, and families.

Gillette Women's Cancer Connection
www.gillettecancerconnect.org

National Alliance of Breast Cancer Organizations (NABCO)
www.nabco.org

National Lymphedema Network
www.lymphnet.org

Online Management of Breast Diseases
www.breastdiseases.com

Susan G. Komen Breast Cancer Foundation
5005 LBJ Freeway, Suite 370
Dallas, TX 75244
800-IM-AWARE
www.komen.com

UCSF Breast Care Center Clinical Trials Search
bcc-ct.his.ucsf.edu

UCSF Carol Franc Buck Breast Care Center
breastcarecenter.his.ucsf.edu

Y-ME National Breast Cancer Organization, Inc.
212 West Van Buren St.
Chicago, IL 60607-3908
800-221-2144
www.yme.org
info@y-me.org

Breast Cancer Activists Websites

Breast Cancer Action
www.bcaction.org

The Breast Cancer Fund
www.breastcancerfund.org

National Breast Cancer Coalition
1707 L St. NW, Suite 1060
Washington, DC 20036
202-296-7477
www.natlbcc.org

Breast Cancer Online Support

Breast Cancer Discussion List

Metastatic Breast Cancer Online Support and Discussions
LISTSERV@MORGAN.UCS.
   MUN.CA
Address to post:
   CANCER@MORGAN.UCS.
   MUN.CA
To subscribe, leave subject blank; in body of message write only:
   subscribe BREAST-CANCER
YourFirstName YourLastName

General Cancer Websites

American Cancer Society
1599 Clifton Road, NE
Atlanta, GA 30329-4251
800-ACS-2345
www.cancer.org

American Society of Clinical Oncologists
www.asco.org

Ask NOAH About Cancer
www.noah.cuny.edu/cancer/
cancer.html

Cancer Care, Inc.
1180 Avenue of the Americas
New York, NY 10036
800-813-HOPE
www.cancercare.org

Cancer Club Online
Christine Clifford
www.cancerclub.com

Cancer Genetics
www.cancergenetics.org

Cancer News on the Net
www.cancernews.com

Cancer Resource Center at UCSF
cc.ucsf.edu/crc

Cancer Resources from LifeCare Concepts, Inc.
LifeCare Concepts, Inc.
www.cancerresources.com

Cancer Supportive Care Programs (CSCP)
www.cancersupportivecare.com

CancerGuide
www.cancerguide.org

Cancerlinks
www.cancerlinks.org

CancerNet & PDQ National Cancer Institute
800-4-CANCER
cancernet.nci.nih.gov

CANSearch: National Coalition for Cancer Survivorship
www.cansearch.org

Guide to Internet Resources for Cancer
www.ncl.ac.uk/~nchwww/guides/
clinks1.htm

Medline
www.nlm.nih.gov/databases/
freemedl.html

National Coalition for Cancer Survivorship
1010 Wayne Ave., Suite 505
Silver Spring, MD 20910
888-650-9127
cansearch.org
info@cansearch.org

National Comprehensive Cancer Network
www.nccn.org

Oncolink
oncolink.upenn.edu

Patient Advocate Foundation
www.patientadvocate.org
Provides education and legal
counseling to cancer patients
concerning managed care,
insurance, and financial issues.

General Health Websites

BlackWomensHealth.com
www.blackwomenshealth.com

Healthfinder
www.healthfinder.gov

HealthGate
www.healthgate.com

Med Help International
www.medhelp.org

Mediconsult
www.mediconsult.com

National Hospice Organization
1901 N. Moore St., Suite 901
Arlington, VA 22209
800-658-8898
www.nho.org
drsnho@cais.com

Needy Meds
www.needymeds.com
Assistance for people who cannot
    afford to purchase necessary
    drugs.

NIH Health Information
www.nih.gov/health

Nutrition Websites

American Dietetic Association
216 W. Jackson Blvd.
Chicago, IL 60606-6995
www.eatright.org

**American Institute for Cancer
Research (AICR)**
1759 R St., NW
Washington, DC 20009
800-843-8114
www.aicr.org
aicrweb@aicr.org

Food and Drug Administration
800-322-0178
www.vm.cfsan.fda.gov

Let's Talk Soy
800-TALKSOY
www.talksoy.com
info@talksoy.com

The Office of Dietary Supplements
odp.od.nih.gov/ods

Soy Com
www.soy.com

U.S. Soyfoods Directory
www.soyfoods.com
info@soyfoods.com

Vegetarian Resource Group
www.veg.org

Locating a Practitioner

Acupressure

**American Oriental Bodywork
Therapy Association**
609-782-1616
www.healthy.net/aobta

Acupuncture

**American Academy
of Medical Acupuncture**
5820 Wilshire Blvd., Suite 500
Los Angeles, CA 90036
800-521-2262

**National Acupuncture and
Oriental Medicine Alliance**
253-851-6896
www.acuall.org

Aromatherapy

American Alliance of Aromatherapy
P.O. Box 309
Depoe Bay, OR 97341
800-809-9850
healthy.net/aaoa
aaoa@wcn.net

**National Association for
Holistic Aromatherapy**
836 Hanely Industrial Court
St. Louis, MO 63144
888-ASK-NAHA
www.naha.org
info@naha.org

Ayurvedic Medicine

Ayurvedic Institute
505-291-9698
www.ayurvedic.com

Biofeedback

**Association for Applied
Psychophysiology and
Biofeedback**
303-422-8436
www.aapb.org

Chiropractic

American Chiropractic Association
800-986-4636
www.amerchiro.org

Guided Imagery

Guided Imagery
P.O. Box 2070
Mill Valley, CA 94942
800-726-2070
www.interactiveimagery.com

Herbal Medicine

**American Holistic Medical
Association**
703-556-9245
www.holisticmedicine.org

Index of Herbalists
www.santabarbarahealth.net

Homeopathy

National Center for Homeopathy
801 N. Fairfax St., Suite 306
Alexandria, VA 22314
703-548-7790
fax: 703-548-7792
www.homeopathic.org
info@homeopathic.org

Hypnotherapy

American Board of Hypnotherapy
800-872-9996
www.aih.cc

**American Society of Clinical
Hypnosis**
2200 E. Devon Ave., #291
Des Plaines, IL 60018

Massage

**American Massage Therapy
Association**
847-864-0123
www.amtamassage.org

Meditation

**American Oriental Bodywork
Therapy Association**
888-532-7686
www.tm.org

Insight Meditation Society
Pleasant St.
Barre, MA 01005
508-868-0970

Spirit Rock
415-488-0164
www.spirit.rock.org

Transcendental Meditation
17301 Sunset Blvd.
Pacific Palisades, CA 90272
310-459-3522

Naturopathy

**American Association of
Naturopathic Physicians**
206-298-0125
www.naturopathic.org

**American Naturopathic
Medical Association**
702-897-7053
www.anma.com

Reflexology

**Ingham Publishing and
International
Institute of Reflexology**
727-343-4811
www.reflexology-usa.net

Rolfing

Rolf Institute
800-530-8875
www.rolf.org

Tai Chi

**American Oriental Bodywork
Therapy Association**
609-782-1616
www.healthy.net/aobta

**Nurse Healers–Professional
Associates International**
215-545-8079
www.therapeutic-touch.org

Traditional Chinese Medicine

**American Association of
Naturopathic Physicians**
601 Valley St., Suite 105
Seattle, WA 98109
206-298-0125
fax: 206-298-0129
www.naturopathic.org

**American Association of
Oriental Medicine**
433 Front St.
Catasauqua, PA 18032
610-433-2448
www.aaom.org

American Herbalist Guild
P.O. Box 70
Roosevelt, UT 84066
435-722-8434
fax: 435-722-8452
www.healthworld.com
ahgoffice@earthlink.net

**American Holistic Medical
Association**
6728 Old McLean Village Drive
McLean, VA 22101-3906
703-556-9728
fax: 703-556-8729
www.holisticmedicine.org

Herb Research Foundation
1007 Pearl St., Suite 200
Boulder, CO 80302
800-748-2617 or 303-449-2265
www.herbs.org

**National Acupuncture and
Oriental Medicine Alliance**
253-851-6896
www.acuall.org

National Cancer Institute Cancer Centers

The three types of cancer centers are ranked based on the degree of specialization of their research activities. The highest ranking centers are designated by the NCI as Comprehensive Cancer Centers. These institutions integrate strong basic science, clinical research, and care with extensive ancillary cancer-related activities such as outreach, education and information dissemination, prevention, control, and population sciences. The generic cancer centers have narrow research agenda that may focus, for example, on basic sciences; the clinical cancer centers usually integrate strong basic science with strong clinical science.

Alabama
UAB Comprehensive Cancer Center
University of Alabama at
   Birmingham
1824 Sixth Ave. South, Room 237
Birmingham, AL 35293-3300
205-934-5077
fax: 205-975-7428
www.ccc.uab.edu
(Comprehensive Cancer Center)

Arizona
Arizona Cancer Center
University of Arizona
1501 N. Campbell Ave.
Tucson, AZ 85724
520-626-7925
fax: 520-626-2284
www.azcc.arizona.edu
(Comprehensive Cancer Center)

California
Beckman Research Institute, City of
   Hope
Needleman Bldg., Room 204
1500 E. Duarte Road
Duarte, CA 91010
626-301-8164

fax: 626-930-5300
www.cityofhope.org
(Comprehensive Cancer Center)

Salk Institute
10010 N. Torrey Pines Road
La Jolla, CA 92037
858-453-4100 x1386
fax: 858-457-4765
www.salk.edu
(Cancer Center)

The Burnham Institute
10901 N. Torrey Pines Road
La Jolla, CA 92037
858-455-6480 x3209
fax: 858-646-3198
www.burnhaminstitute.org
(Cancer Center)

UCSD Cancer Center
University of California at San Diego
9500 Gilman Drive
La Jolla, CA 92093-0658
858-822-1222
fax: 858-822-0207
http://cancer.ucsd.edu
(Clinical Cancer Center)

Jonsson Comprehensive Cancer
  Center
University of California
  Los Angeles
Factor Bldg., Room 8-684
10833 Le Conte Ave.
Los Angeles, CA 90095-1781
310-825-5268
fax: 310-206-5553
www.cancer.mednet.ucla.edu
(Comprehensive Cancer Center)

USC/Norris Comprehensive Cancer
  Center
University of Southern California
1441 Eastlake Ave., Room 815, MS #83
Los Angeles, CA 90033
323-865-0816
fax: 323-865-0102
http://ccnt.hsc.usc.edu
(Comprehensive Cancer Center)

Chao Family Comprehensive Cancer
  Center
University of California at Irvine
101 The City Drive
Bldg. 23, Rt. 81, Room 406
Orange, CA 92868
714-456-6310
fax: 714-456-2240
www.ucihs.uci.edu/cancer
(Comprehensive Cancer Center)

UCSF Cancer Center & Cancer
  Research Institute
University of California
  San Francisco
2340 Sutter St., Box 0128
San Francisco, CA 94115-0128
415-502-1710
fax: 415-502-1712
http://cc.ucsf.edu
(Comprehensive Cancer Center)

Colorado

University of Colorado Cancer
  Center
University of Colorado Health
  Science Center
4200 E. 9th Ave., Box B188
Denver, CO 80262
303-315-3007
fax: 303-315-3304
http://uch.uchsc.edu/uccc
(Comprehensive Cancer Center)

Connecticut

Yale Cancer Center
Yale University School of Medicine
333 Cedar St., Box 208028
New Haven, CT 06520-8028
203-785-4371
fax: 203-785-4116
http://info.med.yale.edu/ycc
(Comprehensive Cancer Center)

District of Columbia

Lombardi Cancer Research Center
Georgetown University Medical
  Center
3800 Reservoir Road, N.W.
Washington, DC 20007
202-687-2110
fax: 202-687-6402
http://lombardi.georgetown.edu
(Comprehensive Cancer Center)

Florida

H. Lee Moffitt Cancer Center &
  Research Institute at the
  University of South Florida
12902 Magnolia Drive
Tampa, FL 33612-9497
813-979-7265
fax: 813-979-3919
www.moffitt.usf.edu
(Clinical Cancer Center)

Hawaii
Cancer Research Center of Hawaii
University of Hawaii at Manoa
1236 Lauhala St.
Honolulu, HI 96813
808-586-3013
fax: 808-586-3052
http://www2.hawaii.edu/crch
(Clinical Cancer Center)

Illinois
University of Chicago Cancer
  Research Center
S. Maryland Ave., MC 1140
Chicago, IL 60637-1470
773-702-6180
fax: 773-702-9311
http://128.135.138.124
(Comprehensive Cancer Center)

Robert H. Lurie Cancer Center
Northwestern University
303 E. Chicago Ave.
Olson Pavilion 8250
Chicago, IL 60611
312-908-5250
fax: 312-908-1372
www.lurie.nwu.edu/
  index.cfm
(Comprehensive Cancer Center)

Indiana
Purdue University Cancer Center
Hansen Life Sciences Research
  Bldg.
S. University St.
West Lafayette, IN 47907-1524
765-494-9129
fax: 765-494-9193
www.pharmacy.purdue.edu/~ccenter
(Cancer Center)

Indiana University Cancer Center
Indiana Cancer Pavilion
535 Barnhill Drive, Room 455
Indianapolis, IN 46202-5289
317-278-0070
fax: 317-278-0074
http://iucc.iu.edu
(Clinical Cancer Center)

Iowa
Holden Comprehensive Cancer
  Center at the University of Iowa
5970 "Z" JPP
200 Hawkins Drive
Iowa City, IA 52242
319-353-8620
fax: 319-353-8988
www.uihealthcare.com/
  DeptsClinicalServices/
  CancerCenter
(Comprehensive Cancer Center)

Maine
The Jackson Laboratory
600 Main St.
Bar Harbor, ME 04609-0800
207-288-6041
fax: 207-288-6044
www.jax.org
(Cancer Center)

Maryland
Johns Hopkins Oncology Center
N. Wolfe St., Room 157
Baltimore, MD 21287-8943
410-955-8822
fax: 410-955-6787
www.hopkinscancercenter.org
(Comprehensive Cancer Center)

Massachusetts
Dana-Farber/Harvard Cancer Center
Dana-Farber Cancer Institute
44 Binney St., Room 1628
Boston, MA 02115
617-632-4266
fax: 617-632-2161
www.dfci.harvard.edu/index.shtml
(Comprehensive Cancer Center)

Center for Cancer Research
Massachusetts Institute of
　Technology
77 Massachusetts Ave., Room
　E17-110
Cambridge, MA 02139-4307
617-253-6422
fax: 617-253-8357
(Cancer Center)

Michigan
Comprehensive Cancer Center
University of Michigan
6302 CGC/0942
1500 E. Medical Center Drive
Ann Arbor, MI 48109-0942
734-936-1831
fax: 734-615-3947
www.cancer.med.umich.edu
(Comprehensive Cancer Center)

Barbara Ann Karmanos Cancer
　Institute
Wayne State University
Operating the Meyer L. Prentis Com-
　prehensive Cancer Center of
　Metropolitan Detroit
540 E. Canfield, Room 1241
Detroit, MI 48201
313-577-1335
fax: 313-577-8777
www.karmanos.org
(Comprehensive Cancer Center)

Minnesota
University of Minnesota Cancer
　Center
MMC 806, 420 Delaware St., S.E.
Minneapolis, MN 55455
612-624-8484
fax: 612-626-3069
www.cancer.umn.edu
(Comprehensive Cancer Center)

Mayo Clinic Cancer Center
Mayo Foundation
200 First St., S.W.
Rochester, MN 55905
507-284-3753
fax: 507-284-9349
www.mayo.edu/cancercenter
(Comprehensive Cancer Center)

Nebraska
University of Nebraska Medical
　Center/Eppley Cancer Center
600 S. 42nd St.
Omaha, NE 68198-6805
402-559-7081
fax: 402-559-4651
www.unmc.edu/cancercenter
(Cancer Center)

New Hampshire
Norris Cotton Cancer Center
Dartmouth-Hitchcock Medical
　Center
One Medical Center Drive, Hinman
　Box 7920
Lebanon, NH 03756-0001
603-650-6300
fax: 603-650-6333
http://nccc.hitchcock.org
(Comprehensive Cancer Center)

New Jersey
The Cancer Institute of New Jersey
Robert Wood Johnson Medical
  School
195 Little Albany St., Room 2002B
New Brunswick, NJ 08901
732-235-8064
fax: 732-235-8094
http://130.219.231.104/html/
  home.html
(Clinical Cancer Center)

New York
Cancer Research Center
Albert Einstein College of Medicine
Chanin Bldg., Room 209
1300 Morris Park Ave.
Bronx, NY 10461
718-430-2302
fax: 718-430-8550
www.aecom.yu.edu/cancer/
  default.htm
(Comprehensive Cancer Center)

Roswell Park Cancer Institute
Elm & Carlton Streets
Buffalo, NY 14263-0001
716-845-5772
fax: 716-845-8261
www.roswellpark.org
(Comprehensive Cancer Center)

Cold Spring Harbor Laboratory
P.O. Box 100
Cold Spring Harbor, NY 11724
516-367-8383
fax: 516-367-8879
www.cshl.org
(Cancer Center)

Kaplan Cancer Center
New York University Medical
  Center
550 First Ave.
New York, NY 10016
212-263-8950
fax: 212-263-8210
http://kccc-www.med.nyu.edu
(Comprehensive Cancer Center)

Memorial Sloan-Kettering Cancer
  Center
1275 York Ave.
New York, NY 10021
212-639-6561
fax: 212-717-3299
www.mskcc.org
(Comprehensive Cancer Center)

American Health Foundation
320 E. 43rd St.
New York, NY 10017
212-953-1900
fax: 212-687-2339
www.ahf.org
(Cancer Center)

Herbert Irving Comprehensive
  Cancer Center
College of Physicians & Surgeons
Columbia University
177 Fort Washington Ave.
6th Floor, Room 435
New York, NY 10032
212-305-8602
fax: 212-305-3035
http://cpmcnet.columbia.edu/dept/
  medicine
(Comprehensive Cancer Center)

North Carolina

UNC Lineberger Comprehensive
  Cancer Center
University of North Carolina Chapel
  Hill
School of Medicine, CB-7295
102 West Drive
Chapel Hill, NC 27599-7295
919-966-3036
fax: 919-966-3015
http://cancer.med.unc.edu
(Comprehensive Cancer Center)

Duke Comprehensive Cancer Center
Duke University Medical Center
Box 3843
Durham, NC 27710
919-684-5613
fax: 919-684-5653
www.canctr.mc.duke.edu
(Comprehensive Cancer Center)

Comprehensive Cancer Center
Wake Forest University
Bowman Gray School of Medicine
Medical Center Boulevard
Winston-Salem, NC 27157-1082
336-716-7971
fax: 336-716-0293
www.bgsm.edu/cancer
(Comprehensive Cancer Center)

Ohio

Ireland Cancer Center
Case Western Reserve University and
  University Hospitals of Cleveland
11100 Euclid Ave., Wearn 151
Cleveland, OH 44106-5065
216-844-8562
fax: 216-844-4975
www.irelandcancercenter.org
(Comprehensive Cancer Center)

Arthur G. James Cancer Hospital &
  Richard J. Solove Research
  Institute
Ohio State University
A455 Staring Loving Hall
300 W. 10th Ave.
Columbus, OH 43210-1240
614-293-7518
fax: 614-293-7520
www.jamesline.com
(Comprehensive Cancer Center)

Oregon

Oregon Cancer Center
Oregon Health Sciences University
3181 S.W. Sam Jackson Park Rd.,
  CR145
Portland, OR 97201-3098
503-494-1617
fax: 503-494-7086
www.ohsu.edu/occ
(Clinical Cancer Center)

Pennsylvania

University of Pennsylvania Cancer
  Center
16th Floor Penn Tower
3400 Spruce St.
Philadelphia, PA 19104-4283
215-662-6065
fax: 215-349-5325
www.cancer.med.upenn.edu
(Comprehensive Cancer Center)

The Wistar Institute
3601 Spruce St.
Philadelphia, PA 19104-4268
215-898-3926
fax: 215-573-2097
www.wistar.upenn.edu
(Cancer Center)

Fox Chase Cancer Center
7701 Burholme Ave.
Philadelphia, PA 19111
215-728-2781
fax: 215-728-2571
www.fccc.edu
(Comprehensive Cancer Center)

Kimmel Cancer Center
Thomas Jefferson University
233 S. 10th St.
BLSB, Room 1050
Philadelphia, PA 19107-5799
215-503-4645
fax: 215-923-3528
www.kcc.tju.edu
(Clinical Cancer Center)

University of Pittsburgh Cancer
    Institute
3471 Fifth Ave., Suite 201
Pittsburgh, PA 15213-3305
412-692-4670
fax: 412-692-4665
www.pci.upmc.edu
(Comprehensive Cancer Center)

Tennessee
St. Jude Children's Research
    Hospital
332 N. Lauderdale
P.O. Box 318
Memphis, TN 38105-2794
901-495-3301
fax: 901-525-2720
www.stjude.org
(Clinical Cancer Center)

Vanderbilt-Ingram Cancer Center
Vanderbilt University
Medical Research Bldg. II
Nashville, TN 37232-6838
615-936-1782
fax: 615-936-1790
www.mc.vanderbilt.edu/cancer
(Clinical Cancer Center)

Texas
M. D. Anderson Cancer Center
1515 Holcombe Boulevard, Box 91
Houston, TX 77030
713-792-6000
fax: 713-799-2210
www.mdanderson.org
(Comprehensive Cancer Center)

San Antonio Cancer Institute
8122 Datapoint Drive, Suite 600
San Antonio, TX 78229-3264
210-616-5580
fax: 210-692-9823
www.ccc.saci.org
(Comprehensive Cancer Center)

Utah
Huntsman Cancer Institute
University of Utah
2000 Circle of Hope
Salt Lake City, UT 84112-5550
801-585-3401
fax: 801-585-6345
www.hci.utah.edu
(Clinical Cancer Center)

Vermont
Vermont Cancer Center
University of Vermont
Medical Alumni Bldg., 2nd Floor
Burlington, VT 05405
802-656-4414
fax: 802-656-8788
www.vtmednet.org/vcc/index.html
(Comprehensive Cancer Center)

Virginia
Cancer Center
University of Virginia, Health
   Sciences Center
Jefferson Park Ave., Room 4015
Charlottesville, VA 22908
804-924-5022
fax: 804-982-0918
www.med.virginia.edu/medcntr/
   cancer/home.html
(Clinical Cancer Center)

Massey Cancer Center
Virginia Commonwealth University
P.O. Box 980037
Richmond, VA 23298-0037
804-828-0450
fax: 804-828-8453
www.vcu.edu/mcc
(Clinical Cancer Center)

Washington
Fred Hutchinson Cancer Research
   Center
1100 Fairview Ave., N.
P.O. Box 19024, D1060

Seattle, WA 98104-1024
206-667-4305
fax: 206-667-5268
www.fhcrc.org
(Comprehensive Cancer Center)

Wisconsin
Comprehensive Cancer Center
University of Wisconsin
600 Highland Ave., Room K4/610
Madison, WI 53792-0001
608-263-8610
fax: 608-263-8613
www.cancer.wisc.edu
(Comprehensive Cancer Center)

McArdle Laboratory for Cancer
   Research
University of Wisconsin
1400 University Ave., Room 1009
Madison, WI 53706-1599
608-262-2177 or 7992
fax: 608-262-2824
http://mcardle.oncology.wisc.edu
(Cancer Center)

Cancer Support Organizations

AMC Cancer Research Center's
Cancer Information and
Counseling Line
800-525-3777

Provides information on cancer and will
mail free publications upon request.
Equipped for deaf and hearing-impaired
callers.

American Brain Tumor
Association
2720 River Road
Des Plains, IL 60018
847-827-9910
800-886-2282

National organization that helps people
with brain tumors. Services include a
listing of support groups, a pen pal
program, a newsletter, information on
treatment facilities, and funding for
research.

American Cancer Society
1599 Clifton Road, N.E.
Atlanta, GA 30329
800-227-2345

Nationwide organization dedicated to research, education, and service. Provides information on support groups, educational materials, financial aid, loans, and medical equipment.

American Pain Society
4700 W. Lake Ave.
Glenview, IL 60025
847-375-4715

APS publishes the *Pain Facilities Directory,* with information on more than 500 specialized pain treatment centers across the country.

Breast Cancer Legal Project
3460 Wilshire Boulevard,
    Suite 1102
Los Angeles, CA 90010
888-774-5200

Provides free legal information and referrals on the full range of legal issues arising from the diagnosis and treatment of breast cancer. Such issues include employment discrimination, getting and keeping insurance, access to treatment, debt collection, and government benefits.

Cancer Care, Inc.
1180 Avenue of the Americas,
    2nd Floor
New York, NY 10036
800-813-HOPE
www.cancercare.org

Dedicated to providing psychological support and information to people with cancer and their families. Provides telephone and on-line support groups, a counseling line, and free teleconferences for patients, families, and friends.

Cancer Hope Network
2 North Road, Suite A
Chester, NJ 07930
877-HOPE-NET
www.cancerhopenetwork.org

Matches cancer patients to survivors. Also has a small database of family members and caregivers of cancer patients.

Cancer Information Service of the
    Canadian Cancer Society
888-939-3333
www.cancer.ca

Provides information service where callers can receive accurate and up-to-date information, in either French or English, on all aspects of cancer from medically approved and complementary therapies to programs and services across Canada.

Cancer Resource Center
UCSF Comprehensive Cancer
   Center
1600 Divisadero, First Floor
San Francisco, CA 94143-1725
415-885-3693
http://cc.ucsf.edu/crc

Provides health information on treatment options and clinical trials, health insurance and benefits counseling, nutrition counseling, support groups, peer support program, and information and referral services in the San Francisco Bay Area.

Cancervive
6500 Wilshire Boulevard, Suite 500
Los Angeles, CA 90048
310-203-9232

Nonprofit organization that helps cancer survivors overcome the challenges of life after cancer. Services include support groups, fund-raising, insurance information and assistance, and advocacy for cancer survivors.

Candlelighters Childhood
Foundation
7910 Woodmont Ave., Suite 460
Bethesda, MD 20814
800-366-CCCF

Organization formed by parents of young cancer patients. An important goal is to help families cope with the emotional stresses of their experiences.

CANHELP
3111 Paradise Bay Road
Port Ludlow, WA 98365
800-565-1732

Prepares detailed, individualized, professional reports to help cancer patients with their treatment options.

Center for Attitudinal Healing
33 Buchanan Drive
Sausalito, CA 94965
415-331-6161

Provides nonsectarian spiritual and emotional support. Services include counseling and support groups, an information and referral service, and a speakers' bureau. Provides information, education, and referrals.

Choice in Dying, Inc.
200 Varick St., 10th Floor,
   Room 1001
New York, NY 10014
800-989-9455
www.choices.org

Provides information that can help people prepare for "end-of-life" decisions. Services include legal assistance, pain management, and a speakers' bureau. Also has a 24-hour counseling/crisis hotline for families concerned about treatments and refusal of treatment situations.

Commonweal
P.O. Box 316
Bolinas, CA 94924
415-868-0970

Center for service and research in health and human ecology. Program helps people seek physical, emotional, and spiritual healing. Offers workshops for people with cancer and for health care providers working with cancer patients.

Corporate Angel Network
Westchester County Airport
Bldg. One
White Plains, NY 10604
914-328-1313

Provides free air transportation for cancer patients traveling to and from recognized treatment centers in the United States without regard to their financial resources. Can book three days to three weeks in advance.

Exceptional Cancer Patients
522 Jackson Park Drive
Meadevilee, PA 16335
814-337-8192

Provides resources and training based on the science of mind-body-spirit medicine to help individuals meet the challenges of a chronic illness and maintain a healthy life.

Healing Choices
144 St. John's Place
Brooklyn, NY 11217
718-636-1679

Provides information and consultation service for people diagnosed with cancer. It provides clear, objective information, with a focus on alternative and complementary treatments. Reports are researched and written by Dr. Moss.

Healing Journeys
P.O. Box 250
Aptos, CA 95001
800-423-9882
www.healingjourneys.com

Sponsors a two-day conference for women with cancer, "Cancer as a Turning Point: From Surviving to Thriving." Conference is free and offered yearly in Northern California.

The Health Resource, Inc.
933 Faulkner St.
Conway, AR 72032
800-949-0090
www.thehealthresource.com

Provides comprehensive, individualized research reports for patients and their families with information on their specific type and stage of breast cancer, as well as other cancers. Annual updates offered, and news bulletin if a new treatment is discovered. Fee for services.

Helpline
50 California St., Suite 200
San Francisco, CA 94111-4696
415-772-HELP

General information and referral services for health and human service agencies in San Francisco and Marin Counties.

Hospice Education Institute
190 Westbrook Road
Essex, CT 06426
800-331-1620

Provides information to the public and professionals about hospice and palliative care. Services include a toll-free information and referral service (Hospice Link), regional seminars, professional education, advice, and assistance.

Latino Coalition for a Healthy
    California
1535 Mission St.
San Francisco, CA 94103
415-431-7430
www.lchc.org

A statewide health policy and advocacy organization dedicated to ensuring the health and well-being of Latino communities in California. The Policy Project provides education, advocacy, and outreach on a variety of health issues, including breast cancer.

Make a Wish Foundation
    of America
100 W. Claredon, Suite 2200
Phoenix, AZ 85013
800-722-WISH

Grants "special wishes" to children up to age 18 who have a life-threatening illness.

Mothers Supporting Daughters
    with Breast Cancer
21710 Bayshore Road
Chestertown, MD 21620
410-778-1982
www.mothersdaughters.org

Offers educational materials and support services for mothers who have daughters with breast cancer. Services include one-on-one support to help mothers cope with their daughters' diagnosis and treatment, and provides constructive help and support to their daughters and their families.

National Alliance of Breast
    Cancer Organizations
9 E. 37th St.
New York, NY 10016
800-719-9154

Nonprofit central resource for education and information about breast cancer. Information for a network of 375 organizations providing detection, treatment, and care.

National Asian Women's
Health Organization
250 Montgomery St. #1510
San Francisco, CA 94104
888-NAWHO-18

National Asian women's health
advocacy and education organization.
Programs in breast and cervical cancer,
sexual and reproductive health. Breast
cancer materials are free and available
in Asian languages.

National Breast Cancer Coalition
1707 L St., N.W., Suite 1060
Washington, DC 20036
800-622-2838

Grassroots advocacy group of more
than 300 member organizations and
thousands of individuals dedicated to
the eradication of breast cancer through
action, advocacy, and public education.

National Cancer Institute
Bldg. 31, Room 10A31
31 Center Drive, MSC 2580
Bethesda, MD 20892-2580
800-4-CANCER

Provides information on cancer
treatments, clinical trials, and services
for patients and their families. Also
provides free publications.

National Center for
Complementary
and Alternative Medicine
NCCAM Clearinghouse
P.O. Box 8218
Silver Spring, MD 20907
888-644-6226

The National Center for Complementary
and Alternative Medicine (NCCAM) at
the National Institutes of Health is
dedicated to exploring complementary
and alternative healing practices in the
context of rigorous science, training
CAM researchers, and disseminating
authoritative information.

National Chronic Pain Outreach
Association
7979 Old Georgetown Road,
Suite 100
Bethesda, MD 20814
301-652-4948

Works to lessen the suffering of people
with chronic pain by educating pain
sufferers, health care professionals, and
the public about chronic pain and its
management.

National Coalition for Cancer
Survivorship
101 Wayne Ave., 5th Floor
Silver Spring, MD 20910
310-650-8868
www.cansearch.org

Acts to help cancer survivors find local
support groups, learn about health
insurance options, prevent employment
bias, obtain health care news, and
speak out on cancer policy. Produces a
quarterly newsletter, is involved in
policy and advocacy issues, and
provides Internet and other resources.

National Family Caregiver
Association
10400 Connecticut Ave., Suite 500
Kensington, MD 20895
800-896-3650

A grassroots organization dedicated to educating, supporting, empowering, and speaking up for the millions of Americans who care for chronically ill, aged, or disabled loved ones.

National Hispanic Council on
Aging (NHCoA)
Breast and Cervical Cancer
Screening Project
2713 Ontario Road N.W.
Washington, DC 20009
202-265-1288
www.nhcoa.org

Dedicated to improving the quality of life for Latino elderly. The Breast and Cervical Cancer Screening Project strives to educate midlife and older Latina women about risk factors, diagnostic methods, and treatment options available. Aims to increase the number of women seeking cancer screening services, while breaking down barriers that limit their access to these services. Services are free.

National Hospice Organization
1901 N. Moore St., Suite 901
Arlington, VA 22209
800-658-8898

Provides information and referrals to local hospice programs via a toll-free number. Other services include patient advocacy and professional education.

National Latina Health
Organization
1900 Fruitvale Ave.,
P.O. Box 7567
Oakland, CA 94601
510-534-1362

Dedicated to establishing bilingual access to quality health care and to the self-empowerment of Latina women through education, political advocacy, and public policy. Free brochures available in Spanish. Offers free services.

National Lymphedema Network
(NLN)
1611 Telegraph Ave., Suite 1111
Oakland, CA 94612
800-541-3259
www.lymphnet.org

Provides education and support to patients, health care professionals, and the public by providing information on prevention and management of primary and secondary lymphedema. Offers a quarterly newsletter, website, and biennial conference.

National Self-Help
  Clearinghouse
Graduate School and University
  Center of the City of New York
365 5th Ave., Suite 3300
New York, NY 10016
212-817-1822
www.selfhelpweb.org

Provides information about regional
self-help services.

National Women's Health
  Network
514 10th St. N.W., Suite 400
Washington, DC 20004
202-347-1140
www.womenshealthnetwork.org

National membership group that
advocates for better federal health policies
for women. Maintains a large array of
information on a broad range of
women's health topics. Newsletter
available in English.

Office of Minority Health
  Resource Center
P.O. Box 37337
Washington, DC 20013-7337
800-444-6472
www.omhrc.gov

Serves as a national resource and
referral service on minority health
issues. Collects and distributes
information on a wide variety of health
topics, including breast cancer
information and referral services.
Publishes and provides a breast cancer
resource guide.

Patient Advocate Foundation
780 Pilot House Drive, Suite 100-C
Newport News, VA 23606
800-532-5274

Serves as an active liaison between
patient and insurer, employer, and/or
creditors to resolve insurance, job
discrimination, and/or debt crisis
matters to help patients maintain access
to care, maintain employment, and
preserve financial stability.

Planetree Health Resource Center
2040 Webster St.
San Francisco, CA 94115
415-923-3680

A health and medical library containing
a wide range of health information from
conventional to alternative therapies.
For a fee, Planetree can provide
information packets on specific medical
topics and diagnoses. Has a lecture
series and a guide to community
referrals.

Pregnant with Cancer Support
  Group
P.O. Box 1243
Buffalo, NY 14220
800-743-6724, ext. 308
www.pregnantwithcancer.org

Provides hope and support to women who are facing a diagnosis of cancer while pregnant. Through a network of women across the country, this group will match a new patient with someone who once faced cancer while pregnant.

R. A. Bloch Cancer Foundation,
Inc.
4400 Main St.
Kansas City, MO 64111
800-433-0464

Matches cancer patients with survivors. Provides a listing of institutions that provide multidisciplinary second opinions for patients if requested within three weeks of diagnosis or recurrence.

RESOLVE, Inc.
1310 Broadway
Somerville, MA 02144
617-623-0744
www.ihr.com/resolve

National organization helping infertile people and the medical infertility community. Services include sexual therapy, support groups, a newsletter, a help line, a physician referral service, medical call-in hours, a member-to-member contact system, and support services through local chapters.

Smith Farm Center
  for the Healing Arts
1229 Fifteenth St., N.W.
Washington, DC 20005
202-483-8601

Nonprofit center for the study and teaching of healing practices, complementary to mainstream medicine, that can lead to life-affirming changes. Its objectives include helping people with cancer, strengthening the community of health professionals who serve those with life-threatening illness, and providing joint learning opportunities for patients and physicians to integrate the best of biomedicine with the best of complementary approaches to healing.

Susan G. Komen Breast
  Cancer Foundation
5005 LBJ Freeway, Suite 370
Dallas, TX 75244
800-IM-AWARE, 800-462-9273
www.breastcancerinfo.com

Dedicated to eradicating breast cancer as a life-threatening illness, by advancing research, education, screening, and treatment. Services include research and program grants, and a toll-free helpline staffed by trained volunteers.

Vietnamese Community Health
  Promotion Project
44 Page St., Suite 500
San Francisco, CA 94102
415-476-0557
www.dgim.ucsf.edu/viet/viet.html

Provides an array of Vietnamese-
language media products, including
posters, brochures, videotapes, and
articles on breast cancer, smoking, and
hepatitis B. Vietnamese spoken.
Products are free.

Wellness Community National
  Headquarters
2716 Ocean Park Boulevard,
  Suite 1040
Santa Monica, CA 90405
310-314-2555

Nonprofit organization whose mission
is to help people with cancer and their
families enhance their health and well-
being by providing a professional
program of emotional support,
education, and hope.

Women's Cancer Resource Center
3023 Shattuck Ave.
Berkeley, CA 94705
510-548-9272 or 510-548-9286

Provides information and referral
services, support groups, peer referral,
library services, and educational
materials.

Women's Information Network
  Against Cancer (WIN ABC)
19325 East Navilla Place
Covina, CA 91723
626-332-2255
www.winabc.org

Provides information, resources, peer
support, and referral sources, free of
charge, for breast cancer patients and
their families through telephone
counseling, mail support, and
community outreach.

Y-Me National Breast Cancer
  Organization
212 W. Van Buren St.,
  5th Floor
Chicago, IL 60607
800-221-2141
www.y-me.org

Provides support to individuals
concerned about or diagnosed with
breast cancer. Services include
counseling, peer-to-peer support,
insurance information, a newsletter,
and a toll-free hotline staffed by trained
counselors and volunteers.

Notes

Foreword

1. Angell M, Kassirer JP. Editorials: Alternative medicine. *N Engl Med* 1998;339(12):839–841.
2. Ornish DM, Scherwitz LW, Doody RS, et al. Effects of stress management training and dietary changes in treating ischemic heart disease. *JAMA* 1983; 249:54–59.
3. Ornish DM, Brown SE, Scherwitz LW, et al. Can lifestyle changes reverse coronary atherosclerosis? The Lifestyle Heart Trial. *Lancet* 1990;336: 129–133.
4. Gould KL, Ornish D, Kirkeeide R, Brown S, et al. Improved stenosis geometry by quantitative coronary arteriography after vigorous risk factor modification. *Am J Cardiol* 1992;69:845–853.
5. Gould KL, Ornish D, Scherwitz L, et al. Changes in myocardial perfusion abnormalities by positron emission tomography after long-term, intense risk factor modification. *JAMA* 1995;274:894–901.
6. Ornish D. Avoiding revascularization with lifestyle changes: The multicenter lifestyle demonstration project. *Am J Cardiol* 1998;82:72T–76T.
7. Ornish D, Scherwitz L, Billings J, et al. Can intensive lifestyle changes reverse coronary heart disease? Five-year follow-up of the Lifestyle Heart Trial. *JAMA* 1998;280:2001–2007.
8. Ornish D. Concise review: Intensive lifestyle changes in the management of coronary heart disease. In: *Harrison's Principles of Internal Medicine* (online), edited by Eugene Braunwald et al., 1999.
9. Spiegel D, Bloom JR, Kraemer HC, Gottheil E. Effect of psychosocial treatment on survival of patients with metastatic breast cancer. *Lancet* 1989;2:888–91.
10. Ornish D. *Love & Survival: The Scientific Basis for the Healing Power of Intimacy.* New York: HarperCollins, 1998.

Chapter 1

1. Spiegel D, Bloom JR, Kraemer HC, Gottheil E. Effect of psychosocial treatment on survival of patients with metastatic breast cancer. *Lancet* 1989; Oct. 14:889–991.

Chapter 4

1. Shi L, Shi P. *Experience in Treating Carcinoma with Traditional Chinese Medicine.* Shandong: Shandong Science and Technology Press, 1990.

2. Xie W. *Cancer = Death?: Treatment of Cancer the Chinese Way.* Beijing: New World Press, 1997.

3. Cheung CS. *Breast cancer supportive management: A collective work from TCM practitioners of China.* Harmonious Sunshine Press, 1999.

4. Zhou M, Wu YH, Liu YD. Integrated Chinese-Western medicine treatments for advanced stage breast cancer: An analysis of 14 cases. *China Integrated Chinese-Western Medicine Journal,* 1995;15:237.

5. Yin XD. An analysis of 32 cases of breast cancer treated with combination of FACT and kang lai te injection. *Ji Lu Tumor Journal* 1999;6:158–59. (Chinese)

6. An analysis of 134 cases of breast cancer treated with Chinese-Western integrated medicine. *Chinese Medicine Journal* 1985;13:111. No author noted. (Chinese)

7. Lei QM, Song JS, Fan DN, et al. Observations on 77 cases of breast cancer treated with the Chinese herb teng huang. *Cancer Prevention Research* 1986;13:111. (Chinese)

8. Yang GJ, Zhao I. Observations on the results of 216 cases of breast cancer treated with combined Chinese-Western medicine. *Intermediate Medical Periodical* 1988;23:48–50. (Chinese)

9. Shen SY, Jiang CY. 14 cases of breast disease treated with a combination of hai zao and gan cao. *Chinese Medical News* 1990;7:40–41. (Chinese)

10. Wang Q, He SJ. 31 cases of breast cancer treated with integrated Chinese-Western medicine. *Cancer* 1990;9:238. (Chinese)

11. Guo T, Xu B, Yan SQ, et al. Neoadjuvant chemotherapy of advanced breast cancer (stage III). Qingdao Tumor Hospital, Shandong, 2000. (Chinese)

12. Niu DL, et al. Curative observation on effects of Chinese herbs and Western drugs applied to quench vomiting caused by tumor chemotherapy. *Ch J Integ TCM-WM* 1995;15:397.

13. Liu M, Yao M, Shen P. Personal experience in herbal treatment of postoperative breast cancer. Affiliated Longhua Hospital, Shanghai College of TCM, 1996. (Translated for the author by Dr. Li PP, Chief, Department of TCM, The School of Oncology, Beijing Medical University, Beijing Institute for Cancer Research, Beijing, China.)

14. Fan C. 30 cases of breast cancer treated by herbal medicines during chemotherapy after surgery. 1996. (Translated for the author by Dr. Li PP, Chief, Department of TCM, The School of Oncology, Beijing Medical University, Beijing Institute for Cancer Research, Beijing, China.)

15. Li P, Wang X, Yu R, et al. A study of breast cancer due to mental depression. Beijing TCM Hospital, 1996. (Translated for the author by Dr. Li PP, Chief, Department of TCM, The School of Oncology, Beijing Medical University, Beijing Institute for Cancer Research, Beijing, China.)

16. Liu S. Lu Deming's experience in treatment of advanced metastatic breast cancer. 1996. (Translated for the author by Dr. Li PP, Chief, Department of TCM, The School of Oncology, Beijing Medical University, Beijing Institute for Cancer Research, Beijing, China.)

17. Ni M (trans.). *The Yellow Emperor's Classic of Medicine.* Boston: Shambhala, 1995.
18. Wu JN (trans.). *Ling Shu or The Spiritual Pivot.* Washington, DC: The Taoist Center, 1993.
19. Unschuld PU. *Medicine in China: A History of Ideas.* Berkeley: University of California Press, 1985:17, 74–75.
20. Harper DJ. *Early Chinese Medical Literature: The Mawangdui Medical Manuscripts.* London: Kegan Paul International, 1998:4–5.
21. Unschuld PU. *Chinese Medicine.* Brookline, MA: Paradigm Publications, 1998.
22. Fu W. *TCM and Pharm.* Beijing: Foreign Language Press, 1985:34–38.
23. Zhang DZ. *The Treatment of Cancer by Integrated Chinese Western Medicine.* Boulder, CO: Blue Poppy Press, 1989:1–2.
24. See note 18, 274.
25. Fu QZ (A.D. 1607–1684). (Yang S, Liu D, trans.) *Fu Qing Zhu's Gynecology.* Boulder, CO: Blue Poppy Press, 1992:248–50.
26. Zhu DX (A.D. 1281–1358). (Yang S, trans.) *The Heart and Essence of Dan-xi's Methods of Treatment.* Boulder, CO: Blue Poppy Press, 1993:313–16.
27. See note 23, 2–13.
28. See note 18, 274.
29. Wiseman N, Feng Y. *A Practical Dictionary of Chinese Medicine.* Brookline, MA: Paradigm Publications, 1998:385–6.
30. Wu X. How Chinese medicine understands breast cancer. In Li P, Zou L (eds.), *The Comprehensive Diagnosis and Treatment of Breast Cancer.* Beijing: China Chinese Medical Publishing House, 1999:16–26. (Chinese)
31. Wu X. Discourse on breast cancer in the classical texts of Chinese medicine. In Li P, Zou L (eds.), *The Comprehensive Diagnosis and Treatment of Breast Cancer.* Beijing: China Chinese Medical Publishing House, 1999:26–32. (Chinese)
32. Zhou W, Guo Y, Xie C. Discussion about the principle of diagnosis and treatment of breast cancer. Tumor Department, Affiliated Hospital Zhejiang College of TCM, 1996. (Translated for the author by Dr. Li PP, Chief, Department of TCM, The School of Oncology, Beijing Medical University, Beijing Institute for Cancer Research, Beijing, China.)
33. See note 23, 81–83.
34. Hsu HY. *Treating Cancer with Chinese Herbs.* Long Beach, CA: Oriental Healing Arts Institute, 1982:82–90.
35. Jia K. *Prevention and Treatment of Carcinoma in TCM.* Hong Kong: Commercial Press, 1985:98–111.
36. Pan M. *Cancer Treatment with Fu Zheng Pei Ben Principle.* Fujian: Fujian Science and Technology Publishing House, 1992:225–38.
37. Zmiewski P, Wiseman N, Ellis A. *Fundamentals of Chinese Medicine.* Brookline, MA: Paradigm Publications, 1985.
38. Maciocia G. *The Foundations of Chinese Medicine.* Edinburgh: Churchill Livingstone, 1989.

39. Kaptchuk T. *The Web That Has No Weaver: Understanding Chinese Medicine*. New York: Congdon and Weed, 1983.
40. Cohen SK. *The Way of Qigong: The Art and Science of Chinese Energy Healing*. New York: Ballantine Books, 1997:3.
41. Ibid., 57–70, 352–53. All the clinical effects of qigong are summarized by Ken Cohen.
42. Sun Q, Zhao L. A clinical observation of qigong as a therapeutic aid for advanced cancer patients. (Presented at First World Conference for Academic Exchange of Medical Qigong, Beijing, 1988), 97–98; in note 40, 71–73.
43. Wu JCH (trans.). *Lao Tzu: Tao Te Ching*. Boston: Shambhala, 1989:17.
44. Li P. A discussion of the task of preventing and treating breast cancer from the point of view of integrated Chinese-Western medicine. In Li P, Zou L (eds.). *The Comprehensive Diagnosis and Treatment of Breast Cancer*. Beijing: Science and Technology Press, 1999.
45. See note 36, 28–35.
46. Cohen I. The treatment of women with breast cancer undergoing adjuvant treatment with adriamycin and cytoxan with Chinese herbal medicine. *California Journal of Oriental Medicine* 1998:19–21.
47. Shukla HS, Melhuish J, Mansel RE, et al. Does local therapy affect survival rates in breast cancer? *Ann Surg Oncol* 1999;6:455–60.
48. Saimura M, Fukutomi T, Tsuda H, et al. Prognosis of a series of 763 consecutive node-negative invasive breast cancer patients without adjuvant therapy: Analysis of clinicopathological prognostic factor. *J Surg Oncol* 1999;71:101–5.
49. Grabau DA, Jensen MB, Blichert-Toft M, et al. The importance of surgery and accurate axillary staging for survival in breast cancer. *Eur J Surg Oncol* 1998; 24:499–507.
50. Hacking EA, Dent DM, Gudgeon CA, et al. Survival after local treatment for early breast cancer. *S Afr Med J* 1985;67:842–44.
51. Montague ED, Ames FC, Schell SR, et al. Conservation surgery and irradiation as an alternative to mastectomy in the treatment of clinically favorable breast cancer. *Cancer* 1984;54(11 Suppl):2668–72.
52. Huang KC. *The Pharmacology of Chinese Herbs*, 2nd ed. Boca Raton, Fla: CRC Press, 1999:28, 376, 93, 95.
53. Zhu YP. *Chinese Materia Medica: Chemistry, Pharmacology and Applications*. Harwood Academic Publishers, 1998:6, 437, 439, 460, 555, 583.
54. Chang HM, But PPH. *Pharmacology and Applications of Chinese Materia Medica*, Vols. I, II. Singapore: World Scientific, 1988:17, 131, 255, 461.
55. Hsu HY. *Oriental Materia Medica: A Concise Guide*. Long Beach, CA: Oriental Healing Arts Institute, 1986:529.
56. Bensky D, Gamble A. *Chinese Herbal Medicine: Materia Medica*. Seattle: Eastland Press, 1986:385, 453.
57. Xing C, Takeo S, Yoshio S, et al. Orally administered panax ginseng extract decreases platelet adhesiveness in 66% hepatectomized rats. *Am J Chin Med* 1999;27:251–56.
58. See note 52, 320.

59. See note 53, 437, 565.
60. See note 54, 374, 533.
61. See note 56, 461.
62. See note 52, 267.
63. See note 53, 437, 588.
64. See note 55, 470.
65. See note 56, 387, 399.
66. See note 52, 294.
67. See note 53, 45–51.
68. See note 54, 1119–1124.
69. See note 55, 53.
70. See note 56, 33.
71. See note 53, 369, 387.
72. See note 54, 659.
73. See note 55, 412.
74. See note 56, 333, 342.
75. See note 53, 137, 233.
76. See note 54, 72, 1030.
77. See note 55, 93, 156.
78. Chang DE, Zhang TL, Flaws B (trans). *Secret Shaolin Formulae for the Treatment of External Injury.* Boulder, CO: Blue Poppy Press, 1987.
79. See note 53, 561.
80. See note 53, 593.
81. See note 53, 437, 460, 470.
82. See note 54, 131, 255, 533.
83. See note 53, 513.
84. See note 54, 1221.
85. Lin JG, Yang SH. Effects of acupuncture on exercise-induced muscle soreness and serum creatine kinase activity. *Am J Chin Med* 1999;27:299–305.
86. Takeshi T, Osamu N, Fukie N, et al. The effects of traditional tonics on fatigue differ from those of antidepressant imipramine: A pharmacological and behavioral study. *Am J Chin Med* 2000;28:97–104.
87. See note 54, 975.
88. See note 54, 1043.
89. See note 54, 852.
90. Cui X, Dai XG, Li WB, et al. Effects of Lu-Duo-Wei capsule on prolonging life span of housefly and *Drosophila melanogaster. Am J Chin Med* 1999;27:407–413.
91. Krishnamurthy R, Whitman GJ, Stelling CB, et al. Mammographic findings after breast conservation therapy. *Radiographics* 1999;Oct:19.
92. Huch RA, Kunzi W, Debatin JF, et al. MR imaging of the augmented breast. *Eur Radiol* 1998;8:371–76.
93. Brenner RJ, Pfaff JM. Mammographic features after conservation therapy for malignant breast disease: Serial findings standardized by regression analysis. *AJR Am J Roentgenol* 1996;167:171–78.

94. See note 53, 451.
95. Cohen I. Preliminary draft on the treatment of breast cancer with integrated Western and Chinese medicine. Presented by Meridian Seminars 1995, 25.
96. Polychemotherapy for early breast cancer: An overview of the randomized trials. Early Breast Cancer Trialists' Collaborative Group. *Lancet* 1998;352: 930–42.
97. Systemic treatment of early breast cancer by hormonal, cytotoxic, or immune therapy: 133 randomized trials involving 31,000 recurrences and 24,000 deaths among 75,000 women. Early Breast Cancer Trialists' Collaborative Group. *Lancet* 1992;339:1–15.
98. Takatsuka Y, Tominaga T. Adjuvant chemotherapy for early breast cancer. *Breast Cancer* 2000;7:358–60.
99. Leong AS. The prognostic dilemma of nodal micrometastases in breast carcinoma. *Gan To Kagaku Ryoho* 2000;27 Suppl 2:315–20.
100. Braun S, Pantel K. Micrometastatic bone marrow involvement: Detection and prognostic significance. *Med Oncol* 1999;16:154–65.
101. Yeatman TJ, Cox CE. The significance of breast cancer lymph node micrometastases. *Surg Oncol Clin N Am* 1999;8:481–96, ix.
102. See notes 96–98.
103. Fisher B, Redmond C. Systemic therapy in node-negative patients: Updated findings from NSABP clinical trials. National Surgical Adjuvant Breast and Bowel Project. *J Natl Cancer Inst Monogr* 1992:105–16.
104. Fisher B, Redmond C, Brown A, et al. Adjuvant chemotherapy with and without tamoxifen in the treatment of primary breast cancer: 5-year results from the National Surgical Adjuvant Breast and Bowel Project Trial. *J Clin Oncol* 1986;4:459–71.
105. Smith I, Bonadonna G, Forrest APM, et al. Part 6: Primary (neoadjuvant) medical therapy for operable breast cancer. In Powles TJ, Smith IE, *Medical Management of Breast Cancer*. London: J. B. Lippincott Company, 1991: 259–87.
106. Fisher B, Brown A, Mamounas E. Effect of preoperative chemotherapy on local-regional disease in women with operable breast cancer: Findings from National Surgical Adjuvant Breast and Bowel Project B-18. *J Clin Oncol* 1997;15:2483–93.
107. See notes 3, 5–8, 10–15.
108. Wang YF, et al. Clinical study on preventing and treating chemotherapy induced nausea and vomiting using supplemented inula-haematite decoction. *Ch J Integ TCM-WM* 1998;18:273–75.
109. Tagliaferri M, Cohen I, Tripathy D. Complementary and alternative medicine in early stage breast cancer. *Semin Oncol* Feb 2001.
110. Li PP. Vomiting treated by TCM. *Beijing Inst. for Cancer Res* 1995.
111. Zhou J, Li Z, Jin P. A clinical study on acupuncture for prevention and treatment of toxic side effects during radiotherapy and chemotherapy. *J TCM* 1999;19:16–21.

112. Liu Z, Sun F, Li J, et al. Application of acupuncture and moxibustion for keeping shape. *J TCM* 1998;18:265–71.
113. Li W, Lien EJ. Fu-zhen herbs in the treatment of cancer. *Orient Healing Arts Int Bull* 1986;11:1–8.
114. Jin H. Ginseng and astragalus combination and the defensive function of the body. *Int J Orient Med* 1999;24:21–23.
115. Yata N, Tanaka O. The effects of saponins in promoting the solubility and absorption of drugs. *Orient Healing Arts Int Bull* 1988;13:13–22.
116. Shen J, Wenger N, Glaspy J, et al. Electroacupuncture for control of myeloablative chemotherapy-induced emesis: A randomized controlled trial. *JAMA* 2000;284:2755–61.
117. See note 6.
118. See note 8.
119. Bosnjak SM, Neskovic-Konstantinovic ZB, Radulovic SS, et al. High efficacy of a single oral dose of ondansetron 8 mg versus a metoclopramide regimen in the prevention of acute emesis induced by fluorouracil, doxorubicin and cyclophosphamide (FAC) chemotherapy for breast cancer. *J Chemother* 2000;12:446–53.
120. Sigsgaard T, Herrstedt J, Christensen P, et al. Antiemetic efficacy of combination therapy with granisetron plus prednisolone plus the dopamine D2 antagonist metopimazine during multiple cycles of moderately emetogenic chemotherapy in patients refractory to previous antiemetic therapy. *Support Care Cancer* 2000; 8:233–7.
121. The Italian Group for Antiemetic Research. Dexamethasone, granisetron, or both for the prevention of nausea and vomiting during chemotherapy for cancer. *N Engl J Med* 1995;332:1–5.
122. Levitt M, Warr D, Yelle L, et al. Odansetron compared with dexamethasone and metoclopramide as antiemetics in the chemotherapy of breast cancer with cyclophosphamide, methotrexate, and fluorouracil. *N Engl J Med* 1993;328:1081–84.
123. Acupuncture. NIH Consensus Statement Online. 1997;Nov 3–5, 15:1–34.
124. Dundee JW, Chestnut WN, Ghaly RG, et al. Traditional Chinese acupuncture: A potentially useful antiemetic? *Br Med J* 1986;293:583–84.
125. Dundee JW, Ghaly RG. Local anaesthesia blocks the antiemetic action of P6 acupuncture. *Clin Pharmacol Ther* 1991;50:78–80.
126. Dundee JW, McMillan C. Positive evidence for P6 acupuncture antiemesis. *Postgrad Med J* 1991;67:417–22.
127. Dundee JW, McMillan C. Some problems encountered in the scientific evaluation of acupuncture antiemesis. *Acupuncture Med* 1992;10:2–8.
128. Dundee JW, Yang J. Prolongation of the antiemetic action of P6 acupuncture by acupressure in patients having cancer chemotherapy. *J Roy Soc Med* 1990;83:360–62.
129. Dundee JW, Ghaly RG, Fitzpatrick KT, et al. Acupuncture prophylaxis of cancer chemotherapy-induced sickness. *J Roy Soc Med* 1989;82:268–71.

130. Dundee JW, Yang J, McMillan C. Non-invasive stimulation of P6 (Neiguan) antiemetic acupuncture point in cancer chemotherapy. *J Roy Soc Med* 1991; 84:210–12.

131. Lewith GT, Vincent C. On the evaluation of the clinical effects of acupuncture: A problem reassessed and a framework for future research. *J Alt Complementary Med* 1996;2:79–90.

132. There are thousands of scientific articles concerning the physiological effect of acupuncture. The following three references summarize what we know so far. Stux G, Hammerschlag R, eds. *Clinical Acupuncture: Scientific Basis.* Berlin: Springer, 2000. This book summarizes the current advances in acupuncture research.

133. Filshie J, White A, eds. *Medical Acupuncture: A Western Scientific Approach.* Edinburgh: Churchill Livingstone, 1998. This book summarizes the current scientific literature and clinical applications of acupuncture.

134. Pomeranz B, Stux G, eds. *Scientific Bases of Acupuncture.* Berlin: Springer-Verlag, 1989.

135. See note 110.

136. See note 53, 56, 352.

137. See note 54, 366.

138. Amadori D, Nanni O, Marangolo M, et al. Disease-free survival advantage of adjuvant cyclophosphamide, methotrexate, and fluorouracil in patients with node-negative, rapidly proliferating breast cancer: A randomized multicenter study. *J Clin Oncol* 2000;18:3125–34.

139. Dees EC, O'Reilly S, Goodman SN, et al. A prospective pharmacologic evaluation of age-related toxicity of adjuvant chemotherapy in women with breast cancer. *Cancer Invest* 2000;18:521–29.

140. Ang P, Cheong WK, Khoo KS. Pseudomembranous colitis in a patient treated with paclitaxel for carcinoma of the breast: A case report. *Ann Acad Med Singapore* 2000;29:132–34.

141. Liaw CC, Wang CH, Chang HK, et al. Prevention of acute and delayed cisplatin-induced nausea and vomiting with intravenous ondansetron plus intravenous dexamethasone. *Changgeng Yi Xue Za Zhi* 2000;23:413–19.

142. Olsen JC, Keng JA, Clark JA. Frequency of adverse reactions to prochlorperazine in the ED. *Am J Emerg Med* 2000;18:609–11.

143. See note 36, 43–44.

144. See note 95, 67.

145. Shibata S, Tanaka O, Shoji J, et al. Chemistry and pharmacology of panax. In Wagner H, Hiniko H, Farnsworth NR, *Economic and Medicinal Plant Research,* Vol. 1. London: Academic Press, 1985:217–84.

146. See note 53, 641.

147. Xiao P, Wang L. Studies on anti-aging Chinese material medica. *Int J Orient Med* 2000;25:12–23.

148. Ping B. The effects of Chinese drugs for supporting healthy energy and removing blood stasis on postoperative metastasis of gastric carcinoma and ornithine decarboxylase. *J TCM* 1998;18:3–6.

149. Wang R, Ren S, Lien EJ. Chemical and clinical investigations of ginseng: A survey. *Int J Orient Med* 1999;24:57–84.
150. Gui S, Yu J, Wei M, et al. Experimental study on the effect of tonifying kidney herbs on pituitary, ovary and adrenal gland in androgen-sterilized rats. *Int J Orient Med* 1998;23:195–99.
151. Jun O. An overview of modern research into traditional anti-aging herbs. *Int J Orient Med* 1995;20:57–62.
152. Yin G, Yin Y. Clinical research into zhuchun capsule's effect on immune and endocrine function in elderly patients with kidney yang deficiency. *Int J Orient Med* 1993;18:100–102.
153. Chen K. *Imperial Medicaments: Imperial Prescriptions Written for Empress Dowager Cixi and Emperor Guangxu, with Commentary.* Beijing: Foreign Language Press, 1996: 37–39.
154. See note 53, 48, 174, 513, 516, 550–51, 655.
155. See note 54, 1119.
156. Wei Z. Clinical observation on therapeutic effect of acupuncture at St 36 for leukopenia. *J TCM* 1998;18:94–95.
157. Sun D, Wu Y, Peng Y. Treatment of 128 cases of leukocytopenia by acupuncture and massage. *Shanghai J Acupuncture Moxibustion* 1999;4:23–26.
158. Zhou J, Li Z, Jin P. A clinical study on acupuncture for prevention and treatment of toxic side effects during radiotherapy and chemotherapy. *J TCM* 1999;19:16–21.
159. See note 156.
160. See note 158.
161. See note 95, 74.
162. Chang M. *Anticancer Medicinal Herbs.* Hunan: Science and Technology Publishing House, 1992:234.
163. Shan B, Shao S. The clinical observation on treating peripheral nerve injury by electroacupuncture. *Shanghai J Acu Moxi* 1999;1:24–26.
164. Zhen H, Li Y, Yuan S. Clinical observation on diabetic peripheral neuropathy treated by needling combined with drug. *Shanghai J Acu Mox* 2000;3:13–16.
165. Li M, Wang X. Clinical observation on treatment of diabetic peripheral neuropathy with refined tianma duzhong capsule. *J TCM* 1999;19:182–84.
166. Goodwin PJ, Ennis M, Pritchard KI, et al. Adjuvant treatment and onset of menopause predict weight gain after breast cancer diagnosis. *J Clin Oncol* 1999;17:120–29.
167. Goodwin PJ, Panzarella T, Boyd NF. Weight gain in women with localized breast cancer: A descriptive study. *Breast Cancer Res Treat* 1988;11:59–66.
168. Goodwin P, Esplen MJ, Butler K, et al. Multidisciplinary weight management in locoregional breast cancer: Results of a phase II study. *Breast Cancer Res Treat* 1998;48:53–64.
169. See note 168.
170. See note 53, 164.
171. Shen J, Hou Q. Clinical observation on curative effect of acupuncture of point jiaji on simple obesity. *Shanghai J Acu Mox* 2000;3:55–56.

172. Goodwin PJ, Ennis M, Pritchard KI, et al. Risk of menopause during the first year after breast cancer diagnosis. *J Clin Oncol* 1999;17:2365–70.

173. Wolberg WH. Adjunctive chemotherapy as an alternative to ovarian ablation in premenopausal women with carcinoma of the breast. *Surg Gynecol Obstet* 1987;165:563–66.

174. Lage A, Rodriguez M, Pascual MR, et al. Factors associated with prognosis in human breast cancer: I. Predictors for rate of evolution and relapse. *Neoplasma* 1983;30:475–83.

175. Mazuhara I, Moishita S. Effects of extract tang-kuei and peony formula on infertility. *Int J Orient Med* 1993;18:85–95.

176. Koyama T, Hagino N, Cothron AW, et al. Neuroendocrine effect of toki-shakuyaku-san on ovulation in rats. *Am J Chin Med* 1989;17:29–33.

177. Ushiroyama T, Tsubokura S, Ikeda A, et al. The effect of unkei-to on pituitary gonadotropin secretion and ovulation in anovulatory cycles of young women. *Am J Chin Med* 1995;23:223–30.

178. Usuki S. Effects of tokishakuyakusan and keishibukuryogan on steroidogenesis by rat preovulatory follicles in vivo. *Am J Chin Med* 1990;18:149–56.

179. Usuki S. Effects of hachimijiogan, tokishakuyakusan, keishibukuryogan, ninjinto and unkeito on estrogen, progesterone secretion in preovulatory follicle incubated in vitro. *Am J Chin Med* 1991;19:65–71.

180. Usuki S, Tanaka J, Kawakura Y, et al. A proposal of ovarian ERAANPS (endothelin-renin-angiotensin-atrial natriuretic peptide system) and effects of tokishakuyakusan, keishibukuryogan and unkeito on the ERAANPS. *Am J Chin Med* 1992;20:65–74.

181. Brezden CB, Phillips KA, Abdolell M, et al. Cognitive function in breast cancer patients receiving adjuvant chemotherapy. *J Clin Oncol* 2000;18:2695–701.

182. Schagen SB, van Dam FS, Muller MJ, et al. Cognitive deficits after postoperative adjuvant chemotherapy for breast carcinoma. *Cancer* 1999;85:640–50.

183. Van Dam FS, Schagen SB, Muller MJ, et al. Impairment of cognitive function in women receiving adjuvant treatment for high-risk breast cancer: High-dose versus standard-dose chemotherapy. *J Nat Cancer Inst* 1998;90:210–18.

184. Tang W, Eisenbrand G. *Chinese Drugs of Plant Origin: Chemistry, Pharmacology and Use in Traditional and Modern Medicine.* Berlin: Springer-Verlag, 1992:555–65.

185. Lin Q. Research on strengthening cerebral function and improving intelligence. *Int J Orient Med* 1989;14:227–32.

186. Sun G, Ren J, Sun Q. Advances in TCM treatment of senile dementia. *J TCM* 1999;19:304–12.

187. Cheng J, Kuang P, Wu W, et al. Effects of transient forebrain ischemia and radix salvia miltorrhizae on extracellular levels of monoamine neurotransmitters and metabolites in the gerbil striatum—an in vivo microdialysis study. *J TCM* 1999;19:135–40.

188. Wu W, Kuang P, Li Z, et al. Protective effect of radix salvia miltorrhizae on apoptosis of neurons during focal cerebral ischemia and reperfusion injury. *J TCM* 1997;17:220–25.

189. Hadden JW. The immunology of breast cancer: Prospects for immunotherapy. *Clin Immunother* 1995;4:249–330.

190. Wiltschke C, et al. Reduced mitogenic stimulation of peripheral blood mononuclear cells as a prognostic parameter for the course of breast cancer: A prospective longitudinal study. *Br J Cancer* 1995;71:1292–96.

191. Early Breast Cancer Trialists' Collaborative Group. Systemic treatment of early breast cancer by hormonal, cytotoxic, or immune therapy: 33 randomized trials involving 31,000 recurrences and 24,000 deaths among 75,000 women. *Lancet* 1992;339:1–15, 71–85.

192. Lin SY, Liu LM, Wu LC. The effect of shen mai injection on immune function in stomach cancer patients after chemotherapy. *Chin J Integrated Trad West Med* 1995;15:451–53.

193. See note 54.

194. See note 53.

195. See note 52.

196. Halstead BW, Hood LL. Natural methods to enhance immunity: Chinese herbs and immunity. *Bull OHAI* 1984;9:391–99.

197. Tang Y, Chen S. Acupuncture moxibustion and the immune system. *Int J Oriental Med* 1999;24:193–98.

198. Tagliaferri M, Cohen I, Tripathy D. Complementary and alternative medicine in early-stage breast cancer. *Semin Oncol* 2001;28:121–34.

199. References for the herbs in the chart are provided in note 198. For information about all the immune effects quoted please refer to Abbas AK, Lichtman AH, Pober JS, *Cellular and Molecular Immunology*, 3rd ed. Philadelphia: W.B. Saunders, 1997; Delves PJ, Roitt IM, Advances in immunology: The immune system. *N Engl J Med* 2000;343:108–17; Delves PJ, Roitt IM, Advances in immunology: The immune system. *N Engl J Med* 2000;343: 37–49.

200. Shen R, Zhan Z. Clinical study of the use of ginseng and tang-kuei ten combination in the treatment of leukopenia. *Int J Orient Med* 1997;22:30–31.

201. Liu JQ, Wu DW. 58 cases of postoperative osteogenic sarcoma treated by chemotherapy combined with Chinese medicinal herbs. *Zhong Guo Zhong Xi Yi Jie He Za Zhi* 1993;13:150–52.

202. See note 53, 354, 455, 554, 643, 649.

203. Hsu H, Ho Y, Lian S, et al. Preliminary study on antiradiation effect of kuei pi tang. *Am J Chin Med* 1991;19:275–84.

204. Hsu H, Hau D, Lin C. Effect of kuei pi tang on cellular immunocompetence of γ-irradiated mice. *Am J Chin Med* 1993;21:151–58.

205. Ben-Hur E, Fulder S. Effect of panax ginseng saponins and eleuthrococcus senticosus on survival of cultured mammalian cells after ionizing radiation. *Am J Chin Med* 1981;9:48–56.

206. Chen W, Hau D, Lee S. Effects of ganoderma lucidum and krestin on cellular immunocompetence in γ-irradiated mice. *Am J Chin Med* 1995;23:71–80.

207. See note 53, 70, 129, 174, 437, 473, 558, 641.

208. See note 53, 159, 354.

209. Zhang D, Zheng X, Wang Q. Clinical study on climacteric syndrome treated by acupuncture and moxibustion. *Shanghai J Acu Mox* 1999;3:29–32.

210. Yan J, Liang J. Auricular-plaster therapy for 89 cases of climacteric syndrome. *Shanghai J Acu Mox* 1998;1:63–64.

211. Wu L, Zhou X. Menopausal syndrome treated by acupuncture. *J Trad Chin Med* 1998;18:259–62.

212. Ganz PA, Desmond KA, Belin TR, et al. Predictors of sexual health in women after breast cancer diagnosis. *J Clin Oncol* 1999;17:2371–80.

213. Rao G. Semen cndii monnieri powder for 204 cases of trichomoniasis and mycotic pudendal itching. *Shanghai J TCM & Medicinals* 1992;9:12. In Flaws B, Chace C, *Recent TCM Research from China* 1991–1994. Boulder, CO: Blue Poppy Press, 1994.

214. Flaws B. *Fire in the Valley—The TCM Diagnosis and Treatment of Vaginal Diseases.* Boulder, CO: Blue Poppy Press, 1991.

215. Dennison E, Cooper C. Epidemiology of osteoporotic fractures. *Horm Res* 2000;54 Suppl S1:58–63.

216. Van der Poest CE, Patka P, Vandormael K, et al. The effect of alendronate on bone mass after distal forearm fracture. *J Bone Miner Res* 2000;15:586–93.

217. Parker MJ. Prediction of fracture union after internal fixation of intracapsular femoral neck fractures. *Injury* 1994;25 Suppl 2:B3–6.

218. Rodan GA, Martin TJ. Therapeutic approaches to bone disease. *Science* 2000;289:1508–14.

219. Liu H, et al. Influence of kidney tonifying formula on estrogen and 1,25-hydroxy-vitamin D_3 of osteoporosis rats induced by dexamethasone. *Chin J Integ Trad West Med* 1993;13:544–45.

220. Shen L, et al. Preliminary clinical study on prevention of bone loss in postmenopausal women with kidney invigoration. *Chin J Integ Trad West Med* 1994;14:515–18.

221. Huang Y, Ye X. Influence of bushen pian on osteoporotic metabolism of round-menopausal women. *Chin J Integ Trad West Med* 1993;13:522–24.

222. Liu H, et al. Influence of kidney tonifying formula on some indexes and bone density in different aged women. *Chin J Integ Trad West Med* 1997; 17:671–72.

223. Liang L, Jiang Z, Liu Z, et al. Osteoporosis treated with Chinese kidney-nourishing medicaments. *J TCM* 1992;33:36–37.

224. See note 53, 384, 608, 610.

225. See note 54, 32, 636, 893, 1125.

226. Liu H, Li E, Cui L, et al. The influence of kidney tonic herbs on relative parameters and BMD in postmenopausal females. *Int J Orient Med* 1998;23:205–7.

227. Early Breast Cancer Trialists' Collaborative Group. Tamoxifen for early breast cancer: An overview of the randomized trials. *Lancet* 1998; 351:1506–7.
228. See note 53, 437, 439, 489, 510, 529, 580, 585, 671.
229. See note 225.
230. See note 52, 478–82.
231. See note 162, 303.
232. See note 5.
233. See note 4.
234. See note 7.
235. Cragg GM, Newman DJ, Snader KM. Natural products in drug discovery and development. *J Nat Products* 1997;60:52–60.
236. Cragg GM, Newman DJ. Discovery and development of antineoplastic agents from natural sources. *Cancer Invest* 1999;17:153–63.
237. See note 162.
238. Ou M, Xu H, Li Y, et al. *An Illustrated Guide to Antineoplastic Chinese Herbal Medicine.* Hong Kong: Commercial Press, 1990.
239. Lien EJ, Wen YL. *Structure Activity Relationship Analysis of Anticancer Chinese Drugs and Related Plants.* Long Beach, CA: Oriental Healing Arts Institute, 1985.
240. See note 228.
241. Zeng J, Zheng D, Dai X. Biotherapeutic effect of anticancer remedies. *Int J Orient Med* 2000;25:71–76.
242. Liu F, Ru X. The immunopharmacological and antitumor effects of rehmannis six formula and the single herb rehmannia. *Int J Orient Med* 1997; 22:152–56.
243. Sun Y. Evaluation of Chinese drugs in the treatment of neoplastic disease. In Zhou J, Liu G, *Recent Advances in Chinese Herbal Drugs: Action and Uses.* Beijing: Science Press, 1991:236–44.
244. Sato A. Cancer chemotherapy with oriental medicine (II): Clinical experiments of Oriental medicine with antitumor drugs. *Int J Orient Med* 1991;16:34–43.
245. Pomeranz B. The scientific basis of acupuncture. In Stux G, Pomeranz B, *Basics of Acupuncture,* 4th ed. New York: Springer-Verlag, 1998:6–17.
246. Whitcomb DC, Block GD. Association of acetaminophen hepatotoxicity with fasting and ethanol use. *JAMA* 1994;272:1845–50.
247. Perneger TV, et al. Risk of kidney failure associated with the use of acetaminophen, aspirin, and nonsteroidal anti-inflammatory drugs. *N Engl J Med* 1994;331:1675–79.
248. He JP, Friedrich M, Ertan AK, et al. Pain-relief and movement improvement by acupuncture after ablation and axillary lymphadenectomy in patients with mammary cancer. *Clin Exp Obstet Gynecol* 1999;26:81–84.
249. Sellick SM, Zaza C. Critical review of 5 nonpharmacologic strategies for managing cancer pain. *Cancer Prevent Control* 1998;2:7–14.

250. Guo R, Zhang L, Gong Y, et al. The treatment of pain in bone metastasis of cancer with the analgesic decoction of cancer and the acupoint therapeutic apparatus. *J Trad Chin Med* 1995;15:262–64.

251. Xu J, Li C, Chen J. Treatment of 15 cases of cancerous pain by electropuncture combined with triple step therapy for stopping pain. *Shanghai J Acu Mox* 1999;4:33–35.

252. Wu Y, Qiu Y. Clinical and experimental research on changes in magnetic quantity of a magnetized needle and analgesic effect. *Shanghai J Acu Mox* 1999;Vol. 2:13–16.

253. Dang W, Yang J. Clinical study on acupuncture treatment of stomach carcinoma pain. *J Trad Chin Med* 1998;18:31–38.

254. Zhang J, Zhang P. Treatment of 56 cases of shingles by point injection therapy. *Shanghai J Acu Mox* 1999;1:23–24.

255. Sun Tzu (Cleary T, trans.). *The Art of War*. Boston: Shambhala, 1988:1.

256. See note 53, 216, 588, 611.

257. See note 53, 643–44, 660.

258. See note 53, 312, 566.

259. See note 53, 354–55.

260. Brink AA, van Den Brule AJ, van Diest P, et al. Re: Detection of Epstein-Barr virus in invasive breast cancers. *J Nat Cancer Inst* 2000;92:655–56.

261. Dixon JM, McDonald C, Elton RA, et al. Risk of breast cancer in women with palpable breast cysts: A prospective study. *Lancet* 1999;353:1742–45.

262. Flaws B, Chace C. *Recent TCM Research from China: 1991–1994*. Boulder, CO: Blue Poppy Press, 1994: 86–99. The author analyzed the various studies.

263. Ye X, Zhang G. Clinical experience in the treatment of 120 cases of mammary neoplasia with ru tong ling (breast pain efficacious remedy). *Tianjin J TCM* 1994;3:6.

264. Tan J, Feng Y. Analysis on 96 cases of masto-hyperplasia treated by point injection. *Chin Acu Mox* 1996; Vol. 7:27–28.

265. Byrne C, Schairer C, Wolfe J, et al. Mammographic features and breast cancer risk: Effects with time, age, and menopause status. *J Nat Cancer Inst* 1995;87:1622–29.

266. Boyd NF, Lockwood GA, Byng JW, et al. Mammographic densities and breast cancer risk. *Cancer Epidemiol Biomarkers Prev* 1998;7:1133–44.

267. Boyd NF, Byng JW, Jong RA, et al. Quantitative classification of mammographic densities and breast cancer risk: Results from the Canadian National Breast Screening Study. *J Nat Cancer Inst* 1995;87:670–75.

268. Saftlas AF, Wolfe JN, Hoover RN, et al. Mammographic parenchymal patterns as indicators of breast cancer risk. *Am J Epidemiol* 1989;129:518–26.

269. Wolfe JN, Saftlas AF, Salane M. Mammographic parenchymal patterns and quantitative evaluation of mammographic densities: A case-control study. *AJR Am J Roentgenol* 1987;148:1087–92.

270. Boyd NF, Lockwood GA, Martin LJ, et al. Mammographic densities and risk of breast cancer among subjects with a family history of this disease. *J Nat Cancer Inst* 1999;91:1404–8.

271. Yin K. Observation on curative effect of xiao he ling applied to treat 460 patients of mastoplasia. *Gansu J TCM* 1995;8:30–1.

Chapter 5

1. Schlosser E. Why McDonald's fries taste so good. *Atlantic Monthly* 2001(Jan):50–56.
2. Cavadini C, Siega Riz AM, Popkin BM. US adolescent food intake trends from 1965 to 1996. *West J Med* 2000;173:378–83.
3. See note 1.
4. Binkley JK, Eales J, Jekanowski M. The relation between dietary change and rising US obesity. *Int J Obes Relat Metab Disord* 2000;24:1032:39.
5. American Institute for Cancer Research & World Cancer Research Fund. *Diet, Nutrition, and Cancer Prevention. Food, Nutrition and the Prevention of Cancer: A Global Perspective.* Washington, D.C.: American Institute for Cancer Research, 1997.
6. Adapted from an analysis by Prentice RL, Kakar F, Hursting S, et al. Aspects of the rationale for the Women's Health Trial. *J Natl Cancer Inst* 1988;80: 802–14.
7. Armstrong B, Doll R. Environmental factors and cancer incidence and mortality in different countries, with special reference to dietary practices. *Int J Cancer* 1975;15:617–31.
8. Marshall JR, Qu Y, Chen J, et al. Additional ecological evidence: Lipids and breast cancer mortality among women aged 55 and over in China. *Eur J Cancer* 1992;28A:1720–27.
9. McMichael AJ, Giles GG. Cancer in migrants to Australia: Extending the descriptive epidemiological data. *Cancer Res* 1988;48:751–56.
10. Freedman LS, Clifford C, Messina M. Analysis of dietary fat, calories, body weight, and the development of mammary tumors in rats and mice: A review. *Cancer Res* 1990;50:5710–19.
11. Hunter DJ, Spiegelman D, Adami HO, et al. Cohort studies of fat intake and the risk of breast cancer: A pooled analysis. *N Engl J Med* 1996;334:356–61.
12. Howe GR, Hirohata T, Hislop TG, et al. Dietary factors and risk of breast cancer: Combined analysis of 12 case-control studies. *J Natl Cancer Inst* 1990;82:561–69.
13. Toniolo P, Riboli E, Shore RE, et al. Consumption of meat, animal products, protein, and fat and risk of breast cancer: A prospective cohort study in New York. *Epidemiology* 1994;5:391–97.
14. Gaard M, Tretli S, Loken EB. Dietary fat and the risk of breast cancer: A prospective study of 25,892 Norwegian women. *Int J Cancer* 1995;63:13–17.
15. Hirayama T. Nutrition and cancer: A large scale cohort study. *Prog Clin Biol Res* 1986;206:299–311.
16. Zheng W, Gustafson DR, Sinha R, et al. Well-done meat intake and the risk of breast cancer. *J Nat Cancer Inst* 1998;90:1724–29.

17. Sinha R, Gustafson DR, Kulldorff M, et al. 2-amino-1-methyl-6-phenylimi-dazo[4,5-b]pyridine, a carcinogen in high-temperature-cooked meat, and breast cancer risk. *J Nat Cancer Inst* 2000;92:1352–54.

18. See note 11.

19. Kelsey JL, Gammon MD, John EM. Reproductive factors and breast cancer. *Epidemiol Rev* 1993;15:36–47.

20. Berkey CS, Gardner JD, Frazier AL. Relation of childhood diet and body size to menarche and adolescent growth in girls. *Am J Epidemiol* 2000; 152: 446–52.

21. Hughes RE, Jones E. Intake of dietary fibre and age of menarche. *Ann Hum Biol* 1985;12:325–32.

22. Sanchez A, Kissinger DG, Phillips RI. A hypothesis on the etiological role of diet on age of menarche. *Med Hypotheses* 1981;7:1339–45.

23. Tretli S, Gaard M. Lifestyle changes during adolescence and risk of breast cancer: An ecologic study of the effect of World War II in Norway. *Cancer Causes Control* 1996;7:507–12.

24. Franceschi S, Favero A, Decarli A, et al. Intake of macronutrients and risk of breast cancer. *Lancet* 1996;347:1351–56.

25. Hems G. The contributions of diet and childbearing to breast cancer rates. *Br J Cancer* 1978;31:118–23.

26. See note 12.

27. Yuan JM, Wang QS, Ross RK. Diet and breast cancer in Shanghai and Tianjin, China. *Br J Cancer* 1995;71:1353–58.

28. Freudenheim JL, Marshall JR, Vena JE, et al. Premenopausal breast cancer risk and intake of vegetables, fruits, and related nutrients. *J Nat Cancer Inst* 1996;88:340–48.

29. Goldin BR, Adlercreutz H, Gorbach SL, et al. Estrogen excretion patterns and plasma levels in vegetarian and omnivorous women. *N Engl J Med* 1982; 307:1542–47.

30. Goodwin PJ, Ennis M, Pritchard KI, et al. Fasting insulin and outcome in early-stage breast cancer: Results of a prospective cohort study. *J Clin Oncol* 2002;20:42–51.

31. Rohan TE, Jain MG, Howe GR, et al. Dietary folate consumption and breast cancer risk. *J Nat Cancer Inst* 2000;92:266–69.

32. Zhang S, Hunter DJ, Hankinson SE, et al. A prospective study of folate intake and the risk of breast cancer. *JAMA* 1999;281:1632–37.

33. Sellers TA, Vierkant RA, Kushi LH, et al. Prospective study of dietary B-vitamin intake and risk of breast cancer: Low folate is a risk factor among alcohol users. *Proc Am Assoc Cancer Res* 2000;41:809.

34. See note 5.

35. Ibid.

36. Ibid.

37. Jacobson JS, Workman SB, Kronenberg F. Research on complementary and alternative medicine for cancer: Issues and methodological considerations. *J Am Med Womens Assoc* 1999;54:177–80.

38. Greenwald P. Role of dietary fat in the causation of breast cancer: Point. *Cancer Epidemiol Biomarkers Prev* 1999;8:3–7.
39. Wynder EL, Cohen LA, Muscat JE, et al. Breast cancer: Weighing the evidence for a promoting role of dietary fat. *J Nat Cancer Inst* 1997;89: 766–75.
40. Shao ZM, Wu J, Shen ZZ, et al. Genistein exerts multiple suppressive effects on human breast carcinoma cells. *Cancer Res* 1998;58:4851–57.
41. Gregorio DI, Emrich LJ, Graham S, et al. Dietary fat consumption and survival among women with breast cancer. *J Natl Cancer Inst* 1985;75:37–41.
42. Hébert JR, Hurley TG, Ma Y. The effect of dietary exposures on recurrence and mortality in early stage breast cancer. *Breast Cancer Res Treat* 1998;51: 17–28.
43. Holm LE, Nordevang E, Hjalmar ML, et al. Treatment failure and dietary habits in women with breast cancer. *J Natl Cancer Inst* 1993;85:32–36.
44. Jain M, Miller AB, To T. Premorbid diet and the prognosis of women with breast cancer. *J Natl Cancer Inst* 1994;86:1390–97.
45. Jain M, Miller AB. Tumor characteristics and survival of breast cancer patients in relation to premorbid diet and body size. *Breast Cancer Res Treat* 1997;42:43–55.
46. Nomura AM, Marchand LL, Kolonel LN, et al. The effect of dietary fat on breast cancer survival among Caucasian and Japanese women in Hawaii. *Breast Cancer Res Treat* 1991;18 Suppl 1:S135–41.
47. Saxe GA, Rock CL, Wicha MS, et al. Diet and risk for breast cancer recurrence and survival. *Breast Cancer Res Treat* 1999; 53(3):241–53.
48. Zhang S, Folsom AR, Sellers TA, et al. Better breast cancer survival for postmenopausal women who are less overweight and eat less fat: The Iowa Women's Health Study. *Cancer* 1995;76:275–83.
49. Hébert JR, Hurley TG, Ma Y. The effect of dietary exposures on recurrence and mortality in early stage breast cancer. *Breast Cancer Res Treat* 1998;51:17–28.
50. See note 41.
51. See note 43.
52. See note 48.
53. Holmes MD, Stampfer MJ, Colditz GA, et al. Dietary factors and the survival of women with breast carcinoma. *Cancer* 1999;86:826–35.
54. See note 47.
55. See note 48.
56. See note 44.
57. See note 43.
58. Rohan TE, Hiller JE, McMichael AJ. Dietary factors and survival from breast cancer. *Nutr Cancer* 1993;20:167–77.
59. Kyoguku S, Hirohata T, Nomura Y, et al. Diet and prognosis of breast cancer. *Nutr Cancer* 1992;17:271–77.
60. See note 46.
61. Ibid.

62. Newman SC, Miller AB, Howe GR, et al. A study of the effect of weight and dietary fat on breast cancer survival time. *Am J Epidemiol* 1986;123:767–74.
63. See note 41.
64. See note 42.
65. See note 43.
66. See note 53.
67. Stoll BA. Alcohol intake and late-stage promotion of breast cancer. *Eur J Cancer* 1999;35:1653–58.
68. Tseng M, Weinberg CR, Umbach DM, et al. Calculation of population attributable risk for alcohol and breast cancer (United States). *Cancer Causes Control* 1999;10:119–23.
69. Rohan TE, Jain M, Howe GR, et al. Alcohol consumption and risk of breast cancer: A cohort study. *Cancer Causes Control* 2000;11:239–47.
70. Longnecker MP. Alcoholic beverage consumption in relation to risk of breast cancer: Meta-analysis and review. *Cancer Causes Control* 1994;5:(1)73–82.
71. Vaeth PA, Satariano WA. Alcohol consumption and breast cancer stage at diagnosis. *Alcohol Clin Exp Res* 1998;22:928–34.
72. Longnecker MP, Newcomb PA, Mittendorf R, et al. Risk of breast cancer in relation to lifetime alcohol consumption. *J Natl Cancer Inst* 1993;85:722–27.
73. Makita M, Sakamoto G. Natural history of breast cancer among Japanese and Caucasian females. *Gan To Kagaku* 1990;17:1239–43.
74. Chlebowski RT, Nixon DW, Blackburn, et al. A breast cancer Nutrition Adjuvant Study (NAS): Protocol design and initial patient adherence. *Breast Cancer Res Treat* 1987;10:21–29.
75. Sakamoto G, Sugano H, Hartman WH. Stage-by-stage survival from breast cancer in the U.S. and Japan. *Japan J Cancer* 1979;25:161–70
76. Wynder EL, Kajitani T, Kuno J, et al. A comparison of survival rates between American and Japanese patients with breast cancer. *Surg Gynec Obstet* 1963;117:196–200.
77. See note 75.
78. Rose DP, Boyar AP, Wynder EL. International comparison of mortality rates for cancer of the breast, ovary, prostate, and colon, and per capita food consumption. *Cancer* 1986;58:2363–71.
79. Hubbard NE, Erickson KL. Enhancement of metastasis from a transplantable mouse mammary tumor by dietary linoleic acid. *Cancer Res* 1987;47:6171–75.
80. Hubbard NE, Erickson KL. Effect of dietary linoleic acid level on lodgement, proliferation and survival of mammary tumor metastasis. *Cancer Lett* 1989;44:117–25.
81. Katz EB, Boylan ES. Stimulatory effect of high polyunsaturated fat diet on lung metastasis from the 13762 mammary adenocarcinoma in female retired breeder rats. *N Natl Cancer Inst* 1987;79:351–58.
82. Katz EB, Boylan ES. Effects of reciprocal changes of diets differing in fat content on pulmonary metastasis from the 13762 rat mammary tumor. *Cancer Res* 1989;40:2477–84.

83. Newman V, Rock CL, Faerber S, et al. Dietary supplement use by women at risk for breast cancer recurrence: The Women's Healthy Eating and Living Study Group. *J Am Diet Assoc* 1998;98:285–92.

84. Pierce JP, Faerber S, Wright FA, et al. Feasibility of a randomized trial of a high-vegetable diet to prevent breast cancer recurrence. *Nutr Cancer* 1997;28:282–88.

85. Rock CL, Newman V, Flatt SW, et al. Nutrient intakes from foods and dietary supplements in women at risk for breast cancer recurrence: The Women's Healthy Eating and Living Study Group. *Nutr Cancer* 1997;29:133–39.

86. See note 73.

87. See note 5.

88. See note 85.

89. See note 5.

90. Ibid.

91. See note 62.

92. Ewertz M, Gillander S, Meyer L, et al. Survival of breast cancer patients in relation to factors which affect the risk of developing breast cancer. *Int J Cancer* 1991;49:526–30.

93. See note 46.

94. See note 59.

95. See note 58.

96. See note 43.

97. Ingram D. Diet and subsequent survival in women with breast cancer. *Br J Cancer* 1994;69:592–95.

98. See note 44.

99. See note 48.

100. See note 45.

101. See note 42.

102. Ibid.

103. See note 47.

104. See note 53.

105. Lerner M. *Choices in Healing: Integrating the Best of Conventional and Complementary Approaches to Cancer.* Cambridge, MA.: MIT Press, 1994.

106. Office of Alternative Medicine. *Alternative Medicine: Expanding Medical Horizons.* Washington, D.C.: U.S. Government Printing Office, 1994.

107. Office of Technology Assessment. *Unconventional Cancer Treatments.* Washington, D.C.: U.S. Government Printing Office, 1990.

108. See note 5.

109. See note 105.

110. Wynder EL. A corner of history: Hufeland. *Prev Med* 1974;3:421–27.

111. Needham J. *Science in Traditional China.* Cambridge, Mass.: Harvard University Press, 1981.

112. Kotzsch RE. *Macrobiotics Yesterday and Today.* New York: Japan Publications, 1985.

113. Kushi M. *The Book of Macrobiotics.* New York: Japan Publications, 1977.

114. Kushi M, Jack A. *The Cancer Prevention Diet: Michio Kushi's Nutritional Blueprint for the Relief and Prevention of Disease.* New York: St. Martin's Press, 1983.

115. Kushi M, Jack A. *One Peaceful World: Michio Kushi's Approach to Creating a Healthy and Harmonious Mind, Home, and World Community.* New York: St. Martin's Press, 1987.

116. See note 107.

117. Kohler JC, Kohler MA. *Healing Miracles from Macrobiotics: A Diet for All Diseases.* West Nyack N.Y.: Parker Publishing, 1979.

118. Sattilaro AJ, Monte T. *Recalled by Life: The Story of My Recovery from Cancer.* Boston, Mass.: Houghton Mifflin, 1982.

119. Kushi M, Jack A. *The Cancer Prevention Diet: Michio Kushi's Macrobiotic Blueprint for the Prevention and Relief of Disease.* New York: St. Martin's Press, 1994.

120. See note 106.

121. See note 107.

122. See note 117.

123. See note 118.

124. Brown PT, Bergan JG. The dietary status of "new" vegetarians. *J Am Diet Assoc* 1975;67:455–59.

125. Kushi LH, Samonds KW, Lacey JM, et al. The association of dietary fat with serum cholesterol in vegetarians: The effect of dietary assessment on the correlation coefficient. *Am J Epidemiol* 1988;128:1054–64.

126. U.S. Department of Agriculture, Human Nutrition Information Service, Nutrition Monitoring Division. *CSFII: Nationwide Food Consumption Survey, Continuing Survey of Food Intake by Individuals. Women 19–50 Years and Their Children 1–5 Years, 4 Days, 1986.* (NFCS, CSFII Report No. 86–3.) Hyattsville, Md.: Human Nutrition Information Service, 1988.

127. See note 5.

128. Sacks FM, Rosner B, Kass EH. Blood pressure in vegetarians. *Am J Epidemiol* 1974;100:390–98.

129. Sacks FM, Castelli WP, Donner A, et al. Plasma lipids and lipoproteins in vegetarians and controls. *N Engl J Med* 1975;292:1148–51.

130. Bergan JG, Brown PT. Nutritional status of "new" vegetarians. *J Am Diet Assoc* 1980;76:151–55.

131. Knuiman JT, West CE. The concentration of cholesterol in serum and in various serum lipoproteins in macrobiotic, vegetarian and non-vegetarian men and boys. *Atherosclerosis* 1982;43:71–82.

132. Sacks FM, Ornish D, Rosner B, et al. Plasma lipoprotein levels in vegetarians: The effect of ingestion of fats from dairy products. *JAMA* 1985;254:1337–41.

133. See note 128.

134. See note 129.

135. Pronczuk A, Kipervarg Y, Hayes KC. Vegetarians have higher plasma alpha-tocopherol relative to cholesterol than do nonvegetarians. *J Am Coll Nutr* 1992;11:50–55.

136. Tartter PI, Papatestas AE, Ioannovich J, et al. Cholesterol and obesity as prognostic factors in breast cancer. *Cancer* 1981;47:2222–27.

137. Hirayama T. Nutrition and cancer: A large scale cohort study. *Prog Clin Biol Res* 1986;206:299–311.

138. Wu AH, Ziegler RG, Nomura AM, et al. Soy intake and risk of breast cancer in Asians and Asian Americans. *Am J Clin Nutr* 1998;68(6 Suppl):1437S–43S.

139. Baggott JE, Ha T, Vaughn WH, et al. Effect of miso (Japanese soybean paste) and NaCl on DMBA-induced rat mammary tumors. *Nutr Cancer* 1990;14: 103–9.

140. Santiago LA, Hiramatsu M, Mori A. Japanese soybean paste miso scavenges free radicals and inhibits lipid peroxidation. *J Nutr Sci Vitaminol* 1992;38: 297–304.

141. Teas J, Harbison ML, Gelman RS. Dietary seaweed (laminaria) and mammary carcinogenesis in rats. *Cancer Res* 1984;44:2758–61.

142. Yamamoto I, Maruyama H, Moriguchi M. The effect of dietary seaweeds on 7,12-dimethylbenz[a]anthracene-induced mammary tumorigenesis in rats. *Cancer Lett* 1987;35:109–18.

143. Messina M, Barnes S. The role of soy products in reducing risk of cancer. *J Natl Cancer Inst* 1991;83:541–46.

144. Adlercreutz H, Höckerstedt K, Bannwart C, et al. Effect of dietary components, including lignans and phytoestrogens, on enterohepatic circulation and liver metabolism of estrogens and on sex hormone binding globulin (SHBG). *J Steroid Biochem* 1987;27:1135–44.

145. Brown V, Stayman S. *Macrobiotic Miracle: How a Vermont Family Overcame Cancer*. New York: Japan Publications, 1984.

146. Nussbaum E. *Recovery from Cancer*. Garden City Park, N.Y.: Avery Publishing Group, 1992.

147. East West Foundation, with A Fawcett and C Smith. *Cancer-Free: 30 Who Triumphed over Cancer Naturally*. New York: Japan Publications, 1991.

148. See note 107.

149. American Cancer Society 1996 Advisory Committee on Diet, Nutrition, and Cancer Prevention. Guidelines on diet, nutrition, and cancer prevention: Reducing the risk of cancer with healthy food choices and physical activity. *CA Cancer J Clin* 1996;46:325–41.

Chapter 6

1. Beaston, GW. On the treatment of inoperable cases of carcinoma of the mamma: Suggestions for a new method of treatment with illustrative cases. *Lancet* 1896:2–104.

2. Feinleib M. Breast cancer and artificial menopause: A cohort study. *J Nat Cancer Inst* 1968;41:315–29.

3. Willet WC, Rockhill B, Hankinson SE, et al. *Epidemiology and Nongenetic Causes of Breast Cancer: Diseases of the Breast*. New York: Lippincott Williams & Wilkins, 2000.

4. Guiochon-Mantel A, Milgrom E. Role of progestins and progestronereceptors in breast cancer biology. In Manni A, *Endocrinology of Breast Cancer.* Totowa, N.J.: Humana Press, 1999:252.

5. See note 3.

6. Longnecker MP, Newcomb PA, Mittendorf R, et al. Risk of breast cancer in relation to lifetime alcohol consumption. *J Natl Cancer Inst* 1993;85:722–27.

7. Wu AH, Ziegler RG, Nomura AM, et al. Soy intake and risk of breast cancer in Asians and Asian Americans. *Am J Clin Nutr* 1998;68(Suppl):1437S–43S.

8. Ziegler RG, Hoover RN, Pike MC, et al. Migration patterns and breast cancer risk in Asian-American women. *J Natl Cancer Inst* 1993;85:1819–27.

9. Wakai K, Egami I, Kato K, et al. Dietary intake and sources of isoflavones among Japanese. *Nutr Cancer* 1999;33:139–45.

10. Matthews G, Ravnikar V. Phytoestrogens and menopause. In *Menopause: Endocrinology and Management.* Totowa N.J.: Humana Press, 1999.

11. Chen Z, Zheng W, Custer LJ, et al. Usual dietary consumption of soy foods and its correlation with the excretion rate of isoflavones in overnight urine samples among Chinese women in Shanghai. *Nutr Cancer* 1999;33: 82–87.

12. Trock B, Butler LW, Clarke R, et al. Meta-analysis of soy intake and breast cancer risk. Abstract, Third International Symposium on the Role of Soy in Preventing and Treating Chronic Disease, Washington, D.C., Oct. 31–Nov. 3, 1999.

13. Horn-Ross PL, Barnes S, Lee M, et al. Assessing phytoestrogen exposure in epidemiologic studies: Development of a database (United States). *Cancer Causes Control* 2000;11:289–98.

14. U.S. Department of Agriculture–Iowa State University Isoflavones Database. www.nal.usda.gov/fnic/foodcomp/Data/isoflav.html.

15. Collaborative Group on Hormonal Factors in Breast Cancer. Breast cancer and hormone replacement therapy: Collaborative reanalysis of data from 51 epidemiological studies of 52,705 women with breast cancer and 108,411 women without breast cancer. *Lancet* 1997;350:1047–59.

16. Schaier C, Lubin J, Troisi R, et al. Menopausal estrogen and estrogen-progestin replacement therapy and breast cancer risk. *JAMA* 2000;283:485–91.

17. Messina MJ, Persky V, Setchell KDR, et al. Soy intake and cancer risk: A review of the *in vitro* and *in vivo* data. *Nutr Cancer* 1994;21:113–31.

18. Aldercreutz H, Mousavi Y, Clark J, et al. Dietary phytoestrogens and cancer: In vitro and In vivo studies. *J Steroid Biochem Molec Biol* 1992;41:331–37.

19. Quella SK, Loprinzi CL, Barton DL, et al. Evaluation of soy phytoestrogens for the treatment of hot flashes in breast cancer survivors: A north central cancer treatment group trial. *J Clin Oncol* 2000;18:1068–74.

20. Murkies AL, Lombard C, Strauss BJ, et al. Dietary flour supplementation decreases post-menopausal hot flashes: Effect of soy and wheat. *Maturitas* 1995;21:189–95.

21. Albertazzi P, Pansini F, Bonaccorsi G, et al. The Effect of dietary soy supplementation on hot flashes. *Obstet Gynecol* 1998;91:6–11.

22. Washburn S, Burke GL, Morgan T, et al. Effect of soy protein supplementation on serum lipoproteins, blood pressure, and menopausal symptoms in perimenopausal women. *Menopause* 1999;6:7–13.

23. Garland M, Hunter DJ, Colditz GA, et al. Menstrual cycle characteristics and history of ovulatory infertility in relation to breast cancer risk in a large cohort of US women. *Am J Epidemiol* 1998;147:636–43.

24. Cassidy A, Bingham S, Setchell K. Biological effects of a diet of soy protein rich in isoflavones on the menstrual cycle of premenopausal women. *Am J Clin Nutr* 1994;60:333–40.

25. Lu LJW, Anderson KE, Grady JJ, et al. Effects of soya consumption for 1 month on steroid hormones in premenopausal women: Implications for breast cancer risk reduction. *Cancer Epidemiol Biomarkers Prev* 1996;5:63–70.

26. Nagata C, Takatsuka N, Inaba S, et al. Effect of soymilk consumption on serum estrogen concentrations in premenopausal Japanese women. *J Natl Cancer Inst* 1998;90:1830–35.

27. Duncan AM, Merz BE, Xu X, et al. Soy isoflavones exert modest hormonal effects in premenopause women. *J Clin Endocrinol Metab* 1999;84:192–97.

28. Lu LJ, Anderson KE, Grady JJ, et al. Decreased ovarian hormones during a soya diet: Implications for breast cancer prevention. *Cancer Res* 2000;60: 4112–21.

29. Kim H, Peterson TG, Barnes S. Mechanisms of action of the soy isoflavone genistein: Emerging role for its effects via transforming growth factor β signaling pathways. *Am J Clin Nutr* 1998;68(Suppl):1418S–25S.

30. Wei H, et al. Inhibition of UV light and Fenton reaction induced oxidative DNA damage by the soybean isoflavone genistein. *Carcinogenesis* 1996;17: 73–77.

31. Ruiz-Larrea MB, et al. Antioxidant activity of phytoestrogenic isoflavones. *Free Radical Res* 1997;26:63–70.

32. Gyorgy P, Murata K, Ikehata H. Antioxidants isolated from fermented soybeans (tempeh). *Nature* 1963;204:870–72.

33. Pratt DE, Di Pietro C, Porter WL, et al. Phenolic antioxidants of soy protein hydrolyzates. *J Food Sci* 1981;47:24–25.

34. Wei H, Bowen R, Cai Q, et al. Antioxidant and antipromotional effects of the soybean isoflavone genistein. *Proc Soc Exp Biol Med* 1995;208:124–30.

35. Bonjean K, Locigno R, Devy L, et al. Genistein and daidzein, two soy derived isoflavones, inhibit angiogenesis. *Proc Am Assoc Cancer Res* 2000;41:647.

36. Fotsis T, Pepper M, Aldercreutz H, et al. Genistein, a derived inhibitor of in vitro angiogenesis. *Proc Natl Acad Sci USA* 1993;90:2690–94.

37. Akiyama T, Ishida J, Nakagawa H, et al. Genistein, a specific inhibitor of tyrosine-specific protein kinases. *J Biol Chem* 1987;262:5592–95.

38. Clark JW, Santos-Moore A, Stevenson LE, et al. Effects of tyrosine kinase inhibitors on the proliferation of human breast cancer cell lines and proteins important in the ras signaling pathway. *Int J Cancer* 1996;65:186–91.

39. See note 12.

40. Lamartiniere CA. Protection against breast cancer with genistein: A component of soy. *Am J Clin Nutr* 2000;71(Suppl):1705S–7S.
41. McMichael-Phillips DF, et al. Effects of soy-protein supplementation on epithelial proliferation in the histologically normal human breast. *Am J Clin Nutr* 1998;68(Suppl):1431S–35S.
42. Hilakivi-Clarke L, Onojafe I, Raygada M, et al. Prepubertal exposure to zearalenone or genistein reduces mammary tumorigenesis. *Br J Cancer* 1999; 80:1682–88.
43. Murrill WB, Brown NM, Zhang JX, et al. Prepubertal genistein exposure suppresses mammary cancer and enhances gland differentiation in rats. *Carcinogenesis* 1996;17:1451–57.
44. Strom BL, Schinnar R, Zeigler EE, et al. Exposure to soy-based formula in infancy and endocrinological and reproductive outcomes in young adulthood. *JAMA* 2001;286:807–14.

Chapter 8

1. Boon H, Stewart M, Kennard MA, et al. The use of complementary/alternative medicine by breast cancer survivors in Ontario: Prevalence and perceptions. *J Clin Oncol* 2000;18:2515–21.
2. Yates P, Beadle G, Clavarino A, et al. Patients with terminal cancer who use alternative therapies: Their beliefs and practices. *Soc Health Illness* 1993;15: 199–217.
3. Lerner IJ, Kennedy BJ. The prevalence of questionable methods of cancer treatment in the United States. *CA-A Cancer J Clinicians* 1992;42:181–91.
4. Cassileth BR, Lusk EJ, Strouse TB, et al. Contemporary unorthodox treatments in cancer medicine. *Ann Intern Med* 1984;101:105–12.
5. Downer SM, Cody MM, McCluskey P, et al. Pursuit and practice of complementary therapies by cancer patients receiving conventional treatment. *Br Med J* 1994;309:86–89.
6. Gray RE, Greenberg M, Fitch M, et al. Perspectives of cancer survivors interested in unconventional therapies. *J Psychosocial Oncol* 1997;15:149–71.
7. Boon H, Brown JB, Gavin A, et al. Breast cancer survivors' perceptions of complementary/alternative medicine (CAM): Making the decision to use or not to use. *Qualitative Health Care* 1999;9:639–53.
8. Ibid.
9. Ibid.
10. Ibid.
11. See note 1.
12. Smith M, Boon H. Counseling cancer patients about herbal medicine. *Patient Education and Counseling* 1999;38:109–20.
13. Kaegi E. Unconventional therapies for cancer. 1. Essiac. *Can Med Assoc J* 1998;158:897–902.
14. Locock RA. Essiac. *Can Pharmaceutical J* 1997;Feb.:18–19, 51.

15. Tamayo C, Richardson M, Diamond S, et al. The chemistry and biological activity of herbs used in Flor-Essence herbal tonic and Essiac. *Phyto Res* 2000;14:1–14.
16. See note 12.
17. See note 13.
18. See note 14.
19. See note 12.
20. See note 13.
21. Essiac International. Essiac Testimonials. 1996.
22. See note 15.
23. See note 12.
24. See note 13.
25. Ernst E, Cassileth B. How useful are unconventional cancer treatments. *Eur J Cancer* 1999;35:1608–13.
26. Stelling K. Essiac. In Chandler F, ed., *Herbs: Everyday Reference for Health Professionals*. Ottawa, Ontario, Canada: Canadian Pharmacists Association/Canadian Medical Association; 2000:110–11.
27. See note 20.
28. See note 21.
29. Kaegi E. Unconventional therapies for cancer. 2. Green tea. *Can Med Assoc J* 1998;158:1033–35.
30. Ahmad N, Mukhtar H. Green tea polyphenols and cancer: Biologic mechanisms and practical implications. *Nutr Rev* 1999;57:78–83.
31. See note 29.
32. Mukhtar H, Ahmad N. Tea polyphenols: Prevention of cancer and optimizing health. *Am J Clin Nutr* 2000;71(6 Suppl):1698S–1702S, 1703S–4S.
33. Mukhtar H, Ahmad N. Green tea in chemoprevention of cancer. *Toxicol Sci* 1999;52(2 Suppl):111–17.
34. Ibid.
35. Gao Y, McLaughlin J, Blot W, et al. Reduced risk of esophageal cancer associated with green tea consumption. *J Int Cancer Inst* 1994;86:855–58.
36. Kinjo Y, Cui Y, Akiba S, et al. Mortality risks of esophageal cancer associated with hot tea, alcohol, tobacco and diet in Japan. *J Epidemiol* 1998;8:235–43.
37. Bushman J. Green tea and cancer in humans: A review of the literature. *Nutr Cancer* 1998;31:151–59.
38. Nakachi K, Suemasu K, Suga K, et al. Influence of drinking green tea on breast cancer malignancy among Japanese patients. *Jap J Cancer Res* 1998;89:254–61.
39. See note 24.
40. See note 12.
41. Centre for Alternative Medicine Research in Cancer (http://www.sph.uth.tmc.edu/utcam/summary/hoxsey.htm). Hoxsey Summary. 1999; accessed 29 Dec 2000.
42. Ibid.

43. Austin S, Baumgartner-Dale E, De Kadt S. Long term follow up of cancer patients using Contreras, Hoxsey and Gerson formulas. *J Naturopathic Med* 1994;5:74–76.
44. Newall CA, Anderson LA, Phillipson JD. *Herbal Medicines. A Guide for Health Care Professionals.* London: Pharmaceutical Press, 1996.
45. Kaegi E. Unconventional therapies for cancer. 3. Iscador. *Can Med Assoc J* 1998;158:1057–59.
46. Ibid.
47. Ibid.
48. Torma J. Complementary and alternative medicine in oncology. *J Pharm Practice* 1999;12:225–39.
49. Kuttan G, Menon L, Antony S, et al. Anticarcinogenic and antimetastatic activity of Iscador. *Anti-Cancer Drugs* 1997;1:S15–16.
50. Kleijnen J, Knipschild P. Mistletoe treatment for cancer: Review of controlled trials in humans. *Phytomedicine* 1994;1:255–260.
51. Keine H. Clinical studies on mistletoe therapy for cancerous diseases, review. *Therapeutikon* 1989;3:347–353.
52. Hajto T, Lanzrein C. Natural killer and antibody-dependent cell mediated cytotoxicity activities and large granular lymphocyte frequencies in *Viscum album* treated breast cancer patients. *Oncology* 1986;43:93–97.
53. See note 50.
54. Grossarth-Maticek R, Kiene H, Baumgartner SM, et al. Use of Iscador, an extract of European mistletoe (*Viscum album*), in cancer treatment: Prospective nonrandomized and randomized matched-pair studies nested within a cohort study. *Alt Therapies Health Med* 2001;7:57–78.
55. See note 54.
56. See note 24.
57. Saunders PR. Reishi. In Chandler F, ed., *Herbs: Everyday Reference for Health Professionals.* Ottawa, Ontario, Canada: Canadian Pharmacists Association/ Canadian Medical Association, 2000:181–84.
58. Ibid.
59. McGuffen M, Hobbs C, Upton R, et al. *American Herbal Products Association's Botantical Safety Handbook.* New York: CRC Press, 1997.
60. Jellin JM, Batz F, Hitchens K. *Pharmacist's Letter/Prescriber's Letter Natural Medicines Comprehensive Database.* Stockton, Calif.: Therapeutic Research Faculty, 1999.
61. See note 55.
62. Jurgens TM. Shiitake mushroom. In Chandler F, ed. *Herbs: Everyday Reference for Health Professionals.* Ottawa, Ontario, Canada: Canadian Pharmacists Association/Canadian Medical Association, 2000:193–95.
63. Taguchi T. Clinical efficacy of lentinan on patients with stomach cancer: End point results of a four-year follow-up survey. *Cancer Detect Prev Suppl* 1987; 1:333–49.
64. Taguchi T, Furue H, Kimura T, et al. Clinical efficacy of lentinan on neoplastic diseases. *Adv Exp Med Biol* 1983;166:181–87.

65. Matsuoka H, Seo Y, Wakasugi H, et al. Lentinan potentiates immunity and prolongs survival time of some patients. *Anticancer Res* 1997;17:2751–56.
66. See note 60.
67. See note 63.
68. MacKinnon S. Shark cartilage. In Chandler F, ed., *Herbs: Everyday Reference for Health Professionals*. Ottawa: Canadian Pharmacists Association/Canadian Medical Association, 2000:191–92.
69. Ibid.
70. Ibid.
71. Mathews J. Media feeds frenzy over shark cartilage as cancer treatment. *J Nat Cancer Inst* 1993;85:1190–91.
72. Miller DR, Anderson GT, Stark JJ, et al. Phase I/II trial of the safety and efficacy of shark cartilage in the treatment of advanced cancer. *J Clin Oncol* 1998;16:3649–55.
73. Centre for Alternative Medicine Research in Cancer (http://www.sph.uth.tmc.edu/utcam/therapies/crtlg.htm). Cartilage. 1999; accessed 29 Dec 2000.
74. Ibid.
75. See note 66.

Chapter 9

1. Cassileth BR, Chapman BA. Alternative cancer medicine: A ten-year update. *Cancer Invest* 1996;14:396–404.
2. Hauser SP. Unproven methods in cancer treatment. *Curr Opin Oncol* 1993;5:646–54.
3. Dwyer JT. Unproven nutritional remedies and cancer. *Nutr Rev* 1992;50(4 Pt 1):106–9.
4. Brigden ML. Unproven (questionable) cancer therapies. *West J Med* 1995;163:463–69.
5. See note 1.
6. Council for Responsible Nutrition. *1992 Overview for the Nutritional Supplement Market*. Washington, D.C., 1993.
7. Eisenberg DM, Davis RB, Ettner SL, et al. Trends in alternative medicine use in the United States, 1990–1997: Results of a follow-up national survey. *JAMA* 1998;280:1569–75.
8. Subar AF, Block G. Use of vitamin and mineral supplements: demographics and amounts of nutrients consumed. The 1987 Health Interview Survey. *Am J Epidemiol* 1990;132(6):1091–1101.
9. Moss AJ, Levy AS, Kim J, et al. *Use of Vitamin and Mineral Supplements in the United States; Current Users, Types of Products, and Nutrients*. Advance Data from Health and Vital Statistics. No. 174. Hyattsville, Md.: National Center for Health Statistics, 1989.
10. Slesinski MJ, Subar AF, Kahle LL. Trends in use of vitamin and mineral supplements in the U.S. *J Am Diet Assoc* 1995;95:921–23.

11. Vitolins MZ, Quandt SA, Case LD, et al. Vitamin and mineral supplement use by older rural adults. *J Gerontol Biol Sci Med Sci* 2000;55:M613–17.

12. Frank E, Bendich A, Denniston M. Use of vitamin-mineral supplements by female physicians in the United States. *Am J Clin Nutr* 2000;72:969–75.

13. Stang J, Story MT, Harnak L, et al. Relationship between vitamin and mineral supplement use, dietary intake, and dietary adequacy among adolescents. *J Am Diet Assoc* 2000;100:905–10.

14. Subar AF, Block G. Use of vitamin and mineral supplements: Demographics and amounts of nutrients consumed. *Am J Epidemiol* 1990;132:1091–1101.

15. Slesinski MJ, Subar AF, Kahle LL. Dietary intake of fat, fiber and other nutrients is related to the use of vitamin and mineral supplements in the United States: The 1992 National Health Interview Survey. *J Nutr* 1996;26:3001–8.

16. Block G, Sinha R, Gridley G. Collection of dietary supplement data and implications for analysis. *Am J Clin Nutr* 1994;359(Suppl):232S–39S.

17. Nogae I, Kikuchi J, Yamaguchi T, et al. Potentiation of vincristine by vitamin A against drug-resistant mouse leukemia cells. *Br J Cancer* 1987;56:267–67.

18. Nakagawa M, Yamaguchi T, Ueda H, et al. Potentiation by vitamin A of the action of anticancer agents against murine tumors. *Jap J Cancer Res* 1985;76:887–94.

19. Sankaranarayanan R, Mathew B. Retinoids as cancer-preventive agents. *IARC Sci Publ* 1996:47–59.

20. Holmes WF, Dawson MI, Soprano RD, et al. Induction of apoptosis in ovarian carcinoma cells by AHPN/CD437 is mediated by retinoic acid receptors. *J Cell Physiol* 2000;185:61–67.

21. Chen Y, Buck J, Derguini F. Anhydroretinol induces oxidative stress and cell death. *Cancer Res* 1999;59:3985–90.

22. Nagy L, Thomazy VA, Heyman RA, et al. Retinoid-induced apoptosis in normal and neoplastic tissues. *Cell Death Differ* 1998;5:11–19.

23. Ratnasinghe D, Forman MR, Tangrea JA, et al. Serum carotenoids are associated with increased lung cancer risk among alcohol drinkers, but not among non-drinkers in a cohort of tin miners. *Alcohol* 2000;35:355–60.

24. Boros LG. Population thiamine status and varying cancer rates between western, Asian and African countries. *Anticancer Res* 2000;20:2245–48.

25. Taper HS, Keyeux A, Roberfroid M. Potentiation of radiotherapy by nontoxic pretreatment with combined vitamin C and K3 in mice bearing solid transplantable tumor. *Anticancer Res* 1996;16:499–503.

26. Song EJ, Yang VC, Chiang CD, et al. Potentiation of growth inhibition due to vincristien by ascorbic acid in resistant human non-small cell lung cancer cell line. *Eur J Pharmacol* 1995;292:119–25.

27. Marian M, Matkovics B. Potentiation of biological activities of daunomycin and adriamycin by ascorbic acid and dimethylsulfoxide. *Experientia* 1982;38:573–74.

28. Babu JR, Sundravel S, Arumugam G, et al. Salubrious effect of vitamin C and vitamin E on tamoxifen treated women in breast cancer with reference to plasma lipid and lipoprotein levels. *Cancer Lett* 2000;151:1–5.

29. Furst P, Albers S, Stehle P. Evidence for a nutritional need for glutamine in catabolic patients. *Kidney Int Suppl* 1989;27:S287–92.
30. Miller, AI. Therapeutic considerations of L-glutamine: A review of the literature. *Alt Med Rev* 1999;4:239–48.
31. Klimberg VS, McClellan JL. Glutamine, cancer, and its therapy. *Am J Surg* 1996;172(5):418–24.
32. Langsjoen PH, Langsjoen AM. Overview of the use of CoQ10 in cardiovascular disease. *Biofactors* 1999;9:273–84.
33. Langsjoen PH, Folkers K, Lyson K, et al. Effective and safe therapy with coenzyme Q10 for cardiomyopathy. *Klin Wochenschr* 1988;66:583–90.
34. Jolliet P, Simon N, Barre J, et al. Plasma coenzyme Q10 concentrations in breast cancer: Prognosis and therapeutic consequences. *Int J Clin Pharmacol Ther* 1998;36:506–9.
35. Okuma K, Furuta I, Ota K. Protective effect of coenzyme Q10 in cardiotoxicity induced by adriamycin. *Jap J Cancer Chemother* 1984;11(3):502–8.
36. Tsubaki K, Horiuchi A, Kitani T, et al. Investigation of the preventive effect of CoQ10 against the side-effects of anthracycline antineoplastic agents. *Jap J Cancer Chemother* 1984;11:1420–27.
37. Reiter RJ. Antioxidant actions of melatonin. *Adv Pharmacol* 1997;38:103–17.
38. Lissoni P, Giani L, Zerbini S, et al. Biotherapy with the pineal immunomodulating hormone melatonin versus melatonin plus aloe vera in untreatable advanced solid neoplasms. *Nat Immun* 1998;16:27–33.
39. Lissoni P, Barni S, Fossati V, et al. A randomized study of neuroimmunotherapy with low-dose subcutaneous interleukin-2 plus melatonin compared to supportive care alone in patients with untreatable metastatic solid tumour. *Support Care Cancer* 1995;3:194–97.
40. Lissoni P, Barni S, Rovelli F, et al. Neuroimmunotherapy of advanced solid neoplasms with single evening subcutaneous injection of low-dose interleukin-2 and melatonin: Preliminary results. *Eur J Cancer* 1993;29A:185–89.
41. Maestroni GJ, Conti A. Melatonin in human breast cancer tissue: Association with nuclear grade and estrogen receptor status. *Lab Invest* 1996;75:557–61.
42. Brzezinski A. "Melatonin replacement therapy" for postmenopausal women: Is it justified? *Menopause* 1998;5:60–64.
43. Lissoni P, Barni S, Brivio F, et al. A biological study on the efficacy of low-dose subcutaneous interleukin-2 plus melatonin in the treatment of cancer-related thrombocytopenia. *Oncology* 1995;52:360–62.
44. Furuya Y, Yamamoto K, Kohno N, et al. 5-Fluorouracil attenuates an oncostatic effect of melatonin on estrogen-sensitive human breast cancer cells (MCF7). *Cancer Lett* 1994;81:95–98.
45. Park KG, Heys SD, Blessing K, et al. Stimulation of human breast cancers by dietary L-arginine. *Clinical Science* 1992;82:413–17.
46. Shen F, Xue X, Weber G. Tamoxifen and genistein synergistically downregulate signal transduction and proliferation in estrogen receptor-negative

human breast carcinoma MDA-MB-435 cells. *Anticancer Res* 1999;19: 1657–62.

47. Weber G, Shen F, Yang H, et al. Amplification of signal transduction capacity and down-regulation by drugs. *Adv Enzyme Reg* 1999;39:51–66.

48. Bracke ME, Depypere HT, Boterberg T, et al. Influence of tangeretin on tamoxifen's therapeutic benefit in mammary cancer. *J Nat Cancer Inst* 1999; 91:354–59.

49. Schwartz JA, Liu G, Brooks SC. Genistein-mediated attenuation of tamoxifen-induced antagonism from estrogen receptor-regulated genes. *Biochem Biophys Res Comm* 1998;253:38–43.

50. Faure H, Coudray C, Mousseau M, et al. 5-Hydroxymethyluracil excretion, plasma TBARS and plasma antioxidant vitamins in adriamycin-treated patients. *Free Radic Biol Med* 1996;20:979–83.

51. Faber M, Coudray C, Hida H, et al. Lipid peroxidation products, and vitamin and trace element status in patients with cancer before and after chemotherapy, including adriamycin: A preliminary study. *Biol Trace Elem Res* 1995;47:117–23.

52. Gao Y, Shimizu M, Yamada S, et al. The effects of chemotherapy including cisplatin on vitamin D metabolism. *Endocr J* 1993;40:737–42.

53. Evans TR, Harper CL, Beveridge IG, et al. A randomised study to determine whether routine intravenous magnesium supplements are necessary in patients receiving cisplatin chemotherapy with continuous infusion 5-fluorouracil. *Eur J Cancer* 1995;31A:174–78.

54. Simone CB. Use of therapeutic levels of nutrients to augment oncology care. In Quillin P, Williams RM, eds., *Adjuvant Nutrition in Cancer Treatment.* Arlington Heights, Ill.: Cancer Treatment Research Foundation/American College of Nutrition, 1993:363–70.

55. Prasad KN. Vitamin E induces differentiation, growth inhibition, and enhances the efficacy of therapeutic agents on cancer cells. In Quillin P, Williams RM, eds., *Adjuvant Nutrition in Cancer Treatment.* Arlington Heights, Ill.: Cancer Treatment Research Foundation/American College of Nutrition, 1993:235–52.

56. Mosienko VS, Khasanova LT, Sukolinskii VN, et al. Effectiveness of combined action of vitamins A, E, and C and cyclophosphane or adriamycin on growth of transplanted tumors in mice. *Eksperimentalnaia Onkologiia* 1990;12:55–57.

57. De Flora S, D'Agostini F, Masiello L., et al. Synergism between N-acetylcysteine and doxorubicin in the prevention of tumorigenicity and metastasis in murine models. *Int J Cancer* 1996;67:842–48.

58. D'Agostini F, Bagnasco M, Giunciuglio D, et al. Inhibition by oral N-acetylcysteine of doxorubicin-induced clastogenicity and alopecia, and prevention of primary tumors and lung micrometastases in mice. *Int J Oncol* 1998;13: 217–24.

59. Israel L, Hajji O, Grefft-Alami A, et al. Vitamin A augmentation of the effects of chemotherapy in metastatic breast cancers after menopause: Randomized trial in 100 patients. *Ann Med Interne* 1985;136:551–54.

60. Clarke R, Brenner N, Katzenellenborgen BS, et al. Progression of human breast cancer cells from hormone-dependent to hormone-independent growth both in vitro and in vivo. *Proc Natl Acad Sci USA* 1989;86:3649–53.
61. See note 55.
62. See note 59.
63. See note 60.
64. Boccardo F, Canobbio L, Resasco M, et al. Phase II study of tamoxifen and high-dose retinyl acetate in patients with advanced breast cancer. *J Cancer Res Clin Oncol* 1990;116:503–6.
65. Schwartz JL. The dual roles of nutrients as antioxidants and prooxidants: Their effects on tumor cell growth. *J Nutr* 1996; 126(4 Suppl):1221S–27S.
66. Schwartz JL, Antoniades DZ, Zhao S. Molecular and biochemical reprogramming of oncogenesis through the activity of prooxidants and antioxidants. *Ann NY Acad Sci* 1993;686:262–78.
67. Chinery R, Brockman JA, Peeler MO, et al. Antioxidants enhance the cytotoxicity of chemotherapeutic agents in colorectal cancer: A p53-independent induction of p21 via C/EBP-beta. *Nat Med* 1997;3:1233–41.
68. Cole WC, Prasad KN. Contrasting effects of vitamins as modulators of apoptosis in cancer cells and normal cells: A review. *Nutr Cancer* 1997;29:97–103.
69. See note 57.
70. See note 58.
71. See note 59.
72. See note 60.
73. See note 64.
74. Recchia F, Sica G, de Filippis S, et al. Interferon-beta, retinoids, and tamoxifen in the treatment of metastatic breast cancer: A phase II study. *J Interferon Cytokine Res* 1995;15:605–10.
75. Recchia F, Rea S, Corrao G, et al. Sequential chemotherapy, beta interferon, retinoids and tamoxifen in the treatment of metastatic breast cancer: A pilot study. *Eur J Cancer* 1995;31A:1887–88.
76. Recchia F, Rea S, Pompili P, et al. Beta-interferon, retinoids and tamoxifen as maintenance therapy in metastatic breast cancer: A pilot study. *Clin Terapeutica* 1995;146:603–10.
77. Recchia F, Frati L, Rea S, et al. Minimal residual disease in metastatic breast cancer: Treatment with IFN-beta, retinoids, and tamoxifen. *J Interferon Cytokine Res* 1998;18:41–47.
78. Schwartz JL. The dual roles of nutrients as antioxidants and prooxidants: Their effects on tumor cell growth. *J Nutr* 1996;126(4 Suppl):1221S–27S.
79. Schwartz JL, Antoniades DZ, Zhao S. Molecular and biochemical reprogramming of oncogenesis through the activity of prooxidants and antioxidants. *Ann NY Acad Sci* 1993;686:262–78.
80. See note 67.
81. See note 68.
82. Bold RJ, Termuhlen PM, McConkey DJ. Apoptosis, cancer and cancer therapy. *Surg Oncol* 1997;6:133–42.

83. Lamson DW, Brignall MS. Antioxidants in cancer therapy; their actions and interactions with oncologic therapies. *Altern Med Rev* 1999 Oct;4:304–29.

84. Cameron E, Campbell A. The orthomolecular treatment of cancer: II. Clinical trial of high-dose ascorbic acid supplements in advanced human cancer. *Chem Biol Interact* 1974;9:285–315.

85. Cameron E, Pauling L. Supplemental ascorbate in the supportive treatment of cancer: Reevaluation of prolongation of survival times in terminal human cancer. *Proc Nat Acad Sci USA* 1978;75:4538–42.

86. Morishige F, Murata A. Prolongation of survival times in terminal human cancer by administration of supplemental ascorbate. *J Int Acad Prev Med* 1979;5:47–52.

87. Murata A, Morishige F, Yamaguchi H. Prolongation of survival times of terminal cancer patients by administration of large doses of ascorbate. *Int J Vitamin Nutr Res Suppl* 1982;23:103–13.

88. Cameron E, Campbell A. Innovation vs. quality control: An "unpublishable" clinical trial of supplemental ascorbate in incurable cancer. *Med Hypotheses* 1991;36:185–89.

89. Hoffer A, Pauling L. Hardin Jones biostatistical analysis of mortality data for a second set of cohorts of cancer patients with a large fraction surviving at the termination of the study and a comparison of survival times of cancer patients receiving large regular oral doses of ascorbic acid and other nutrients with similar patients not receiving these doses. *J Orthomolecular Med* 1993;8:157–64.

90. Prasad KN, Kumar R. Effect of individual and multiple antioxidant vitamins on growth and morphology of human nontumorigenic and tumorigenic parotid acinar cells in culture. *Nutr Cancer* 1996;26:11–19.

91. Prasad KN, Hernandez C, Edwards-Prasad J, et al. Modification of the effect of tamoxifen, cis-platin, DTIC, and interferon-alpha 2b on human melanoma cells in culture by a mixture of vitamins. *Nutr Cancer* 1994;22:233–45.

92. Evangelou A, Kalpouzos G, Karkabounas S, et al. Dose-related preventive and therapeutic effects of antioxidants-anticarcinogens on experimentally induced malignant tumors in Wistar rats. *Cancer Lett* 1997;115:105–11.

93. Morozkina TS, Sukolinskii VN, Strelnikov AV. The selective effect of vitamin E, A, and C complexes on antioxidant protection in neoplastic and normal tissues. *Voprosy Meditsinskoi Khimii* 1991;37:59–161.

94. Poydock ME, Fardon JC, Gallina D, et al. Inhibiting effect of vitamins C and B_{12} on the mitotic activity of ascites tumors. *Exp Cell Biol* 1979;47:210–17.

95. Pavelic K. L-ascorbic acid-induced DNA strand breaks and cross links in human neuroblastoma cells. *Brain Res* 1985;342:369–73.

Chapter 10

1. Inohara H, Raz A. Effects of natural complex carbohydrate (citrus pectin) on murine melanoma cell properties related to galectin-3 functions. *Glycoconj J* 1994;11:527–32.

2. Castronovo V, Van Den Brule FA, et al. Decreased expression of galectin-3 is associated with progression of human breast cancer. *J Pathol* 1996;179:43–48.

3. Warfield, PR, Makker PN, et al. Adhesion of human breast carcinoma to extracellular matrix proteins is modulated by galectin-3. *Invasion Metastasis* 1997;17:101–12.

4. Nangia-Makker P, Sarvis R, et al. Galectin-3 and L1 retrotransposons in human breast carcinomas. *Breast Cancer Res Treat* 1998;49:171–83.

5. Platt D, Raz A. Modulation of the lung colonization of B16-F1 melanoma cells by citrus pectin. *J Natl Cancer Inst* 1992;84:438–42.

6. Pienta KJ, Naik H, et al. Inhibition of spontaneous metastasis in a rat prostate cancer model by oral administration of modified citrus pectin [see comments]. *J Natl Cancer Inst* 1995;87:348–53.

7. Folkers K, Osterborg A, et al. Activities of vitamin Q10 in animal models and a serious deficiency in patients with cancer. *Biochem Biophys Res Commun* 1997;234:296–9.

8. Jolliet P, Simon N, et al. Plasma coenzyme Q10 concentrations in breast cancer: Prognosis and therapeutic consequences. *Int J Clin Pharmacol Ther* 1998;36:506–9.

9. Gaby AR. The role of coenzyme Q10 in clinical medicine: part I. *Alt Med Rev* 1996;1:11–17.

10. Gaby AR. What is the best coenzyme Q10 supplement? *Nutr Healing* 1998(March): 7–8.

11. Lockwood K, Moesgaard S, et al. Progress on therapy of breast cancer with vitamin Q10 and the regression of metastases. *Biochem Biophys Res Commun* 1995;212:172–77.

12. Lockwood K, Moesgaard S, et al. Partial and complete regression of breast cancer in patients in relation to dosage of coenzyme Q10. *Biochem Biophys Res Commun* 1994;199:1504–8.

13. Takimoto M, Sakurai T, et al. [Protective effect of CoQ 10 administration on cardial toxicity in FAC therapy]. *Gan To Kagaku Ryoho* 1982;9:116–21.

14. Okuma K, Furuta I, et al. [Protective effect of coenzyme Q10 in cardiotoxicity induced by adriamycin]. *Gan To Kagaku Ryoho* 1984;11:502–8.

15. See note 9.

16. Kaikkonen J, Nyyssonen K, et al. Effect of oral coenzyme Q10 supplementation on the oxidation resistance of human VLDL+LDL fraction: Absorption and antioxidative properties of oil and granule-based preparations. *Free Radic Biol Med* 1997;22:1195–1202.

17. See note 10.

18. Karpatkin S, Pearlstein E. Role of platelets in tumor cell metastases. *Ann Intern Med* 1981;95:636–41.

19. Kandil O. Garlic and the immune system in humans: Its effect on natural killer cells. *Fed Proc* 1987;46:441.

20. Ibid.

21. Kandil O. Potential role of Allium sativum in natural killer cytotoxicity. *Arch AIDS Res* 1988;1:230–31.

22. Weber ND, Andersen DO, et al. In vitro virucidal effects of Allium sativum (garlic) extract and compounds. *Planta Med* 1992;58:417–23.

23. Prasad K, Laxdal VA, et al. Antioxidant activity of allicin, an active principle in garlic. *Mol Cell Biochem* 1995;148:183–89.

24. Koch HP, Lawson LD. *Garlic: The Science and Therapeutic Applications of Allium Sativum L. and Related Species.* 2nd ed. Baltimore: Williams & Wilkins, 1996:1–24.

25. Lau BHS, Tadi PP, et al. Allium sativum (garlic) and cancer prevention. *Nutrition Res* 1990;10:937–48.

26. Liu J, Lin RI, et al. Inhibition of 7,12-dimethylbenz[a]anthracene-induced mammary tumors and DNA adducts by garlic powder. *Carcinogenesis* 1992;13:1847–51.

27. Sundaram SG, Milner JA. Impact of organosulfur compounds in garlic on canine mammary tumor cells in culture. *Cancer Lett* 1993;74:85–90.

28. Sigounas G, Hooker JL, et al. S-allylmercaptocysteine, a stable thioallyl compound, induces apoptosis in erythroleukemia cell lines. *Nutr Cancer* 1997; 28:153–59.

29. Dausch JG, Nixon DW. Garlic: A review of its relationship to malignant disease. *Prev Med* 1990;19:346–61.

30. Lea MA. Organosulfur compounds and cancer. *Adv Exp Med Biol* 1996;401:147–54.

31. Wargovich MJ, Uda N, et al. Allium vegetables: Their role in the prevention of cancer. *Biochem Soc Trans* 1996;24:811–14.

32. Craig WJ. Phytochemicals: Guardians of our health. *J Am Diet Assoc* 1997;97(10 Suppl 2):S199–204.

33. Riggs DR, DeHaven JI, et al. Allium sativum (garlic) treatment for murine transitional cell carcinoma. *Cancer* 1997;79:1987–94.

34. Steinmetz KA, Potter JD. Vegetables, fruit, and cancer: I. Epidemiology. *Cancer Causes Control* 1991;2:325–57.

35. See note 23.

36. Hu X, Benson PJ, et al. Glutathione S-transferases of female A/J mouse liver and forestomach and their differential induction by anti-carcinogenic organosulfides from garlic. *Arch Biochem Biophys* 1996;336:199–214.

37. Kim SG, Surh YJ, et al. Inhibition of vinyl carbamate-induced hepatotoxicity, mutagenicity, and tumorigenicity by isopropyl-2-(1,3-dithietane-2-ylidene)-2-[N-(4- methylthiazol-2-yl)carbamoyl]acetate (YH439). *Carcinogenesis* 1998; 19:687–90.

38. Challier B, Perarnau JM, et al. Garlic, onion and cereal fibre as protective factors for breast cancer: A French case-control study. *Eur J Epidemiol* 1998;14:737–47.

39. Levi F, Franceschi S, et al. Dietary factors and the risk of endometrial cancer. *Cancer* 1993;71:3575–81.

40. See note 38.

41. Agarwal KC. Therapeutic actions of garlic constituents. *Med Res Rev* 1996; 16:111–24.
42. See note 24.
43. Lawson LD. Effect of garlic on serum lipids [letter]. *JAMA* 1998;280:1568.
44. Lawson LD, Wang ZJ, et al. Identification and HPLC quantitation of the sulfides and dialk(en)yl thiosulfinates in commercial garlic products. *Planta Med* 1991;57:363–70.
45. Song K, Milner JA. Heating garlic inhibits its ability to suppress 7, 12-dimethylbenz (a)anthracene-induced DNA adduct formation in rat mammary tissue. *J Nutr* 1999;129:657–61.
46. Kroning F. Garlic as an inhibitor for spontaneous tumors in mice. *Acta Unio Int Cancrum* 1964;61(20):855–56 (Chem Abst 15 206).
47. See note 29.
48. Hertog MG, Kromhout D, et al. Flavonoid intake and long-term risk of coronary heart disease and cancer in the seven countries study [published erratum appears in *Arch Intern Med* 1995;155:1184]. *Arch Intern Med* 1995;155:381–86.
49. Wei YQ, Zhao X, et al. Induction of apoptosis by quercetin: Involvement of heat shock protein. *Cancer Res* 1994;54:4952–57.
50. Plaumann B, Fritsche M, et al. Flavonoids activate wild-type p53. *Oncogene* 1996;13:1605–14.
51. Balabhadrapathruni S, Thomas TJ, et al. Effects of genistein and structurally related phytoestrogens on cell cycle kinetics and apoptosis in MDA-MB-468 human breast cancer cells. *Oncol Rep* 2000;7:3–12.
52. Singhal RL, Yeh YA, et al. Quercetin down-regulates signal transduction in human breast carcinoma cells. *Biochem Biophys Res Commun* 1995;208: 425–31.
53. Verma AK, Johnson JA, et al. Inhibition of 7,12-dimethylbenz(a)anthracene- and N-nitrosomethylurea-induced rat mammary cancer by dietary flavonol quercetin [published erratum appears in *Cancer Res* 1989;1549:1073]. *Cancer Res* 1988;48:5754–58.
54. Rodgers EH, Grant MH. The effect of the flavonoids, quercetin, myricetin and epicatechin on the growth and enzyme activities of MCF7 human breast cancer cells. *Chem Biol Interact* 1998;116:213–28.
55. See note 53.
56. Garcia-Closas R, Gonzalez CA, et al. Intake of specific carotenoids and flavonoids and the risk of gastric cancer in Spain. *Cancer Causes Control* 1999;10:71–75.
57. Huang Z, Fasco MJ, et al. Inhibition of estrone sulfatase in human liver microsomes by quercetin and other flavonoids. *J Steroid Biochem Mol Biol* 1997;63:9–15.
58. Miodini P, Fioravanti L, et al. The two phyto-oestrogens genistein and quercetin exert different effects on oestrogen receptor function. *Br J Cancer* 1999;80:1150–55.

59. Scambia G, Ranelletti FO, et al. Quercetin potentiates the effect of adriamycin in a multidrug-resistant MCF-7 human breast-cancer cell line: P-glycoprotein as a possible target [see comments]. *Cancer Chemother Pharmacol* 1994;34:459–64.
60. Hirose M, Fukushima S, et al. Effect of quercetin on two-stage carcinogenesis of the rat urinary bladder. *Cancer Lett* 1983;21:23–27.
61. Pizzorno J, Murray M. *Textbook of Natural Medicine*. Kenmore, Wash.: Churchill Livingston Press, vol. II, 2000.
62. Graefe EU, Derendorf H, et al. Pharmacokinetics and bioavailability of the flavonol quercetin in humans. *Int J Clin Pharmacol Ther* 1999;37:219–33.
63. Shao ZM, Wu J, et al. Genistein exerts multiple suppressive effects on human breast carcinoma cells. *Cancer Res* 1998;58:4851–57.
64. Zhou JR, Mukherjee P, et al. Inhibition of murine bladder tumorigenesis by soy isoflavones via alterations in the cell cycle, apoptosis, and angiogenesis. *Cancer Res* 1998;58:5231–38.
65. Jiang C, Jiang W, et al. Selenium-induced inhibition of angiogenesis in mammary cancer at chemopreventive levels of intake. *Mol Carcinog* 1999;26:213–25.
66. Rose DP, Connolly JM. Antiangiogenicity of docosahexaenoic acid and its role in the suppression of breast cancer cell growth in nude mice. *Int J Oncol* 1999;15:1011–15.
67. Zhou JR, Gugger ET, et al. Soybean phytochemicals inhibit the growth of transplantable human prostate carcinoma and tumor angiogenesis in mice. *J Nutr* 1999;129:1628–35.
68. Mantell DJ, Owens PE, Bundred NJ, et al. 1 alpha,25-dihydroxyvitamin D(3) inhibits angiogenesis in vitro and in vivo. *Circ Res* 2000;87:214–20.
69. Breitmeyer JB. Immunotherapy of breast cancer. *Cancer Treat Res* 1992;60: 331–56.
70. Dean JH, Connor R, et al. The relative proliferation index as a more sensitive parameter for evaluating lymphoproliferative responses of cancer patients to mitogens and alloantigens. *Int J Cancer* 1977;20:359–70.
71. Early Breast Cancer Trialists' Collaborative Group. Systemic treatment of early breast cancer by hormonal, cytotoxic, or immune therapy: 33 randomised trials involving 31,000 recurrences and 24,000 deaths among 75,000 women. *Lancet* 1992;339:1–15, 71–85.
72. Reiter RJ, Melchiorri D, et al. A review of the evidence supporting melatonin's role as an antioxidant. *J Pineal Res* 1995;18:1–11.
73. Blask DE, Hill SM. Effects of melatonin on cancer: Studies on MCF-7 human breast cancer cells in culture. *J Neural Transm Suppl* 1986;21: 433–49.
74. Cos S, Fernandez R, et al. Influence of melatonin on invasive and metastatic properties of MCF-7 human breast cancer cells [in process citation]. *Cancer Res* 1998;58:4383–90.

75. Hill SM, Spriggs LL, et al. The growth inhibitory action of melatonin on human breast cancer cells is linked to the estrogen response system. *Cancer Lett* 1992;64:249–56.
76. Wilson ST, Blask DE, et al. Melatonin augments the sensitivity of MCF-7 human breast cancer cells to tamoxifen in vitro. *J Clin Endocrinol Metab* 1992;75:669–70.
77. Subramanian A, Kothari L. Melatonin, a suppressor of spontaneous murine mammary tumors. *J Pineal Res* 1991;10:136–40.
78. Lissoni P, Paolorossi F, et al. A phase II study of tamoxifen plus melatonin in metastatic solid tumour patients. *Br J Cancer* 1996;74:1466–68.
79. Lissoni P, Tancini G, et al. Treatment of cancer chemotherapy-induced toxicity with the pineal hormone melatonin. *Support Care Cancer* 1997;5:126–29.
80. Lissoni P, Barni S, et al. Modulation of cancer endocrine therapy by melatonin: A phase II study of tamoxifen plus melatonin in metastatic breast cancer patients progressing under tamoxifen alone. *Br J Cancer* 1995;71:854–56.
81. Yokoe T, Iino Y, et al. HLA antigen as predictive index for the outcome of breast cancer patients with adjuvant immunochemotherapy with PSK. *Anticancer Res* 1997;17:2815–18.
82. Toi M, Hattori T, et al. Randomized adjuvant trial to evaluate the addition of tamoxifen and PSK to chemotherapy in patients with primary breast cancer: 5-year results from the Nishi-Nippon Group of the Adjuvant Chemoendocrine Therapy for Breast Cancer Organization. *Cancer* 1992;70: 2475–83.
83. Morimoto T, Ogawa M, et al. Postoperative adjuvant randomised trial comparing chemoendocrine therapy, chemotherapy and immunotherapy for patients with stage II breast cancer: 5-year results from the Nishinihon Cooperative Study Group of Adjuvant Chemoendocrine Therapy for Breast Cancer (ACETBC) of Japan [published erratum appears in *Eur J Cancer* 1996;32A:1264]. *Eur J Cancer* 1996;32A:235–42.
84. Whiteside TL, Herberman RB. The role of natural killer cells in human disease. *Clin Immunol Immunopathol* 1989;53:1–23.
85. Peters C, Lotzerich H, et al. Influence of a moderate exercise training on natural killer cytotoxicity and personality traits in cancer patients. *Anticancer Res* 1994;14:1033–36.
86. Young M-S, Sexton DL. A retrospective investigation of the relationship between aerobic exercise and quality of life in women with breast cancer. *Oncol Nurs Forum* 1991;18:751–57.
87. Dwivedi C, Downie AA, et al. Modulation of chemically initiated and promoted skin tumorigenesis in CD-1 mice by dietary glucarate. *J Environ Pathol Toxicol Oncol* 1989;9:253–59.
88. Blondell JM. Pesticides and breast cancer, popcorn and colorectal cancer: Innovation versus fashion in dietary epidemiology. *Med Hypotheses* 1983;12:191–94.

89. Falck F Jr., Ricci A Jr., et al. Pesticides and polychlorinated biphenyl residues in human breast lipids and their relation to breast cancer. *Arch Environ Health* 1992;47:143–46.

90. Wolff MS, Toniolo PG, et al. Blood levels of organochlorine residues and risk of breast cancer [see comments]. *J Natl Cancer Inst* 1993;85:648–52.

91. Guttes S, Failing K, et al. Chlororganic pesticides and polychlorinated biphenyls in breast tissue of women with benign and malignant breast disease. *Arch Environ Contam Toxicol* 1998;35:140–47.

92. Olaya-Contreras P, Rodriguez-Villamil J, et al. Organochlorine exposure and breast cancer risk in Colombian women. *Cad Saude Publica* 1998;14 Suppl 3:125–32.

93. Stellman SD, Djordjevic MV, et al. Relative abundance of organochlorine pesticides and polychlorinated biphenyls in adipose tissue and serum of women in Long Island, New York [see comments]. *Cancer Epidemiol Biomarkers Prev* 1998;7:489–96.

94. Crinnion WJ. Results of a decade of naturopathic treatment for environmental illnesses: A review of clinical records. *J Naturopathic Med* 1997; 7:21–26.

95. Morabia A, Szklo M, et al. Thyroid hormones and duration of ovulatory activity in the etiology of breast cancer. *Cancer Epidemiol Biomarkers Prev* 1992; 1:389–93.

96. Smyth PP. Thyroid disease and breast cancer. *J Endocrinol Invest* 1993;16: 396–401.

97. Clur A. Di-iodothyronine as part of the oestradiol and catechol oeastrogen receptor: The role of iodine, thyroid hormones and melatonin in the aetiology of breast cancer. *Med Hypotheses* 1988;27:303–11.

98. Blomhoff R, ed. *Vitamin A in Health and Disease*. New York, Basel, Hong Kong: Marcel Dekker, 1994.

99. Israel L, Hajji O, et al. Vitamin A augmentation of the effects of chemotherapy in metastatic breast cancers after menopause. Randomized trial in 100 patients. *Ann Med Interne Paris* 1985;136:551–54.

100. Ito Y, Gajalakshmi KC, et al. A study on serum carotenoid levels in breast cancer patients of Indian women in Chennai (Madras), India. *J Epidemiol* 1999;9:306–14.

101. Jumaan AO, Holmberg L, et al. Beta-carotene intake and risk of postmenopausal breast cancer. *Epidemiology* 1999;10:49–53.

102. McKeown N. Antioxidants and breast cancer. *Nutr Rev* 1999;57:321–24.

103. Gandini S, Merzenich H, et al. Meta-analysis of studies on breast cancer risk and diet. The role of fruit and vegetable consumption and the intake of associated micronutrients. *Eur J Cancer* 2000;36:636–46.

104. Graham S, Hellman R, Marshall J, et al. Nutritional epidemiology of postmenopausal breast cancer in western New York. *Am J Epidemiol* 1991;Sep 15;134:552–66.

105. Santamaria LA, Santamaria AB. Cancer chemoprevention by supplemental carotenoids and synergism with retinol in mastodynia treatment. *Med Oncol Tumor Pharmacother* 1990;7:153–67.

106. Santamaria L, Bianchi S-A, et al. Carotenoids in cancer, mastalgia, and AIDS: Prevention and treatment—an overview. *J Environ Pathol Toxicol Oncol* 1996;15:89–95.

107. Albanes D, Heinonen OP, et al. Effects of alpha-tocopherol and beta-carotene supplements on cancer incidence in the Alpha-Tocopherol Beta-Carotene Cancer Prevention Study. *Am J Clin Nutr* 1995;62(6 Suppl): 1427S–30S.

108. Rapola JM, Virtamo J, et al. Effect of vitamin E and beta carotene on the incidence of angina pectoris: A randomized, double-blind, controlled trial [see comments] [published erratum appears in *JAMA* 1998;279:1528]. *JAMA* 1996;275:693–98.

109. Redlich CA, Chung JS, et al. Effect of long-term beta-carotene and vitamin A on serum cholesterol and triglyceride levels among participants in the Carotene and Retinol Efficacy Trial (CARET) [corrected and republished in *Atherosclerosis* 1999;145:425–32]. *Atherosclerosis* 1999;143:427–34.

110. Paiva SA, Russell RM. Beta-carotene and other carotenoids as antioxidants [see comments]. *J Am Coll Nutr* 1999;18:426–33.

111. van Het Hof KH, West CE, et al. Dietary factors that affect the bioavailability of carotenoids. *J Nutr* 2000;130:503–6.

112. Zhu Z, Parviainen M, et al. Vitamin E concentration in breast adipose tissue of breast cancer patients (Kuopio, Finland). *Cancer Causes Control* 1996;7:591–95.

113. Charpentier A, Simmons M-M, et al. RRR-alpha-tocopheryl succinate enhances TGF-beta 1, -beta 2, and -beta 3 and TGF-beta R-II expression by human MDA-MB-435 breast cancer cells. *Nutr Cancer* 1996;26:237–50.

114. Gogos CA, Ginopoulos P, et al. Dietary omega-3 polyunsaturated fatty acids plus vitamin E restore immunodeficiency and prolong survival for severely ill patients with a generalized malignancy: A randomized control trial. *Cancer* 1998;82:395–402.

115. Wu AH, Ziegler RG, et al. Tofu and risk of breast cancer in Asian-Americans. *Cancer Epidemiol Biomarkers Prev* 1996;5:901–6.

116. Martin PM, Horwitz KB, Ryan DS, McGuire WL. Phytoestrogen interaction with estrogen receptors in human breast cancer cells. *Endocrinology* 1978;103: 1860–67.

117. Molteni A, Brizio-Molteni L, et al. In vitro hormonal effects of soybean isoflavones. *J Nutr* 1995;125(3 Suppl):751S–56S.

118. Gustafsson JA. Therapeutic potential of selective estrogen receptor modulators. *Curr Opin Chem Biol* 1998;2:508–11.

119. Mazur W. Phytoestrogen content in foods. *Baillieres Clin Endocrinol Metab* 1998;12:729–42.

120. Thompson LU. Experimental studies on lignans and cancer. *Baillieres Clin Endocrinol Metab* 1998;12:691–705.

121. Welshons WV, Murphy CS, et al. Stimulation of breast cancer cells in vitro by the environmental estrogen enterolactone and the phytoestrogen equol. *Breast Cancer Res Treat* 1987;10:169–75.

122. Phipps WR, Martini MC, et al. Effect of flaxseed ingestion on the menstrual cycle. *J Clin Endocrinol Metab* 1993;77:1215–19.

123. Orcheson LJ, Rickard SE, et al. Flaxseed and its mammalian lignan precursor cause a lengthening or cessation of estrous cycling in rats. *Cancer Lett* 1998;125:69–76.

124. Aldercreutz H. Does fiber-rich food containing animal lignan precursors protect against both colon and breast cancer? An extension of the "fiber hypothesis." *Gastroenterology* 86(Apr.):761–64.

125. Aldercreutz H, Fotsis T, et al. Determination of urinary lignans and phytoestrogen metabolites, potential antiestrogens and anticarcinogens, in urine of women on various habitual diets. *J Steroid Biochem* 1986;25:791–97.

126. Adlercreutz H, Hockerstedt K, et al. Effect of dietary components, including lignans and phytoestrogens, on enterohepatic circulation and liver metabolism of estrogens and on sex hormone binding globulin (SHBG). *J Steroid Biochem* 1987;27:1135–44.

127. Martin ME, Haourigui M, et al. Interactions between phytoestrogens and human sex steroid binding protein. *Life Sci* 1996;58:429–36.

128. Schottner M, Gansser D, et al. Lignans from the roots of Urtica dioica and their metabolites bind to human sex hormone binding globulin (SHBG). *Planta Med* 1997;63:529–32.

129. Adlercreutz H, Fotsis T, et al. Excretion of the lignans enterolactone and enterodiol and of equol in omnivorous and vegetarian postmenopausal women and in women with breast cancer. *Lancet* 1982;2:1295–99.

130. Wang C, Makela T, Hase T, Aldercreutz H, Kurzer MS. Lignans and flavonoids inhibit aromatase enzyme in human preadipocytes. *J Steroid Biochem Mol Biol* 1994;50:205.

131. Thompson LU, Seidl MM, et al. Antitumorigenic effect of a mammalian lignan precursor from flaxseed. *Nutr Cancer* 1996;26:159–65.

132. Thompson LU, Rickard SE, et al. Flaxseed and its lignan and oil components reduce mammary tumor growth at a late stage of carcinogenesis. *Carcinogenesis* 1996;17:1373–76.

133. Baltrusch HJ, Stangel W, et al. Stress, cancer and immunity. New developments in biopsychosocial and psychoneuroimmunologic research. *Acta Neurol Napoli* 1991;13:315–27.

134. Levy SM, Herberman RB, et al. Perceived social support and tumor estrogen/progesterone receptor status as predictors of natural killer cell activity in breast cancer patients. *Psychosom Med* 1990;52:73–85.

135. Ginsberg A, Price S, et al. Life events and the risk of breast cancer: A case-control study. *Eur J Cancer* 1996;32A:2049–52.

136. Spiegel D, Bloom JR, et al. Effect of psychosocial treatment on survival of patients with metastatic breast cancer. *Lancet* 1989;2(Oct 14.):P888–91.

137. Lemon HM, Rodriguez-Sierra JF. Timing of breast cancer surgery during the luteal menstrual phase may improve prognosis [corrected and republished article originally printed in *Nebr Med J* 1996 Mar;81:73–8]. *Nebr Med J* 1996;81:110–15.

138. Cooper LS, Gillett CE, et al. Survival of premenopausal breast carcinoma patients in relation to menstrual cycle timing of surgery and estrogen receptor/progesterone receptor status of the primary tumor. *Cancer* 1999;86: 2053–58.

139. Taper HS, G.-J. de, et al. Non-toxic potentiation of cancer chemotherapy by combined C and K3 vitamin pre-treatment. *Int J Cancer* 1987;40:575–79.

140. Huang EY, Leung SW, et al. Oral glutamine to alleviate radiation-induced oral mucositis: A pilot randomized trial. *Int J Radiat Oncol Biol Phys* 2000;46: 535–39.

141. Decker-Baumann C, Buhl K, et al. Reduction of chemotherapy-induced side-effects by parenteral glutamine supplementation in patients with metastatic colorectal cancer. *Eur J Cancer* 1999;35:202–7.

142. Duker EM, Kopanski L, et al. Effects of extracts from Cimicifuga racemosa on gonadotropin release in menopausal women and ovariectomized rats. *Planta Med* 1991;57:420–24.

143. Liske E. Therapeutic efficacy and safety of Cimicifuga racemosa for gynecologic disorders. *Adv Ther* 1998;15:45–53.

144. Dixon-Shanies D, Shaikh N. Growth inhibition of human breast cancer cells by herbs and phytoestrogens. *Oncol Rep* 1999;6:1383–87.

145. Freudenstein J, Bodinet C. Influence of an isopropanolic aqueous extract of Cimicifuga racemosae rhizoma on the proliferation of MCF-7 cells. Presented at the 23rd International Symposium on Phytoestrogens, University of Ghent, Belgium, January 15, 1999.

146. Jensen T, Stender S, et al. Partial normalization by dietary cod-liver oil of increased microvascular albumin leakage in patients with insulin-dependent diabetes and albuminuria. *N Engl J Med* 1989;321:1572–77.

147. Okuda Y, Mizutani M, et al. Long-term effects of eicosapentaenoic acid on diabetic peripheral neuropathy and serum lipids in patients with type II diabetes mellitus. *J Diabetes Complications* 1996;10:280–87.

Chapter 11

1. Osler W. *A Way of Life*. Baltimore: Remington-Putnam, 1932.

2. Osler W. *Aequanimitas: With Other Addresses to Medical Students, Nurses, and Practitioners of Medicine*. Philadelphia: P. Blakiston, 1904.

3. Thoreau H. *Walden*. New York: Random House, 1937:101.

4. Eliot T. Little Gidding. In *Four Quartets*. New York: Harcourt Brace, 1943:59.

5. Rilke R. *Selected Poems of Rainer Maria Rilke* (trans. Robert Bly). New York: Harper & Row, 1981:31.

6. Clemow L, Hébert JR, Massion AO, Fowke J, Druker S, Kabat-Zinn J. A meditation-based stress reduction intervention for younger women with breast cancer. *Ann Behav Med* 1997;19:77.

7. Speca M, Carlson LE, Goodey E, Angen M. A randomized, wait-list controlled clinical trial: The effect of a mindfulness meditation-based stress reduction program on mood and symptoms of stress in cancer outpatients. *Psychosomatic Med* 2000;62:613–22.

8. Clemow L, Hébert J, Massion A, Fowke J, Druker S, Kabat-Zinn J. A meditation-based stress reduction intervention for women with breast cancer: Outcome and 1-year follow-up. *Ann Behav Med* 1998;20:52S.

9. Saxe GA, Hébert JR, Carmody JF, Kabat-Zinn J, Rosenzweig PH, Jarzobski D, Reed GW, Blute RD. Can diet, in conjunction with stress reduction, affect the rate of increase in prostate-specific antigen after biochemical recurrence of prostate cancer? *J Urol* 2001;166:2202–7.

10. Kabat-Zinn J. An out-patient program in behavioral medicine for chronic pain patients based on the practice of mindfulness meditation: Theoretical considerations and preliminary results. *Gen Hosp Psychiatry* 1982;4:33–47.

11. Kabat-Zinn J, Lipworth L, Burney R. The clinical use of mindfulness meditation for the self-regulation of chronic pain. *J Behav Med* 1985;8:163–90.

12. Kabat-Zinn J, Lipworth L, Burney R, et al. Four year follow-up of a meditation-based program for the self-regulation of chronic pain: Treatment outcomes and compliance. *Clin J Pain* 1986;2:159–73.

13. Kabat-Zinn J, Chapman-Waldrop A. Compliance with an outpatient stress reduction program: Rates and predictors of program completion. *J Behav Med* 1988;11:333–52.

14. Kabat-Zinn J, Massion A, Kristeller J, et al. Effectiveness of a meditation-based stress reduction program in the treatment of anxiety disorders. *Am J Psychiatry* 1992;149:936–43.

15. Miller J, Peterson L, Fletcher K, et al. Three-year follow-up and clinical implication of a mindfulness meditation-based stress reduction intervention in the treatment of anxiety disorders. *Gen Hosp Psychiatry* 1995;17:192–200.

16. Bindemann S, Soukop M, Kaye S. Randomised controlled study of relaxation training. 1991;27:170–74.

17. Davis H. Effects of biofeedback and cognitive therapy on stress in patients with breast cancer. *Psychol Rep* 1986;59:967–74.

18. Cunningham A, Tocco E. A randomized trial of group psychoeducational therapy for cancer patients. *Patient Ed Counseling* 1989;14:101–14.

19. Spiegel D, Bloom J. Group therapy and hypnosis reduce metastatic breast carcinoma pain. *Psychosoma Med* 1983;45:333–39.

20. Burish T, Jenkins R. Effectiveness of biofeedback and relaxation training in reducing the side effects of cancer chemotherapy. *Health Psychol* 1992; 11:17–23.

21. Burish T, Snyder S, Jenkins R. Preparing patients for cancer chemotherapy: Effect of coping preparation and relaxation interventions. *J Consult Clin Psychol* 1991;59:518–25.

22. Carey M, Burish T. Providing relaxation training to cancer chemotherapy patients: A comparison of three delivery techniques. *J Consult Clin Psychol* 1987;55:732–37.
23. Burish T, Carey M, Krozely M, et al. Conditioned side effects induced by cancer chemotherapy: Prevention through behavioral treatment. *J Consult Clin Psychol* 1987;55:42–48.
24. Lyles J, Burish T, Krozely M, et al. Efficacy of relaxation training and guided imagery in reducing the aversiveness of cancer chemotherapy. *J Consult Clin Psychol* 1982;50:509–24.
25. Redd W. Management of anticipatory nausea and vomiting. In Holland J, Rowland J, eds., *Handbook of Psychooncology: Psychological Care of the Patient with Cancer.* New York: Oxford University Press, 1989;423–33.
26. Redd W, Jacobsen P, Die-Trill M, et al. Cognitive/attentional distraction in the control of conditioned nausea in pediatric cancer patients receiving chemotherapy. *J Consult Clin Psychol* 1987;55:391–95.
27. Redd W, Andresen G, Minagawa R. Hypnotic control of anticipatory nausea in patients undergoing cancer chemotherapy. *J Consult Clin Psychol* 1982; 50:14–19.
28. Morrow G, Morrill B. Behavioral treatment for the anticipatory nausea and vomiting induced by cancer chemotherapy. *N Eng J Med* 1982;307:1476–80.
29. Vasterling J, Jenkins R, Tope D, et al. Cognitive distraction and relaxation training for the control of side effects due to cancer chemotherapy. *J Behavioral Med* 1993;16:65–80.
30. Decker T, Cline-Elsen J, Gallaher M. Relaxation therapy as an adjunct in radiation oncology. *J Clin Psychol* 1992;48:388–93.
31. Troesch L, Rodehaver C, Delaney E, et al. The influence of guided imagery on chemotherapy-related nausea and vomiting. 1993;20:1179–85.
32. Bridge L, Benson P, Pietroni P, et al. Relaxation and imagery in the treatment of breast cancer. *Br Med J* 1988;297:1169–72.
33. Fawzy F, Fawzy N, Arndt L, et al. Critical review of psychosocial interventions in cancer care. *Arch Gen Psychiatry* 1995;52:100–113.
34. Zachariae R, Kristensen J, Hokland P, et al. Effect of psychological intervention in the form of relaxation and guided imagery on cellular immune function normal healthy subjects. *Psychother Psychosom* 1990;54:32–39.
35. Jasnoski M, Kugler J. Relaxation, imagery, and neuroimmunomodulation. *Ann NY Acad Sci* 1987;496:722–30.
36. McGrady A, Conran P, Dickey D, et al. The Effects of biofeedback-assisted relaxation on cell-mediated immunity, cortisol, and white blood cell count in healthy adult subjects. *J Behav Med* 1992;15:343–54.
37. Peavey B, Lawlis G, Goven A. Biofeedback-assisted relaxation: Effects on phagocytic capacity. *Biofeedback Self-Regulations* 1985;10:33–47.
38. Rider M, Achterberg J. Effect of music-assisted imagery on neutrophils and lymphocytes. *Biofeedback Self Regulation* 1989;14:247–57.
39. Kiecolt-Glaser J, Glaser R, Williger D, et al. Psychosocial enhancement of immunocompetence in a geriatric population. *Health Psychol* 1985;4:25–41.

40. Kiecolt-Glaser J, Glaser R. Psychological influences on immunity. *Psychosomatics* 1986;27:621–24.

41. Van Rood Y, Bogaards M, Goulmy E, et al. The effects of stress and relaxation on the in vitro immune response in man: A meta-analytic study. *J Behav Med* 1993;16:163–81.

42. Taylor D. Effects of a behavioral stress-management program on anxiety, mood, self-esteem, and T-cell count in HIV-positive men. 1995;76:451–57.

43. Guerrero J, Reiter R. A brief survey of pineal gland-immune system interrelationships. *Endocrine Res* 1992;18:91–113.

44. Maestroni G. The immunoneuroendocrine role of melatonin. *J Pineal Res* 1993;14:1–10.

45. Blask D. Melatonin in oncology. In Yu H-S, Reiter R, eds., *Melatonin: Biosynthesis, Physiological Effects, and Clinical Applications*. Boca Raton, Fla.: CRC Press, 1993:447–75.

46. Massion A, Teas J, Hébert J, et al. Meditation, melatonin, and breast/prostate cancer: Hypothesis and preliminary data. *Med Hypotheses* 1995;44:39–46.

47. Epstein M, Lieff J. Psychiatric complications of meditation practice. In Wilber K, Engler J, Brown DP, *Transformation of Consciousness*. Boston: New Science Library, 1986:53–63.

48. Miller J. The unveiling of traumatic memories and emotions through mindfulness and concentration meditation: Clinical implications and three case reports. *J Transpers Psychol* 1993;25:169–80.

49. Bandura A. Self-efficacy: Toward a unifying theory of behavioral change. *Psychol Rev* 1977;84:191–215.

Chapter 12

1. VandeCreek L, Lester J. Use of alternative therapies among breast cancer outpatients compared with the general population. *Alternative Ther* 1999; 5:71–76.

2. Feher S, Maly RC. Coping with breast cancer in later life: The role of religious faith. *Psychooncology* 1999;8:408–16.

3. Poloma MM. *The Charismatic Movement: Is There a New Pentecost?* Boston and New York: Twayne, 1982.

4. Poloma MM. *The Assemblies of God at the Crossroads: Charisma and Institutional Dilemmas*. Knoxville: University of Tennessee Press, 1989.

5. Poloma MM, Pendleton BF. *Exploring Neglected Dimensions of Religion in Quality of Life Research*. Lewiston, NY: Edwin Mellen Press, 1991.

6. Gallup G Jr. *Religion in America: 50 years: 1935–1985*. Gallup Report, 236 (May), 1985.

7. Gallup G Jr, Jones S. *100 Questions and Answers: Religion in America*. Princeton, N.J.: Princeton Religion Research Center, 1989.

8. Poloma MM, Gallup G Jr. *Varieties of Prayer: A Survey Report*. Philadelphia: Trinity Press International, 1991.

9. See note 5.

10. Levin J, Larson DB, Puchalski CM. Religion and spirituality in medicine: Research and education. *JAMA* 1997;278:792–93.
11. Oxman T, Freeman DH, Manheimer ED. Lack of social participation or religious strength and comfort as risk factors for death after cardiac surgery in the elderly. *Psychosomatic Med* 1995;57:5–15.
12. Pressman P, Larson DB, Strain JJ. Religious belief, depression, and ambulation status in elderly women with broken hips. *Am J Psychiatry* 1990;147: 758–60.
13. Koenig HG, George LK, Hays JC, et al. Attendance at religious services, interleukin-6, and other biological parameters of immune function in older adults. *Int J Psychiatry Med* 1997;27:233–50.
14. Larson DB, Koenig HG. Is God good for your health? The role of spirituality in medical care. *Cleve Clin J Med* 2000;67,80:83–84.
15. Benor D. *Healing Research: Holistic Medicine and Spiritual Healing*. Munich: Helix Verlag, 1993.
16. Solfvin J. Mental healing. In Krippner S, ed., *Advances in Parapsychological Research*. Jefferson, NC: McFarland & Co, 1984, Vol. 4:31–63.
17. Dossey L. *Healing Words: The Power of Prayer and the Practice of Medicine*. San Francisco: Harper San Francisco, 1993.
18. May E, Vilenskaya L. Some aspects of parapsychological research in the former Soviet Union. *Subtle Energies* 1994;3:1–24.
19. Grad B. Some biological effects of the "laying on of hands": A review of experiments with animals and plants. *J Am Soc Psychical Res* 1965;59: 95–127.
20. Nash C. Psychokinetic control of bacterial growth. *J Am Soc Psychical Res* 1982;51:217–21.
21. Grad B. Healing by the laying on of hands: Review of experiments and implications. *Pastoral Psychol* 1970;21:19–26.
22. Grad B, Cadoret RJ, Paul GI. The influence of an unorthodox method of treatment on wound healing in mice. *Int J Parapsychol* 1961;3:5–24.
23. Grad B. The biological effects of the "laying on of hands" on animals and plants: Implications for biology. In Schmeidler G, ed., *Parapsychology: Its Relations to Physics, Biology, Psychology and Psychiatry*. Metuchen, NJ: Scarecrow Press, 1976:75–89.
24. Wirth D. Unorthodox healing: The effect of noncontact therapeutic touch on the healing rate of full thickness dermal wounds. Presented at the 32nd Annual Parapsychology Association Convention, San Diego, 1989.
25. Braud W, Schlitz M. Psychokinetic influence on electrodermal activity. *J Parapsych* 1983;47:95–119.
26. Schlitz M, Braud W. Distant intentionality and healing: Assessing the evidence. *Alt Ther* 1997;3:62–73.
27. Utts J. Replication and meta-analysis in parapsychology. *Stat Sc* 1991;6: 363–403.
28. Honorton C, Ferrari DC. "Future telling": A meta-analysis of forced-choice precognition experiments, 1935–1987. *J Parapsychology* 1989;53:281–308.

29. Byrd R. Positive therapeutic effects of intercessory prayer in a coronary care unit population. *South Med J* 1988;81:826–29.
30. Harris W, Gowda M, Kolb JW, et al. A randomized, controlled trial of the effects of remote intercessory prayer on outcomes in patients admitted to the coronary care unit. *Arch Intern Med* 1999;159:2273–78.
31. Krucoff M. Randomized integrative therapies in interventional patients with unstable angina: The monitoring and actualization of noetic training. *Circulation* 1998;98:17.
32. Sicher F, Targ E, Moore D, et al. A randomized double-blind study of the effect of distant healing in a population with advanced AIDS: Report of a small scale study. *West J Med* 1998;169:356–63.
33. Walker SR, Miller WR, Comer S, et al. Intercessory prayer in the treatment of alcohol abuse and dependence: A pilot investigation. *Alt Ther Health Med* 1997;3:79–86.
34. Grad B. Reichian connection to healing by touch. Presented at the Mobius Society Healing Conference, Esalen, July 1987.
35. Benford MS, Doss DB, Boosey S, et al. Gamma radiation fluctuations during alternative healing therapy. *Alt Ther Health Med* 1999;5:51–56.
36. Stapp H. Theoretical model of a purported empirical violation of the predictions of quantum theory. *Am Physical Soc* 1994;50:18–22.
37. Stokes D. Theoretical parapsychology. In Krippner S, ed., *Advances in Parapsychology Research,* Vol. 5. Jefferson, NC: McFarland Press, 1987:77–189.

Chapter 13

1. Glanz K, Lerman C. Psychosocial impact of breast cancer: A critical review. *Ann of Behav Med* 1992;14:204–12.
2. Derogatis LR, Morrow GR, Fetting S. The prevalence of psychiatric disorders among cancer patients. *JAMA* 1983;249:751–57.
3. Speigel D, Bloom JR, Kraemer HC, Gottheil E. Effect of psychosocial treatment on survival of patients with metastatic breast cancer. *Lancet* 1989;14: 889–991.
4. Adler S. Complementary and alternative medicine use among women with breast cancer. *Med Anthropol Q* 1999;3:214–22.
5. Doan BD. Alternative and complementary therapies. In Holland J, ed., *Psychooncology.* New York: Oxford University Press, 1998:817–27.
6. Eisenberg DM, Kessler RC, Foster C, et al. Unconventional medicine in the United States. *N Engl J Med* 1993;328:246–52.
7. Cassileth BR, Lusk EJ, Strause TB, et al. Contemporary unorthodox treatments in cancer medicine. *Ann Intern Med* 1984;101:105–12.
8. Gordon N, Sobel DS, Tarazona E. Use of and interest in alternate therapies among adult primary care clinicians and adult members in a large health maintenance organization. *West J Med* 1998;169:153–61.

9. Astin JA. Why patients use alternative medicine: Results of a national study. *JAMA* 1998;279:1548–52.

10. Miller WR. Spirituality: The silent dimension in addiction research. *Drug Alcohol Rev* 1990;9:259–66.

11. Maugans TA, Wadland WC. Religion and family medicine: A survey of physician and patients. *J Fam Practice* 1991;31:210–13.

12. Koenig HG, Cohen HJ, Blazer DG, et al. Religious coping and depression among elderly hospitalizes medically ill men. *Am J Psychiatry* 1992;149: 1693–1706.

13. Benson H. Faith heals. In *Timeless Healing: The Power of Biology and Belief.* New York: Scribner, 1996.

14. Dossey L. *Healing Words: The Power of Prayer and the Practice of Medicine.* San Francisco: HarperCollins, 1993.

15. Cotton, Levine, Fitzpatrick, et al. Spirituality, quality of life and psychological adjustment in women with breast cancer. Presented at the American Psychological Association annual meeting, San Francisco, August 1998.

16. LeShan L. *Cancer as a Turning Point.* New York: E.P. Dutton, 1989.

17. Sicher F, Targ E, Moore D, et al. A randomized double blind study of distant healing in a population with advanced AIDS. *West J Med* 1998;169:356–63.

18. Harris WS, et al. A randomized, controlled trial of the effects of remote, intercessory prayer on outcomes in patients admitted to the coronary care unit. *Arch Intern Med* 1999;159:2273–78.

19. Kabat-Zinn J, Massion AO, Hébert JR, et al. Meditation. In Holland J, ed., *Psychooncology.* New York: Oxford University Press, 1998:676–79.

20. Taylor E. *The Physical and Psychological Effects of Meditation: A Review of Contemporary Research.* Sausalito, Calif.: Institute of Noetic Sciences, 1996.

21. See note 17.

22. Kabat-Zinn J. Mindfulness meditation: health benefits of an ancient Buddhist practice. In Goleman and Gurion, eds. *Mind/Body Medicine.* New York: Consumer Reports, 1993.

23. Kabat-Zinn J. *Full Catastrophe Living.* New York: Dell, 1990.

24. Kabat-Zinn J. An outpatient program in behavioral medicine for chronic pain patients based on the practice of mindfulness meditation. *Gen Hosp Psychiatry* 1982;4:33–47.

25. Kabat-Zinn J, Lipworth L, Burney R. The clinical use of mindfulness meditation for the self-regulation of chronic pain. *J Behav Med* 1985;8:163–90.

26. Kabat-Zinn J, Chapman-Waldrop A. Compliance with an outpatient stress reduction program: Rates and predictors of program completion. *J Behav Med* 1988;11:333–52.

27. Lerner M, Remen R. Trade craft of the Commonweal cancer help program. *Advances* 1987;4:11–25.

28. Ornish D. *Dr. Dean Ornish's Program for Reversing Heart Disease.* New York: Random House, 1990.

29. See note 19.

30. Benson H, Alexander S, Feldman CL. Decreased premature ventricular contractions through use of the relaxation response in patients with stable ischemic heart disease. *Lancet* 1975;2:380–82.

31. Delmonte MM. Anxiety, defensiveness, and physiological responsivity in novice and experienced meditators. *Int J Eclectic Psychother* 1985;4:1–13.

32. Achterberg J, Dossey B, Kolkmeier L. *Rituals of Healing.* New York: Bantam Books, 1994.

33. Baider L, Uziely B, De-Nour AK. Progressive muscle relaxation and guided imagery in cancer patients. *Gen Hosp Psychiatry* 1994;16:340–47.

34. Siegel B. *Love, Medicine and Miracles.* New York: Harper and Row, 1986.

35. Naparstek B. *Staying Well with Guided Imagery.* New York: Warner Books, 1994.

36. Doan BD. Alternative and complementary therapies. In Holland J, ed., *Psychooncology.* New York: Oxford University Press, 1998:817–27.

37. Gruber BL, Hall NR, Hersh SP, et al. Immune system and psychological changes in metastatic cancer patients using relaxation and guided imagery: A pilot study. *Scand J Behav Ther* 1988;17:25–45.

38. Lyles JN, Burish TG, Krozely MG, et al. Efficacy of relaxation training and guided imagery in reducing the aversiveness of cancer chemotherapy. *J Consult Clin Psychol* 1982;50:509–24.

39. Morris K. Meditating on yogic science. *Lancet* 1998;351:1038.

40. Schell FJ, Allolio B, Schonecke OW. Physiological and psychological effects of hatha-yoga exercise in healthy women. *Int J Psychosomat* 1994;41:46–52.

41. Nespor K. Pain management and yoga. *Int J Psychosomat* 1991;38:76–80.

42. See note 26.

43. Zimmerman J, Coyle V. *The Way of Council.* Bearsville, N.Y.: Bramble Books, 1996.

Chapter 14

1. Siegel, Gluhoski, Gorey. Age-related distress among young women with breast cancer. *J Psychosocial Oncol* 1999;17:1–20.

Index